Closed-Circuit System and Other Innovations in Anaesthesia

Edited by
R. Droh and R. Spintge

With 167 Figures

Springer-Verlag Berlin Heidelberg New York
London Paris Tokyo

Dr. med. Roland Droh
Chefarzt der Anaesthesiologie
Ärztlicher Direktor des
Krankenhauses für Sportverletzte
Hellersen
Paulmannshöher Straße 17

D-5880 Lüdenscheid

Dr. med. Ralph Spintge
Krankenhaus für Sportverletzte
Hellersen
Paulmannshöher Straße 17

D-5880 Lüdenscheid

ISBN-13: 978-3-540-16691-7 e-ISBN-13: 978-3-642-71328-6
DOI: 10.1007/978-3-642-71328-6

Library of Congress Cataloging in Publication Data.
Closed-circuit system and other innovations in anaesthesia.
"Papers presented at the II. International Symposium on Innovations in Management, Technology and Pharmacology held on 26–28 May 1984 in Lüdenscheid" – Pref.
Includes bibliographies and index.
1. Anesthesiology – Apparatus and instruments – Congresses. 2. Anesthesia – Congresses.
I. Droh, R. (Roland). II. Spintge, R. III. International Symposium on Innovations in Management Technology, and Pharmacology (2nd : 1984 : Lüdenscheid, Germany)
[DNLM: 1. Anesthesiology – instrumentation – congresses. WO 240 C645 1984]
RD78.8.C56 1986 617'.96 86-21959
ISBN 0-387-16691-2 (U.S.)

Typesetting: Brühlsche Universitätsdruckerei, Giessen
Offsetprinting: Saladruck, Berlin. Bookbinding: B. Helm, Berlin

2119/3020-543210

Contributors

J. Chrubasik, Dept. of Anaesthesia, University Hospital, Hugstetter Straße 55, 7800 Freiburg, Federal Republic of Germany

J. C. Dorlas, Institute of Anaesthesiology, AZG, Oostersingel 59, 9713 EZ Groningen, The Netherlands

R. Droh, Anaesthesiologie, Sportkrankenhaus Hellersen, 5880 Lüdenscheid, Federal Republic of Germany

W. L. den Dunnen, Dept. of Anaesthesia, Municipal Hospital Dordrecht, Dordrecht, The Netherlands

W. Erdmann, Dept. of Anaesthesia, Erasmus University, 3000 DR Rotterdam, The Netherlands

C. E. Essed, Dept. of Pathology I, Erasmus University, 3000 DR Rotterdam, The Netherlands

N. S. Faithfull, Dept. of Anaesthesia, Erasmus University, 3000 DR Rotterdam, The Netherlands

M. Fennema, Dept. of Anaesthesia, Erasmus University, 3000 DR Rotterdam, The Netherlands

K. W. Fritz, Institut für Anaesthesiologie, Medizinische Hochschule Hannover, 3000 Hannover

G. Garcia, Institute of Bloodless Medicine and Surgery, 707 E. Chapman Ave., Fullerton, CA 92631, USA

G. Jibelian, Medical Research, Institute of San Francisco, 2200 Webster Street, San Francisco CA 94115, USA

T. Jin, Anaesthesia Division, Akita Red Cross Hospital, Akita, Japan

H. Jshihara, Dept. of Anaesthesiology, Hirosaki University, School of Medicine, Hirosaki Aomori-Ken, Japan

D. Klaus, Dept. of Cardiology, Städtische Krankenanstalten Dortmund, 4600 Dortmund, Federal Republic of Germany

G. Klein, ZAW, Klinikum der J. W. Goethe-Universität, 6000 Frankfurt, Federal Republic of Germany

A. Kok, Dept. of Anaesthesia and Pathology I, Erasmus University, 3000 DR Rotterdam, The Netherlands

S. Kunke, Max-Planck-Straße 60, 6500 Mainz

B. Lachmann, Dept. of Anaesthesiology, Erasmus University, 3000 DR Rotterdam, The Netherlands

R. Lapin, Institute of Bloodless Medicine and Surgery, 707 E. Chapman Ave., Fullerton CA 92631, USA

R. Lemke, Dept. of Cardiology, Städtische Krankenanstalten Dortmund, 4600 Dortmund, Federal Republic of Germany

B. Lemmer, Center of Pharmacology, J. W. Goethe University, Theodor-Stern-Kai 70, 6000 Frankfurt/Main 70, Federal Republic of Germany

C. Y. Lin, University of Chicago, Dept. of Anaesthesiology, 5841 South Maryland Ave., Box 428, Chicago Illinois 60637, USA

D. W. Lübbers, Max-Planck-Institute, Rheinlanddamm 201, 4600 Dortmund, Federal Republic of Germany

K. Lundin, Medizinische Hochschule Hannover, Dept. of Anaesthesia, Section 1, 3000 Hannover

T. Mostert, Dept. of Anaesthesia, Municipal Hospital Dordrecht, Dordrecht, The Netherlands

J. Mottner, Justus Liebig-Universität Gießen, Dept. of Anaesthesia, 6300 Gießen, Federal Republic of Germany

T. Murakawa, Anaesthesia Division, Akita Red Cross Hospital, Akita, Japan

T. Oyama, Dept. of Anaesthesia, Hirosaki University, School of Medicine, Hirosaki, Japan

M. Paloheimo, Dept. of Anaesthesia, Helsinki University, Central Hospital, 00290 Helsinki 29, Finland

D. Patschke, Justus Liebig-Universität Gießen, Dept. of Anaesthesia, 6300 Gießen, Federal Republic of Germany

G. Rolly, Dept. of Anaesthesia, University of Ghent, Academic Hospital, De Pintelaan 185, 9000 Ghent, Belgium

R. Spintge, Anaesthesiologie, Sportkrankenhaus Hellersen, 5880 Lüdenscheid, Federal Republic of Germany

M. Tabbert, Justus Liebig-Universität Gießen, Dept. of Anaesthesia, 6300 Gießen, Federal Republic of Germany

B. Taylor, Medical Research Institute of San Francisco, 2200 Webster Street, San Francisco CA 94115, USA

A. Varenne, 03 Cardiology, 6 Rue Spitailerie, 06000 Nice, France

L. Versichelen, Dept. of Anaesthesia, University of Ghent, Academic Hospital, De Pintelaan 185, 9000 Ghent, Belgium

P. D. Wagner, Dept. of Medicine M-23, Section of Physiology, University of California, San Diego, La Jolla, CA 92093, USA

C. F. Wallroth, Dräger-Werk AG, Moislinger Allee 53, 2400 Lübeck, Federal Republic of Germany

C. Wright, Institute of Bloodless Medicine and Surgery, 707 E. Chapman Ave., Fullerton CA 92631, USA

M. Yamashita, Dept. of Anaesthesia, Ibaraki Children's Hospital, Futabadai, Mito 311–41, Japan

G. Yates, Medical Research, Institute of San Francisco, 2200 Webster Street, San Francisco CA 94115, USA

T. van der Zee, Dept. of Anaesthesia, Albany Medical College, Albany, NY 12208, USA

K. Zettergren, Dept. of Anaesthesia, Justus Liebig-Universität Gießen, 6300 Gießen, Federal Republic of Germany

M. Zia, Institute of Bloodless Medicine and Surgery, 707 E. Chapman Ave., Fullerton CA 92631, USA

Preface

This volume contains the lectures and discussion papers presented at the II. International Symposium on Innovations in Management, Technology and Pharmacology held on 26–28 May 1984 in Lüdenscheid. This symposium delt with further developments in the sector of the closed-circuit system; non-invasive measurement and monitoring systems; new aspects of cardiovascular and pulmonary physiology; oxygen-transporting substances; and particular questions in pharmacology. The purpose of this meeting was to allow a mutual international exchange of news on interesting new developments, particularly as these relate to the closed-circuit system, and the encouragement of further scientific developments.

It must be made clear that the large-scale introduction of the closed-circuit system has to be the occasion of completely new quality standards both in anesthesia and in all related technological sectors, combined with the highest demands in terms of precision and measuring techniques. The conventional and still quite crude clinical anesthetic procedures will have to make way for much more physiological, micromolecular precision techniques, which will compare with our present methods rather in the same way as a microelectrode to a spear and will allow new levels of achievement in anesthesiology. All our tasks will need to be rethought and thoroughly understood from these aspects. Some anesthesists, physiologists and engineers already see the closed-circuit system as a challenge, while for others this system will still mean a great deal of work and creativity before the problems are finally solved in the future. Those who meet this challenge with an attitude of full acceptance, however, will soon fall under its particular spell and will thus find new joy and satisfaction in the practice of anesthesia in all its subspecialties.

R. Droh

Contents

The Closed-Circuit Anaesthesia System

The Closed Circuit: Past and Future

R. Droh

In more than 12 years, the closed-circuit system has proved its worth in over 60 000 patients in our department of anesthesiology. From its first simple beginnings up to the present day we have used it throughout the years to our patients' benefit with complete safety and with no sort of untoward incidents. To reach this standard, we expended a great deal of effort over the years 1972–1984 on building up the system step by step and then refining and improving it. During this process we soon became aware that this system would allow far-reaching improvements in all subspecialties of anesthesiology, including intensive care and resuscitation.

It also soon became clear to us that with this system we were introducing substantially higher qualitative specifications for industry, which were no longer comparable with the standards current with the conventional systems. One consequence of this throughout the past years has been an understandably very hesitant attitude of industry in this sector.

So far, expansion of the clinical potential and our knowledge in this area has been curbed only by the quality of our instruments, and in particular that of the measuring and metering instruments. We had to spend a great deal of time just on the problems involved in getting the circuits leak-proof, refining the rotameters to allow metering of extremely small volumes of gas (ml/min), and designing evaporators that would be suitable for these small gas flows and measuring instruments for determination of the concentrations of CO_2, O_2 and the volatile anesthetic agents.

It is not possible for a completely new philosophy to take the place of hitherto accepted systems with no teething troubles or delays. This is especially true in this case, since in the past decades of modern anesthesia, after all, many hundreds of millions of patients all over the world have been so successfully treated with the systems accepted so far. Thus, it is appropriate that we cite a great deal of clinical experience to counter the clinical reservations to this system, especially as the closed-circuit system was rejected as hazardous for some generations precisely because of the inadequate technical facilities.

The catalog of advantages of the closed-circuit system has meanwhile become longer. We have presented these advantages and described the clinical application of the system in detail in publications and lectures over the past few years. To save time the reader is referred at this point to the list of advantages given below, so that I can then concentrate on presenting future developments that are meanwhile taking definite shape for us in more detail.

The closed circuit is *Superior* to conventional systems insofar as:

1. The anesthetic gases and vapors are per se warm.
2. The anesthetic gases contain the optimum degree of moisture by definition.
3. The oxygen consumption per unit of time or per inspiration can by definition be measured precisely without further elaborate auxiliary devices.
4. a) The CO_2 resulting from the oxygen consumption per unit of time or per inspiration can be calculated and measured quantitatively with no great difficulty.
   b) Pathological changes in metabolism or metabolic conditions become apparent spontaneously with this system. This means that the anesthetist is no longer dependent on clinical signs developing secundarily to such changes or conditions for recognition of the primary causes.
   c) Changes in the pH of the circulating blood become apparent from the measurements of gases in the system with no necessity for auxiliary instruments, and can therefore be corrected at once.
5. The uptake of a volatile anesthetic agent, e.g., halothane or isoflurane, can be precisely measured.
6. The ratio of the gaseous concentrations of oxygen to laughing gas can be adjusted to the O_2 concentration of the normal respiratory air with no problem, since within the circuit both the O_2 consumption and the resultant CO_2 can be precisely determined and kept within the normal range.
7. Ventilation of the patient can be accomplished as genuine normal ventilation in a simplified manner with each inspiration, monitored by way of the O_2 uptake and CO_2 output. If necessary, however, it is also possible to carry out accurately controlled hypo- or hyperventilation.
8. a) The level of anesthesia can currently be determined and controlled more precisely with the technique of the closed-circuit system than with any other.
   b) The degree of muscle relaxation can also be assessed from the O_2 consumption and the CO_2 production with no auxiliary instruments.
9. The elimination of excess anesthetic gases and vapors is unnecessary except for insignificant residues during the induction and recovery phases of anesthesia.
10. Changes in the pulmonary perfusion and diffusion can be quickly recognized.
11. Changes in the cardiac output quickly become apparent.
12. Environmental pollution resulting from constant transfer of excess gases and vapors, such as N_2O, halothane, and isoflurane, to the atmosphere, in particular by way of leaks in the circuits themselves, is not only virtually null and therefore negligible in the operating theaters, but is also subsequently drastically lower in the larger atmosphere outside the operating theaters.
13. There is no silent aspiration, since the system has to be quite tight in itself.
14. There is no imperceptible N_2O transfer into the cuff of the tube when porous tubes are used, since changes in the degree of tightness are picked up at once.
15. Any error in intubation is recognized at once, since in such cases there is neither O_2 uptake nor CO_2 output.

16. Injuries to the gastrointestinal tract during laparoscopy become apparent because gases can escape from the gastrointestinal tract through the mouth, in addition to the completely unaffected gaseous exchange in the closed-circuit system.
17. All these advantages, and this is ultimately the most amazing feature of all this, are obtained without extra expense and even with a financial saving. This system is thus not only much better and much safer and superior to all other systems current at present, but also much more economical.
18. This is the one system that will admit of complete and computer-assisted automation with much greater benefit to the patient than with any other system.

Normal ventilation achieved by way of monitoring the O_2 consumption *and* the CO_2 released with *warm* and *moist respiratory gases* is just as important for our work in all sectors as the creation of ways of making it possible to measure the *cardiac output* and the *pulmonary perfusion* and *diffusion*, for example, with this procedure, which is so economical in terms of both *time* and *money*.

Resuscitation can be much better and more simply monitored just *because of* the simple continuous determination of *O_2 consumption* and the simultaneous check on the *CO_2* developing from this O_2 consumption, and it is therefore something that can be *basically* improved. This dual determination does not of course replace the determination of blood gases, measurement of pulse and blood pressure or the ECG trace. It is, however, of at least equal importance and in many critical situations even far superior, since the parameters O_2 consumption and CO_2 production can be determined with no technical problems, and at present even more easily than the others named.

Up to a few months ago we also still had a problem insofar as none of the *respirators* was anywhere near sufficiently leak-proof for the system, which means that none was safe enough. With the use of a Roling Seal and an integrated computer unit (see papers by Schepp and Erdmann and Spintge and Droh, this volume) this gap in the clinical applicability of the closed-circuit system for mechanical ventilation has now been closed for the first time.

With rapid further development of measuring instruments and computer units the closed-circuit system could soon also be applied in the treatment of shock, in intensive care, and in resuscitation.

In addition to the concept of *normal ventilation* – and here I mean genuine normal ventilation and not the pseudonormal ventilation still described as normal ventilation in many clinical studies – we have introduced the *O_2 pulse* as a cardiocirculatory parameter to complement *blood pressure, pulse pressure curve,* and *ECG*. Together with the O_2 transport capacity/heartbeat it gives us a good insight into the cardiac output as to the N_2O uptake and/or washout curves. This makes it possible to correlate the hemoglobin content in the corresponding erythrocytes, blood pressure, pulse, and pulse pressure curves with the cardiac output and to use all this for finer adjustment of anesthesia, treatment of shock, resuscitation and intensive care.

With this closed-circuit system we aim to improve techniques for the noninvasive measurement of alveolar ventilation, pulmonary diffusion and perfusion, functional residual capacity (FRC) and dead space or, in short, the total gas exchange between lung and blood. Our current need is for highly advanced technical facilities for the determination of O_2, N_2, N_2O, CO_2 and volatile anesthetic agents, combined with the ability to analyze a single breath and the availability of sufficiently fine metering units to administer the gases and anesthetic agents to the patient in precisely predetermined amounts breath by breath; once all this is achieved we hope to have insights allowing us to expand our knowledge of cardiocirculatory and pulmonary processes.

We are also hoping to gain more insight from the explanation of the clinical significance of the *nitrogen* in the gaseous mixture. So far, contrary to all theoretical forecasts, in clinical practice the presence of nitrogen in our oxygen–laughing gas mixture in the closed-circuit system has proved to be a sound principle. With this system, in contrast to the open and half-closed systems, we have at least had no pulmonary complications throughout the years.

Our present closed-circuit systems, which are still derived from the systems used hitherto, with the philosophy of continuous large-volume gas flows, will certainly have to be replaced by systems based on completely new technologies with gas volumes delivered intermittently.

With this system, in addition to clinical monitoring, a fully automated computerized system of anesthesia analysis with multiple feedback can also be integrated; this means that the patient can be monitored by multiple systems, the respiration can be more finely controlled, and treatment is even much safer and more effective than with present-day systems.

Thus, we are also expecting to obtain new insights into the gas exchange capabilities of blood substitutes in micro, and on the basis of these to expand our knowledge of these substances and also of the blood, the endogenous proteins and many humoral factors.

Let me just outline with reference to one example how far our conceptions can already go.

Example

A *nonanesthetized slim young patient* at rest consumes aproximately 3.5 ml oxygen per kg (body weight) in 1 min. If we assume a body weight of 70 kg for this patient, he will consume aproximately 240 ml oxygen/min. At a rate of 12 inspirations/min he will take up 20 ml oxygen of this per inspiration, and at 60 heartbeats/min this means that with every heartbeat the heart supplies the 70 kg body weight of the patient with 4 ml oxygen to burn up. This means in turn that according to a crude calculation, each Kilogram of this body weight metabolizes 0.057 ml O_2 per heartbeat, or in other words, 1 mg (body weight) metabolizes 1428 million molecules of O_2 per heartbeat. It can be calculated that of this 4 ml O_2 per heartbeat, 1.056 ml is metabolized in the liver; 0.732 ml in the brain; 0.368 ml in the heart; 0.288 ml in the kidneys; and 1.024 ml in the skeletal muscles. This 4 ml O_2 per heartbeat can be transported by about 2.9 g Hb in 100 ml plasma. Up to 22 ml O_2 can be taken up for transport by 16 g Hb in 100 ml plasma. In the above example, however, 16 g hemoglobin is transporting only 4 ml O_2 or, expressed in molecules, $2.505946 \times 4 \times 10^{16}$ molecules of O_2 in 5×10^{11} erythrocytes.

Thus, with increasing refinement of our methods for measurement, analysis and correlation in the closed-circuit system, we shall be able to determine the level of anesthesia with increasing precision even from the O_2 uptake and the CO_2 output, and it will be possible to improve this further by accurate determination of the uptake and/or output of anesthetic agent. For the deeper the level of anesthesia the more the metabolism and, in turn, the O_2 consumption are slowed down, and conversely when the level of anesthesia flattens off the O_2 consumption increases by a comparable degree.

In the presence of hyperthyroidism the O_2 consumption is above the calculated values from the start. In the presence of hyperthermia the O_2 consumption rises extremely rapidly during anesthesia.

During the depolarization phase caused by succinyldicholine or after relief of a barrier causing partial blood deficiency the oxygen requirement is increased in the short term. Once a phase of this kind is over, however, the increased oxygen requirement returns rapidly to the normal value.

It should be remarked at this point that in the presence of hypothermia the oxygen consumption falls as a function of the temperature, as might be expected.

In the presence of a *pulmonary embolism* the respiratory capacity must be increased in keeping with the extent of the embolism, so that the same volume of oxygen can be taken up. In this case, then, wie can determine changes in the pulmonary perfusion and pulmonary diffusion, the alveolar ventilation, and the dead space directly with no additional measuring instruments, and can rapidly take account of these in our clinical decision-making.

It is true that the closed-circuit system involves the disadvantage that expired metabolites can accumulate in the respiratory gases, but conversely, it also incorporates the opportunity of tracing metabolites quantitatively and qualitatively, for analysis of their effectivity and toxicity. A concentration of undesired metabolites in the system can be avoided by flushing with fresh gases or by the insertion of special filters (e.g., charcoal filters).

When a closed-circuit anesthetic system is used it is possible to determine the cardiac output in addition to the $avDO_2$ in the pulmonary circulation, since the cardiac output can be calculated:

1. From the O_2 consumption and the $avDO_2$ according to Fick's law
2. From the washin and washout curves for N_2O.

Thus, by way of the oxygen consumption and by way of the N_2O uptake or release it is possible to determine the cardiac output and the $avDO_2$ in the lung and/or to monitor the gaseous exchange.

The closed-circuit system thus by definition opens up many new possibilities with increasing refinements of our capacity for measurement, analysis and correlation within this system. In the future it will no longer be necessary for us to compare doubtful volume percentages of volatile anesthetic agents and gas flows with pulse and blood pressure over long periods; we shall be able to take measurements in the molecule and micrometer ranges, from respiration to respiration and from heartbeat to heartbeat, and to adjust the treatment accordingly. In this way, in future we shall no longer have to tag along behind a reaction that is already long since over and react to it ourselves with a long time lag, but shall be able to react at once, since we shall always be aware of the current status.

So far, I have attempted to give some idea of the program I see ahead for the next few years. We can realize this quickly if we all work together. I hope that further international symposia on innovations in anesthesia, clinical physiology and pharmacology and in technology and management will make it possible for us to join forces so that we can reach this objective in the forseeable future for the benefit of our patients.

Practical Application of the Closed-Circuit System

R. Droh

Premedication

Premedication is accomplished in the same way as with the open or semi-open and semi-closed circuit systems. We prefer to give atropine 0.01–0.0065 mg/kg (body weight) and pancuroniumbromide 1 mg/50–90 kg (body weight) i.v. immediately before starting the general anesthesia.

Induction of Anesthesia

The techniques used for induction are the same as have been used hitherto for the open or semi-open and semi-closed systems. As a rule we begin with thiopentone 5–10 mg/kg (body weight) i.v. or ketamine 2–3 mg/kg (body weight) i.v. or with hypnomidate 0.2–0.4 mg/kg (body weight) i.v.

For intubation we give 1–2 mg succinyldicholine/kg (body weight) i.v. as a relaxant.

Ventilation is achieved manually by way of a mask up to the point of intubation, with a mixture of laughing gas and oxygen at a ratio of 1:3.5 or 1.5:4.5 (l/min), and halothane delivery by way of a Dräger halothane vaporizer (vapor) with the valve virtually fully open and with constant monitoring of its end-expiratory concentrations. We choose to use this method of metering oxygen and laughing gas with a completely open halothane valve while the circuit valve is completely closed to ensure that the whole of the circuit will quickly fill up with the anesthetic gases and vapors at the beginning. Up to the point of intubation the supply of oxygen and laughing gas is adjusted to suit the tightness of the mask.

After intubation and once the circuit has filled up, further gas delivery is tailored to the patient's actual requirements, with a totally closed circuit that as a whole has no leaks, and anesthesia is then accomplished with the various volatile anesthetic agents or with neuroleptanesthesia or other anesthetic techniques.

Management of General Anesthesia and Description of the Instruments

The Anesthetic Circuit

We use the normal commercial circuits supplied by Dräger [1], which now must certainly already be leak-proof when purchased and which must be handled and

[1] Fa. Dräger, Moislinger Allee 53–57, 2400 Lübeck, FRG.

cared for with maticulous care if full advantage is to be taken of the superiority of this system over the open and semi-closed systems, which includes in particular its safety. Anesthetic circuits that leak from a few hundred milliliters up to several liters per minute cannot of course be used for the closed-circuit system. They cannot really be used for the open or semi-closed systems either, since leaks of this kind allow the anesthetic gases supplemented by the anesthetic vapors to pass directly into the atmosphere in the operating theatre; the suction exhaust devices cannot provide any protection against this, since they only remove excess gases released in the area of the excess pressure valves, and not those that escape along the length of the whole circuit. The consequence of this for the manufacturer is that from now on the parts of the instruments need to be produced and assembled very precisely. In the future, however, the creation of new designs for the circuit will be unavoidable.

Breathing Tubes

The breathing tubes should have a smooth internal surface and should insulate the gases effectively against temperature losses. Since the anesthetic gases in the closed-circuit system are saturated with water vapor, as anesthesia continues water collects in the system. In tubes with smooth internal surfaces it is no problem for this water of condensation to collect at the lowest point of the tube, from where it is simple to remove it by way of water traps. In pleated tubes the water of condensation collects in the troughs of individual pleats, so that little water can collect at the lowest point of the breathing tube, which means it can easily happen that water collects on the measuring sounds inserted in the system. Measurement of CO_2, N_2O and O_2, however, is critically impaired by the presence of even very small water vapor particles in the measuring chambers.

Bacteria Filters

The use of bacteria filters is advisable not only to reduce the amount of time needed for cleaning and sterilizing the circuits and for keeping the measuring systems clean, but also to stabilize the gas flows in the expiration and inspiration limbs.

Delivery of Volatile Anesthetic Agents

Volatile anesthetic agents are delivered to the system with vaporizers supplied by Dräger, Lübeck. As the consequence of low gas flows is that only small volumes of the anesthetic vapors from the vaporizers can be taken up by the carrier gases per unit of time, we prefer instruments that can reach an end-concentration of 7 vol.%, or we connect two conventional vaporizers in tandem, each of which allows an end-concentration of only 4 vol.%, that is to say 8 vol.% together. Delivery is most simply achieved by continuous monitoring of the end-inspiratory and end-expiratory concentrations of the volatile anesthetic agent. In this way delivery of the volatile anesthetic agents can be determined breath by breath during the course of anesthesia and so the steady state is reached; during this process the amounts of anesthetic agents needed fall continuously, as might be expected.

In clinical practice it is adequate to determine the end-expiratory concentration of volatile anesthetic agents. The halothane values, for example, are about

0.6 vol.% for aged patients and between 0.7 and 0.9 vol.% for young, fit patients.

If the end-expiratory concentration of halothane cannot be reached or maintained because of low gas flow, it is permissible to go over to semi-closed operation until the required end-expiratory concentration of the volatile anesthetic agent is reached; this is usually only necessary for a few breaths.

Determination of the Concentration of Volatile Anesthetic Agents

For this purpose both the measuring instruments supplied by Engström [2] (Emma) and those supplied by Datex [3] (Normac) are suitable. The fact that the absolute values that can be obtained with these instruments are relativized by measuring errors has little significance for clinical work, since sensitivity to anesthetic agents varies widely from patient to patient in any case. In clinical everyday use, however, these instruments are of inestimable worth for good control of anesthesia.

Delivery of Fresh Oxygen and Laughing Gas

At present the delivery of fresh gases is accomplished by way of rotameters. We use special instruments manufactured by Dräger, Lübeck, graduated from 20 up to 500 ml/min in 10-ml increments, from 550 up to 1000 ml/min in 50-ml increments, from 1000 up to 1500 ml/min in 100-ml increments, from 2 up to 5 liters/min in 500-ml increments and from 5 up to 10 liters/min in 1-liter increments.

We first make a crude calculation of the patient's oxygen requirement using 3.5 ml oxygen/kg (corrected body weight). We make a rough calculation of the laughing gas requirement, initially using 1.5 ml/kg (corrected body weight). The formulas we use for corrected body weight are: for males, body height in centimeters minus 100 = body weight in kilograms; for females, body height in centimeters minus 100 minus 10% = body weight in kilograms.

We then set the metering instruments to these calculated values for oxygen and laughing gas inflow per minute as soon as intubation of the patient is complete and the circuit has filled up with the mixture of oxygen and laughing gas specified above.

If we are not able to meet the patient's requirement with the gas inflow volumes calculated in this way, that is if the amount of gas in the respiration bag declines or the bag becomes overfull, or also if the desired gas concentrations change, we reduce the inflow of oxygen or of laughing gas very slightly or increase it very slightly, thus adjusting precisely to consumption.

If neuroleptanesthesia is intended the induction procedure is altered:

Up to intubation, i.e., as long as the patient is breathing through the mask, the patient receives *pure* oxygen, *without* delivery of any laughing gas, in a semi-closed system with a gas inflow of 6–9 liters oxygen/min, depending of course on the tightness of the mask and the degree of fullness of the system.

Overall, in this induction phase we ventilate for about 3–5 min with pure oxygen, until N_2 washout from the lung is achieved, so as subsequently, to achieve high N_2O concentrations rapidly by administration of large amounts of N_2O, thus reinforcing the analgesic effect of fentanyl.

---

[2] Fa. Engström, Elektromedizin GmbH, Heiglhofstr. 1, 8000 München, FRG.

[3] Fa. Datex, Instrumentarium Corp., Elimäenkatu 22, Helsinki/Finland.

Monitoring of the Anesthetic Gas Concentration

In our hospital the concentrations of anesthetic gases are monitored with the aid of the O_2 gas concentration-measuring instruments supplied by Dräger, Lübeck (Oxycom); Instrumentation Laboratory (IL 402/404 and 408/409); Engström (Eliza Duo-instruments); and Datex (Normocap). In keeping with the principle of multiple technical safety factors we measure the O_2 concentration of the anesthetic gases continuously with various measuring techniques in both the inspiratory and the expiratory limbs of the closed-circuit system.

Ventilation

To be on the safe side we still ventilate manually, since conventional ventilation machines also have considerable leaks, which together with the closed-circuit system constitute a potentially fatal hazard for the patient. When a suitable coupling is used that can separate the anesthetic circuit from the ventilation system absolutely, mechanical ventilation can also be performed with no risks. In this case the ventilation machines can even have quite large leaks, since the anesthetic system is unaffected and remains tight. The absolute tightness of the anesthetic circuit is thus the point on which the closed-circuit anesthetic system turns, while ever the ventilation system is not fully integrated into the anesthetic system. An example of one of these couplings is the Rolling Seal supplied by Mijnhardt, Odijk.

Control of Respiration

Respiration is controlled by way of the end-expiratory CO_2 and the tidal volume.

If the CO_2 is measured breath by breath and the end-expiratory values are between 4 and 5.6 vol.% and the tidal volumes between 500 and 800 ml (for adults), this is referred to as normal ventilation. For the sake of simplicity we set the end-expiratory CO_2 at 4.8 vol.% and the tidal volume at 800 ml. We take care to avoid any deviation from these values in either direction. It goes without saying that the tidal volumes must also be adjusted for disturbed gas exchange in the lung.

It is therefore easy to monitor normal ventilation in the closed-circuit system

1. By the O_2 uptake
2. By the CO_2 release
3. By the tidal volumes

Measurement of End-expiratory CO_2

We use measuring instruments supplied by Siemens, Engström and Datex, which work on the principle of ultrared absorption.

In the closed-circuit system the only problem with the use of these instruments for CO_2 measurements arises from the saturation of the circulating gases with water vapor; this can be avoided by

1. Water traps in the expiratory and inspiratory limbs, at the lowest point in each case
2. Watertraps before the inlet to the measuring chambers

3. Respiratory tubes with smooth inner walls
4. Adequately heated measuring chambers

Measurement of Tidal Volume

We perform these measurements with the mechanical volumetric meters supplied by Dräger, Lübeck.

Respiratory Rate

When the respiratory control system described above is used, the *respiratory rate* results from the *tidal volume* and *end-expiratory* CO_2. It is only a resultant parameter.

Ventilation Pressures

The ventilation pressures are determined in the same way in the closed-circuit system as in the semi-closed or semi-open systems. We use the pressure meters supplied by Dräger, Lübeck, for this purpose.

Soda Lime

It must be borne in mind with the closed-circuit anesthetic system that

1. Dry soda lime binds the volatile anesthetic agents and the water, and because of this together with the low gas inflow rates the necessary concentrations of the anesthetic agents can be reached only with considerable delay.
2. With the rising water vapor saturation, the volatile anesthetic agent is in turn expelled from the soda lime, and because of this, conversely, the concentration of the volatile anesthetic agents subsequently rises rapidly. This, however, becomes apparent at once from the measurements of end-expiratory concentration and can be balanced out by adjustment of the vapors.

Temperature of the Anesthetic Gases

The measuring instruments supplied by Yellow Springs Instruments[4] can be used to determine the temperatures of the anesthetic gases in both the inspiratory and the expiratory limbs.

Recovery Phase

This phase can be controlled very well from the time aspect by the delivery of pure oxygen. Thus, the *recovery phase can be extended* by keeping the circuit closed, discontinuing the delivery of volatile anesthetics and of laughing gas, and adjusting the oxygen delivery to only just correspond to the oxygen requirement. *This phase can be shortened* if in addition to discontinuation of the delivery of laughing gas and the volatile anesthetic agents the system is opened and flushed with large volumes of oxygen. The duration of the recovery phase can be adjusted to anything between these two extremes, with maintainance of the normal ventilation described above.

---

[4] Yellow Springs Instruments, Yellow Springs, Ohio 45387, USA.

Closed-Circuit Anaesthesia in Gynaecology and Obstetrics

R. Spintge and G. Rothmann

Gynaecology

For surgery of the breasts, abdominal surgery and vaginal surgery, the same regime always has to be followed (cf. also Droh, previous chapter).

General Checkpoints

1. Tight system
2. Correct working vaporizer
3. Correct working monitors
4. Calculation of $\dot{V}_{O_2}$ and $\dot{V}_{N_2O}$

Premedication

Premedication is carried out e.g. 1–2 mg flunitrazepam orally the evening before the operation and 1–2 mg flunitrazepam i.m. 60 min prior to anaesthesia.

Induction

Induction is carried out as usual, e.g. 0.5 mg atropine + 1.0 mg pancuronium i.v., 350–500 mg thiopentone i.v. (5–7.5 mg/kg) and 70–100 mg succinyl i.v. (1–2 mg/kg). Ventilation is by mask in the semiclosed system.

Gas flow is 1 litre/min O_2 and 3 litres/min N_2O. Intubation is carried out and a closed system is used.

Maintenance

The gas flows are adjusted to the calculated values, so that inspiratory O_2 = 25 vol.%, expiratory O_2 = 21 vol.%, inspiratory N_2O = 75 vol.% and expiratory $N_2O \leqq 75$ vol.%.

The vaporizer is adjusted to the gas flow, so that end expiratory halothane = 0.3–1.2 vol.%.

The ventilation is adjusted so that end expiratory CO_2 = 4.8 vol.%. Muscle relaxants are administered as usual.

Special Considerations Concerning Laparoscopy

During insertion of the Verres-Needle the excess gas valve is briefly opened. During injection of CO_2 into the abdomen end expiratory CO_2 is carefully monitored. If the end expiratory CO_2 concentration suddenly rises, this could be due to CO_2

gas embolism through intravasal placement of the needle. The ECG is also carefully monitored for signs of gas embolism.

Termination

At first only the halothane is stopped. Then the N_2O is also stopped. The O_2 concentration is slowly increased by increasing the O_2 flow up to 500 ml/min. In this way anaesthesia can be prolonged for 20 min after the termination of halothane. Attention should be paid as usual to muscle relaxants and respiratory depression.

Obstetrics: Caesarian Section

General Checkpoints

1. Tight system
2. Correct working vaporizer
3. Correct working monitors
4. Calculation of $\dot{V}_{O_2}$ und $\dot{V}_{N_2O}$

Premedication

For elective surgery 1 mg flunitrazepam + 800 mg cimetidine are given orally the evening before the section. 10 mg metoclopramide are administered 60 min prior to anaesthesia. For emergency surgery there is no premedication.

After premedication there are two possible regimes: one with halothane and the second without halothane.

Using Halothane

Induction
1. 0.5 mg atropine + 1.0 mg pancuronium i.v.
2. 125–250 mg thiopentone i.v. (1.5–3.5 mg/kg)
3. 70–100 mg succinyl i.v. (1–2 mg/kg)

Breathing is by mask in the semiclosed system with a gas flow of *2 liters/min O_2 only*. Intubation is carried out and a closed system is used.

Maintenance. Nitrous oxide is added and gas flows are adjusted to the calculated values, slightly increasing O_2 flow, so that inspiratory O_2 = 30 vol.%, end expiratory O_2 = 25 vol.%, inspiratory N_2O = 70 vol.% and end expiratory $N_2O \leqq$ 70 vol.%. The vaporizer is adjusted to the gas flows, so that end expiratory halothane = 0.3–0.6 vol.%.

The ventilation is adjusted so that end expiratory CO_2 = 4.2 vol.%.

These values are kept until the peritoneum is incised.

After incision of the peritoneum the semiclosed system is used again. O_2 flow is increased to 2 liters/min and N_2O and halothane are stopped.

End expiratory CO_2 is maintained at 4.2 vol.%. As soon as the *umbilical cord* has been *cut* the system is closed again. The gas flows are changed to the calculated values, so that inspiratory O_2 = 25 vol.%, end expiratory O_2 = 21 vol.%, inspiratory N_2O = 75 vol.%, and end expiratory $N_2O \leqq$ 75 vol.%.

The vaporizer is adjusted to the gas flow, so that end expiratory halothane = 0.3–1.2 vol.%. The end expiratory CO_2 is always kept at 4.2 vol.%. Muscle relaxants are used as usual.

Termination. At first only the halothane is stopped. Then the N_2O is also terminated. The O_2 concentration is slowly increased by increasing the O_2 flow up to 500 ml/min. In this way anaesthesia can be prolonged for 20 min from the termination of halothane. Attention should be paid as usual to muscle relaxants and respiratory depression.

Without Using Halothane

Induction

1. 10 mg metoclopramide i.v.
2. 1.0 mg pancuronium i.v.
3. 75–100 mg ketamine i.v. (1.25–2 mg/kg)
4. 75–100 mg thiopentone i.v. (1.2–2 mg/kg)
5. 100 mg succinyl i.v. (1.5–2 mg/kg)

Breathing is by mask in the semiclosed system with only *2 liters* O_2*/min.* Intubation is carried out and the closed system is used.

Maintenance. Nitrous oxide is added and gas flows of O_2 and N_2O are adjusted to the calculated values, slightly increasing O_2 flow, so that inspiratory O_2 = 30 vol.%, end expiratory O_2 = 25 vol.%, inspiratory N_2O = 70 vol.% and end expiratory $N_2O \leqq 70$ vol.%. The ventilation is adjusted so that end expiratory CO_2 = 4.2 vol.%. These values are maintained until the peritoneum is incised.

After Incision of the Peritoneum, the semiclosed system is used again. O_2 flow is increased to 2 liters/min. N_2O is stopped.

End expiratory CO_2 is maintained at 4.2 vol.%.

As soon as the *umbilical cord* has been cut the system is closed again.

The gas flows are changed to the calculated values, so that inspiratory O_2 = 25 vol.%, end expiratory O_2 = 21 vol.%, inspiratory N_2O = 75 vol.% and end expiratory $N_2O \leqq 75$ vol.%.

End expiratory CO_2 is always maintained at 4.2 vol.% and 0.1–0.2 mg fentanyl is injected. Muscle relaxants are used as usual.

Termination. Nitrous oxide is stopped and O_2 concentration is slowly increased by increasing O_2 flow up to 500 ml/min. In this way anaesthesia usually can be prolonged for 15–20 min from the last injection of 0.1 mg fentanyl. Attention should be paid as usual to muscle relaxants and respiratory depression.

First Clinical Experiences with the Narcocon in Completely Computerized On-Demand Closed-Circuit Ventilation

R. Spintge, R. Droh, and G. Rothmann

The many advantages of closed-circuit-ventilation systems (CCV) are well known (Droh 1985).

To perform automatic CCV in clinical practice, e.g. for general anaesthesia and long-term ventilation in intensive care units, some basic preconditions must be fulfilled:

1. A completely *closed and absolutely airtight patient circuit* must be used.
2. The ventilator must have settings for:
   (a) Respiratory rate,
   (b) Tidal volume, and
   (c) Airway pressure;
   with low and high limits for these parameters.
3. There must be *permanent monitoring* of:
   (a) Inspired concentration of O_2
   (b) End expired concentration of CO_2
   (c) End expired concentration of volatile anaesthetics (halothane, isoflurane, ethrane) and
   (d) Heart rate and ECG.
   Besides these essential parameters it is desirable to monitor:
   (e) Inspired and expired concentration of N_2O
   (f) Inspired and expired concentration of N_2
   (g) Inspired and expired gas temperature
   (h) Oxygen consumption
   (i) O_2 pulse/O_2 availability
   (j) Ventilatory minute-volume
   (k) Humidity of the system
4. Furthermore, there should be a completely computerized *on-demand delivery* of anaesthetic gases.
5. The rebreathing circuit of the patient and the ventilation circuit of the ventilator should be *completely separated,* so that the ventilation can be driven by any commonly used ventilator in every clinic.

We will report about our first clinical experiences with a CCV system which fulfills nearly all of the above-listed requirements.

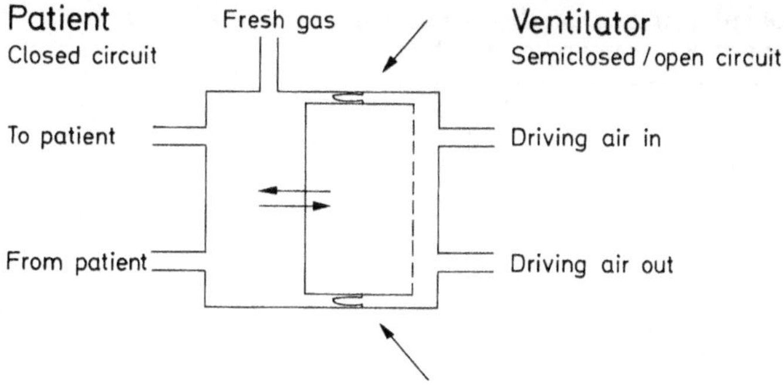

Fig. 1. The rolling seal separates the closed patient circuit from the ventilator circuit

Method

Concerning the method of inducing and maintaining closed-circuit anaesthesia we refer to the paper: "Practical Application of the Closed-Circuit-System" (Droh, this volume).

The machine we used for computerized on-demand delivery of the anaesthetic gases is the Narcocon from Mijnhardt/Hellige. The Narcocon links together the *completely closed patient circuit* and any *pressure-controlled ventilator*. This is achieved by the *"rolling seal rebreathing respirometer"*.

We used the Narcocon together with two old ventilators, the Dräger Pulmomat and the Dräger Asistor, and with one of the most sophisticated modern ventilators, the Bennett 7200.

In the Narcocon the volume loss through gas uptake is determined by a piston not reaching its end position. This loss is replaced via electronic feedback control with N_2O and O_2, keeping inspired oxygen concentration and total volume constant at a predetermined level. That means, before the start of anaesthesia we programme into the Narcocon:

1. The precalculated values of O_2 and N_2O uptake
2. The desired inspired O_2 and N_2O concentration
3. The respiratory rate and airway pressure

We will restrict our presentation to our initial clinical experiences and some basic technical information.

Results

1. Technology
   a) The Narcocon works.
   b) It is easy programmable.
   c) The control of the anaesthetic gas-mixture with additional monitors (Datex "Normocap", Engström "Eliza", Dräger "Oxycom") showed that the delivery and the constancy of concentration of the anaesthetic gases is quickly achieved and reliable.

Table 1. Postoperative evaluation of the anaesthesia protocol and the postoperative subjective questionnaire ($n=221$)

Recovery time until extubation	
Mean	8 min
Maximum	35 min
Stay in recovery room	
Mean	80 min
Maximum	270 min
Postoperative vomiting	
None	
Patient's subjective feeling	
Comfortable	76%
Uncomfortable	4%
No answer	20%

d) No technical failure has so far occurred.

e) The different ventilators mentioned above are easily adaptable to the Narcocon and so to CCV.

2. Clinical results

a) So far 221 patients have been "treated" with automatic computerized ventilation in closed-circuit anaesthesia (May 1984). All of them underwent some orthopaedic surgery of the extremities. The distribution of age and sex were:

Mean age	34 years
Maximum	68 years
Minimum	15 years
Male	66%
Female	34%

b) The intraoperative values of blood pressure and heart rate are unchanged compared with manual ventilation:

Blood pressure (Riva Rocci) (mm Hg)		Heart rate (beats/min)	
Mean RR	130/70	Mean	74
Systolic: maximum	180	maximum	122
minimum	100	minimum	48
Diastolic: maximum	100		
minimum	40		

c) No critical incidences or undesired side effects occurred.

d) The postoperative evaluation from the anaesthesia protocol and the postoperative subjective questionnaire are shown in Table 1.

All parameters are quite similar to the results from our usual manual ventilation.

Summary

On the whole there are still some improvements that are desirable, for instance, the possibility of switching from automatic to manual ventilation.

But the question: "Is completely computerized automatic closed-circuit ventilation possible now?" can be clearly answered: "Yes!"

Reference

Droh R (1985) The closed-circuit anaesthesia system. In: Droh R, Erdmann W, Spintge R (eds) Anaesthesia-Innovations in management. Springer, Berlin Heidelberg New York Tokyo, pp 3–9

Closed-Circuit Anaesthesia for Cardiac Patients

C.-Y. Lin

Closed-circuit anaesthesia itself is not a new technique or concept. It was practised for a long time when cyclopropane was used, purely for economic reasons. With the use of new potent inhalation anaesthetics such as halothane, the introduction of the concept of *minimum alveolar concentration* (MAC) and limited knowledge about the uptake of inhalation anaesthetics, there was a tendency to employ excessive flows of anaesthetic gas to maintain the inspired anaesthetic concentration. Consequently, the closed-circuit system was replaced by the current, very popular semiclosed system. In recent years, the practice of closed-circuit anaesthesia, or the low-flow or minimal-flow technique, attracted the attention of anaesthesiologists because of the inherent advantage of closed-circuit anaesthesia and the publicity on the dangers of anaesthetic pollution.

In order to practise closed-circuit anaesthesia, one should fully understand the mechanism of anaesthetic uptake. During closed-circuit anaesthesia, it is necessary only to supply the amount of anaesthetic vapour which the patient requires or absorbs; otherwise, the patient may be overdosed or underdosed. In the past several years, we have developed a new concept of uptake which differs from previously published concepts, and which provides a better understanding and an easy method of application of closed-circuit anaesthesia.

There are several ways of practising closed-circuit anaesthesia, from very simple to very complicated, fully automated methods. But the most practical method should be one that is simple to apply and safe for the patients. From a practical standpoint, several questions may arise: (1) Can closed-circuit anaesthesia be practised starting from time zero? If not, how soon can one start? (2) Does uptake of inhalation anaesthetics follow a power function, or is it best approximated by a power function? (3) How carefully should the system be monitored, and what basic monitoring is required during closed-circuit anaesthesia?

Can Closed-Circuit Anaesthesia Be Practised Starting from Time Zero? Closed-circuit anaesthesia can seldom be practised from time zero, because of the existence of the functional residual capacity and the large anaesthetic circuit volume. When anaesthetic gases are introduced into the circuit, volume-to-volume gas exchange occurs between the anaesthetic gas and gases pre-existing in the lung and anaesthetic circuit. Administration of high concentrations of nitrous oxide provides a large volume of gas, but not all of the nitrous oxide will be absorbed on a breath-by-breath basis. Consequently, some of the anaesthetic gas provided will need to escape from the circuit; otherwise, it will continually increase the pressure in the circuit with each expiration. Thus, it is impossible to conduct closed-circuit anaesthesia starting from the beginning when a high concentration of anaesthetic gas or a large volume of an anaesthetic such as nitrous oxide is used. The use of a lower volume of a potent inhalation anaesthetic with 100% oxygen certainly is an alternative method; but with a large circuit volume and functional residual capacity, as is present in the closed circuit, this requires efficient circulation in order to eliminate the possible bolus effect or transient extremely high inspired concentration of potent inhalation anaesthetics.

Time Course of Uptake of Inhalation Anaesthetics. Since Severinghaus's publication on nitrous oxide in 1954 [4] many investigators of inhalation anaesthetics have expressed anaesthetic uptake over time as a power function. For example, the rate of nitrous oxide uptake, according to Severinghaus, is expressed by 1000 (ml) $t^{-1/2}$ and the rate of halothane uptake, according to Lowe and Mapleson [5, 6], is given by 50 (ml) $t^{-1/2}$. However, the approximations made in the derivation of the $t^{-1/2}$ function, in fact, do not separate the *functional residual capacity* (FRC) wash-in from the true body uptake. When one uses 80% nitrous oxide at the beginning of wash-in a total of 2400 ml nitrous oxide must be administered to fill the average 3000 ml FRC before uptake begins. Severinghaus's measurements do not take this wash-in volume into account. During wash-in of certain anaesthetic gases into the FRC, especially with a large volume or high concentration of an anaesthetic gas such as nitrous oxide, exchange with gases preexisting in the FRC takes place on a volume-by-volume basis.

If the rate of uptake of inhalation anaesthetics does not follow the square root of time (power function) during the period of wash-in, then what is the time

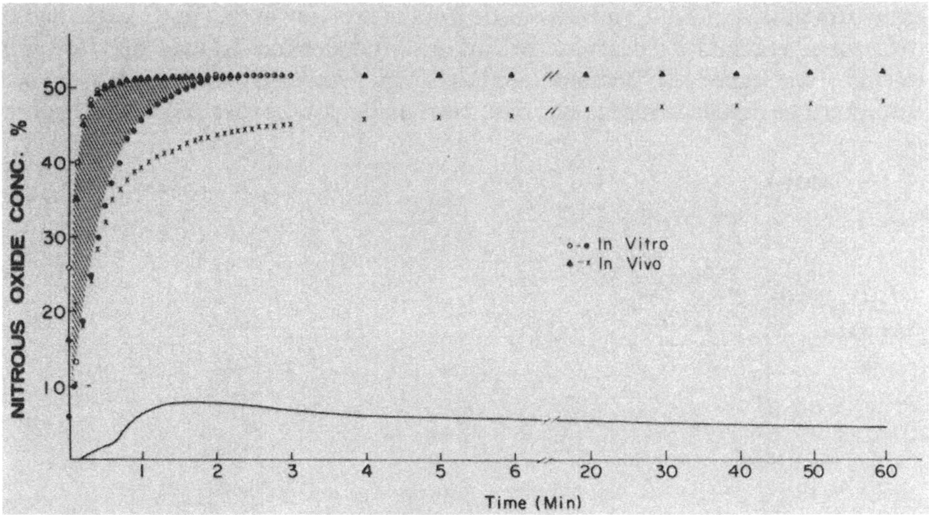

Fig. 1. Results of an experiment conducted in vitro and in vivo, designed to demonstrate the near-constancy of nitrous oxide uptake following FRC wash-in. The *shaded area* indicates in vitro wash-in in an experiment with the FRC of the patient matched by a reservoir bag. Subtraction of the nitrous oxide wash-in into this simulated lung from the tracing obtained in vivo yields the net body uptake, which is plotted *at the bottom*. This demonstrates the near-constant uptake of nitrous oxide over a 1-h period. In the beginning, the anaesthetic gas mixture is washed into the FRC and must be exchanged with existing gases in the FRC. This produces only limited uptake, because the anaesthetic gas has not reached its peak inspiratory concentration due to dilution by gases pre-existing in the lung

course of uptake of inhalation anaesthetics? Because of the higher solubility partition coefficient of anaesthetic gases, it was believed in the past that no membrane barrier existed for uptake of inhalation anaesthetics. However, we have demonstrated in several experiments that: (1) a membrane barrier does exist; (2) uptake is at its peak at the end of FRC wash-in and remains near-constant for a given inspired anaesthetic concentration; and (3) uptake depends on inspired concentration – if the inspired concentration increases, uptake increases.

To separate the FRC wash-in from the total uptake measured at the mouthpiece, we performed an experiment in which we used a subtraction method. During constant-volume ventilation, inspiratory-expiratory concentration differences represent uptake if one assumes that complete mixing of gases occurred in the lungs. For nitrous oxide uptake, we obtained inspiratory and expiratory nitrous oxide concentration curves when nitrous oxide and oxygen were introduced into a circle system with a patient attached. With the same ventilatory rate, ventilatory volume and fresh-gas flow, we then carried out an in vitro wash-in experiment with the FRC of the patient matched by a reservoir bag. Subtraction of the expired nitrous oxide concentration during wash-in into the simulated lung from the expired concentration measured in vivo yielded the net nitrous oxide concentration difference due to actual body uptake of the gas across the alveolar membrane. As shown at the bottom of Fig. 1, nitrous oxide uptake by the blood in the 1st min is less than that in the 2nd or 3rd min. This can be explained by the fact that the inspired concentration of anaesthetic cannot immediately reach a peak at the alveolar level because the anaesthetic gas is diluted by the gases pre-existing in the FRC.

With a similar experimental method, nitrous oxide uptake was measured clinically. As shown in Fig. 2, nitrous oxide uptake was low in the first 2 min; the rate of uptake reached its peak at the 3rd min and declined slowly over the next 60 min. The figure also demonstrated that a 60% inspired nitrous oxide concentration gave a higher average rate of nitrous oxide uptake than did a 50% inspired

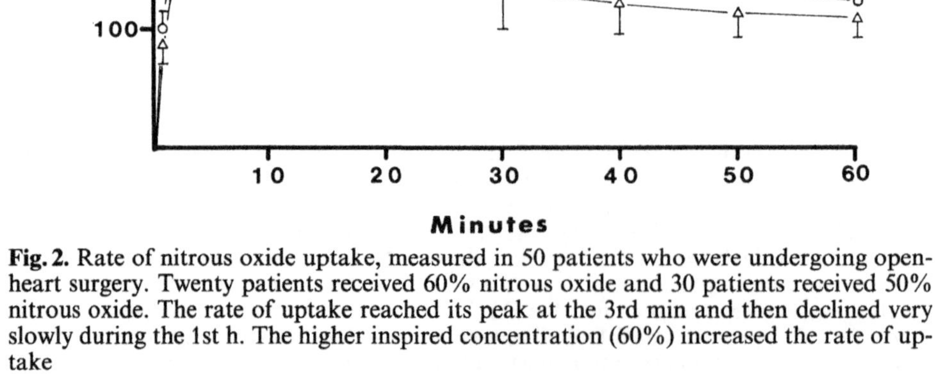

Fig. 2. Rate of nitrous oxide uptake, measured in 50 patients who were undergoing open-heart surgery. Twenty patients received 60% nitrous oxide and 30 patients received 50% nitrous oxide. The rate of uptake reached its peak at the 3rd min and then declined very slowly during the 1st h. The higher inspired concentration (60%) increased the rate of uptake

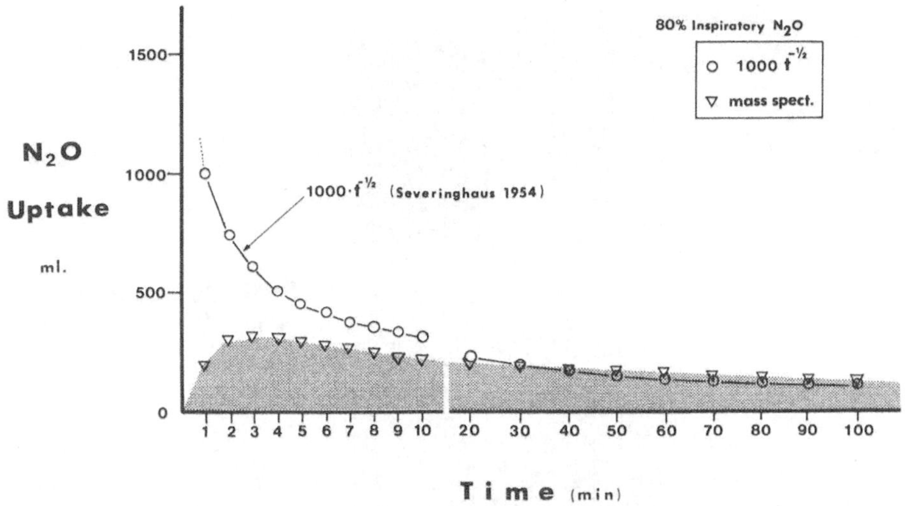

Fig. 3. Schematic comparison of rates of nitrous oxide uptake as measured by mass spectrometry and as approximated with the $t^{-1/2}$ function (Severinghaus), at an inspiratory nitrous oxide concentration of 80%. The discrepancy during the initial phase indicates that the power function approximation overestimates the uptake of nitrous oxide because of failure to separate FRC wash-in from true body uptake. (*Shaded area* represents uptake)

concentration. In Fig. 3, a comparison is made between Severinghaus's power function approximation of the rate of nitrous oxide uptake and our measured values. A great difference in uptake of nitrous oxide during the first 10 min is demonstrated. This discrepancy again reflects that, when an anaesthetic gas mixture is washed into the FRC, it must be exchanged with the gases in the FRC. During the initial time of this exchange, the blood will absorb some of the anaesthetic gas mixture from the lungs, but only to a limited degree, because the anaesthetic has not reached its peak inspiratory concentration. In Fig. 4, it is further shown indirectly from measurements on a patient that, initially, nitrous oxide uptake is limited in amount because of the existence of the FRC and the alveolar membrane. After complete preoxygenation, 1500 ml/min nitrous oxide and 250 ml/min oxygen were introduced. After 6 min at this level, the nitrous oxide concentration at the expiratory side of the circuit reached 60%. With 1500 ml/min nitrous oxide introduced into 3000 ml FRC and 6000 ml circuit volume (a total of 9000 ml), after one time constant of 6 min the nitrous oxide concentration will be 63% if none was absorbed. This indicates that very limited nitrous oxide uptake occurred in this 6-min period. If nitrous oxide uptake is a function of the square root of time, there should be a slower rise in the expired concentration of the gas.

In Fig. 5, we illustrate an experiment which we carried out during anaesthesia to demonstrate the existence of a membrane barrier to the uptake of anaesthetic from the lung. The fresh-gas nitrous oxide concentration was increased five times, at 5-min intervals, in steps of 10%; at a total fresh-gas flow of 10 000 ml/min, and then was decreased in equal steps every 5 min. With constant-volume ventilation, as was used here, inspiratory-expiratory differences in nitrous oxide concentration again represent uptake of the gas after each brief period of FRC wash-in. The figure shows that, when the inspired nitrous oxide concentration rises, the uptake

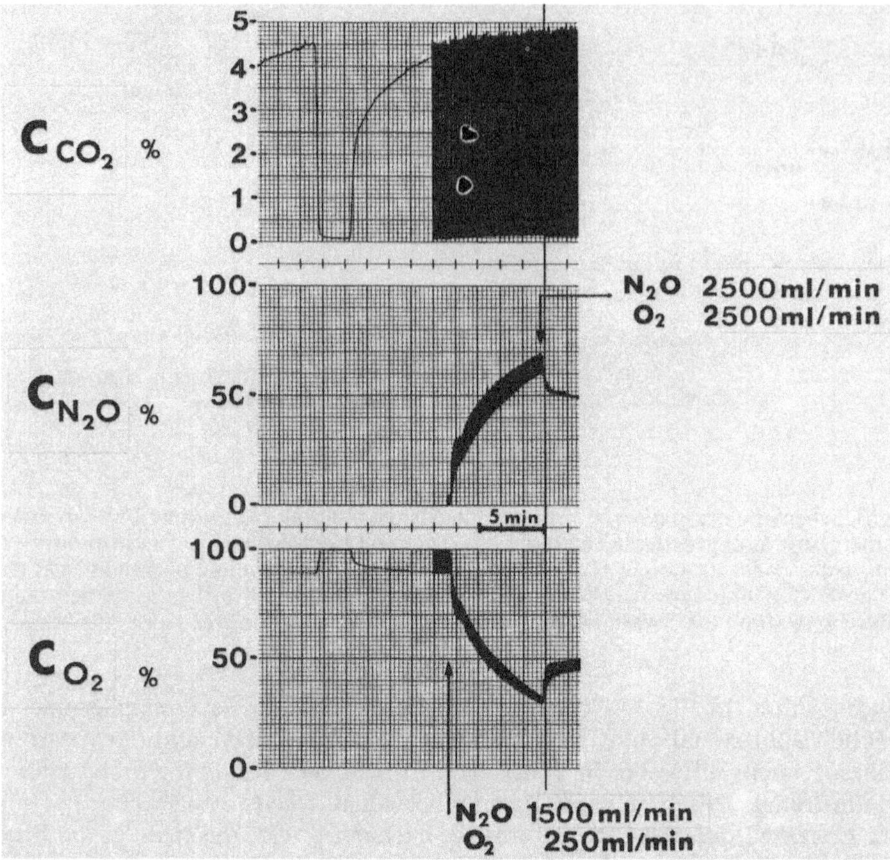

Fig. 4. Mass spectrometric tracing from a patient, showing that the increase in nitrous oxide concentration almost matches the wash-in time constant (6 min) during nitrous oxide administration; this is indicative of limited nitrous oxide uptake in the beginning. 3000 ml FRC plus 6000 ml of circuit equals 9000 ml with 1500 ml/min of nitrous oxide; after 1 time constant of 6 min, the nitrous oxide concentration will reach 63% if there is no uptake across the alveolar membrane

rises. This indicates that, provided the cardiac output, ventilatory rate and solubility partition coefficient remain constant, the partial pressure gradient across the alveolar membrane is the sole factor controlling the rate of uptake. This same phenomenon can be demonstrated with other inhalation anaesthetics such as halothane (Fig. 6). When the inspired halothane concentration was raised from 0.5% to 1.5% in 0.5% increments at 15-min intervals, the uptake, again measured as the inspiratory-expiratory concentration difference, doubled at 1% inspired concentration and tripled at 1.5% inspired concentration.

The uptake of an anaesthetic gas through the alveolar membrane commonly follows the Fick principle of diffusion:

$$\text{Rate of penetration} = (C_{\text{out}} - C_{\text{in}})\, DAK/x,$$

where C_{out} = concentration outside the membrane, C_{in} = concentration inside the membrane, D = diffusion constant, A = area of membrane, K = partition coefficient and x = thickness of membrane.

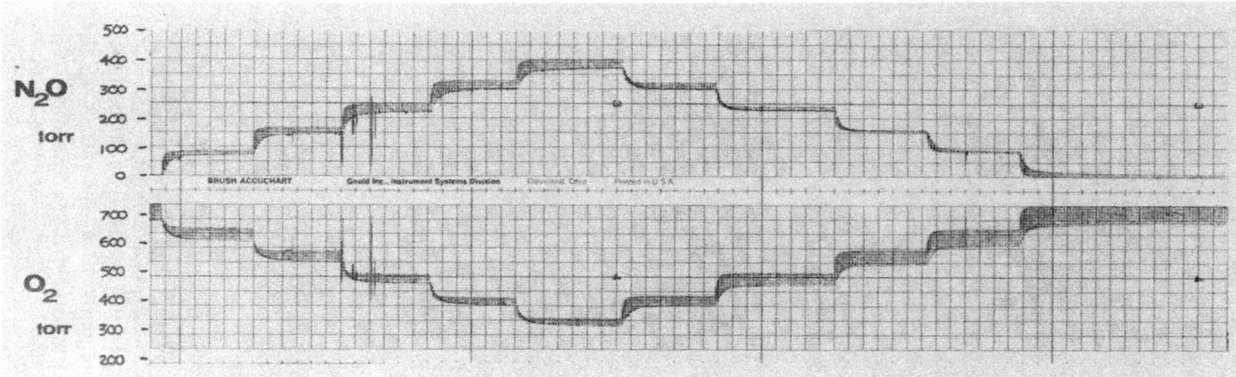

Fig. 5. An experiment was conducted to demonstrate inspiratory-concentration-dependent uptake of nitrous oxide in a patient. The nitrous oxide concentration was increased five times, at 5-min intervals in steps of 10%, at a total fresh-gas flow of 10000 ml/min, and then decreased in equal steps. With constant-volume ventilation, inspiratory-expiratory concentration differences represent the uptake of N_2O after each brief period of FRC wash-in. As the inspired concentration rises, uptake also rises

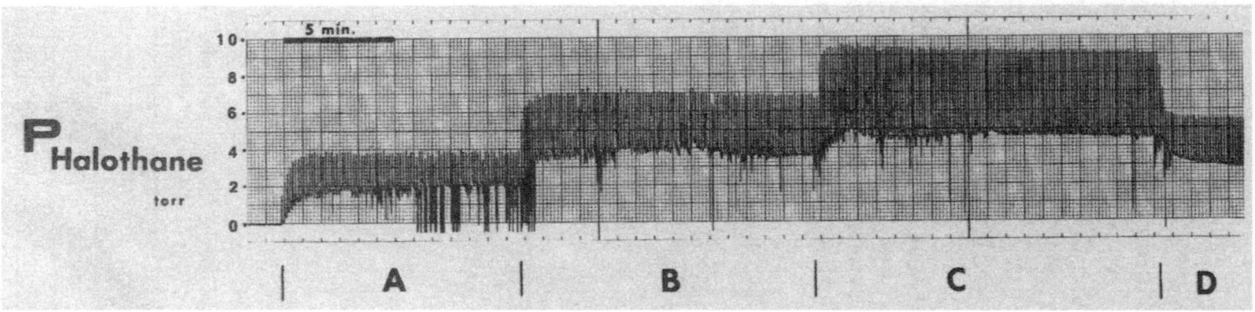

Fig. 6. An experiment was conducted to demonstrate inspiratory-concentration-dependent uptake of halothane in a patient. The halothane concentration was increased three times, at 10- to 15-min intervals, in steps of 0.5% (3.5 torr), at a total fresh-gas flow of 10000 ml/min. With constant-volume ventilation, inspiratory-expiratory concentration differences represent the uptake of halothane after each brief period of FRC wash-in. As the inspired concentration rises, uptake also rises

The quotient DAK/x is frequently called the permeability constant, P, of the system. Thus, we can rewrite this equation as

$$\text{Rate of uptake} = (C_{out} - C_{in})\,P.$$

The permeability constant, P, is mainly determined by the solubility coefficient of the gas, and in the past it was commonly neglected in consideration of the cardiac output, or, strictly speaking, the pulmonary capillary flow together with diffusion. In Pipper's [7] simple, but useful, model for analyses of blood gas equilibration in the lung, the pulmonary capillary blood is separated from the gas space by a "membrane" representing resistance to diffusion. The degree of equilibration, expressed as the ratio of the alveolar-to-arterial pressure difference to the alveolar-to-mixed-venous pressure difference, is a function of the ratio D/BQ (D = diffusion capacity, B = capacitance coefficient, Q = pulmonary capillary blood flow). In the case of anaesthetic gases, no equilibration deficit exists at the membrane ($D/BQ \rightarrow$) and the gas transfer is mainly perfusion-limited.

In the past, the rate of uptake was believed to be very high in the beginning, and no barrier to initial uptake was postulated, so that the mixed venous concentration was thought to rise very rapidly because of rapid equilibration of blood-rich organs. In contrast to this viewpoint, one should recognize that the membrane factor exists, and that uptake is not diffusion-limited, but perfusion-limited in the case of inhalation anaesthetics.

In view of these changes in the concept of uptake of inhalation anaesthetics, let us further examine the relationship between end-expiratory or alveolar con-

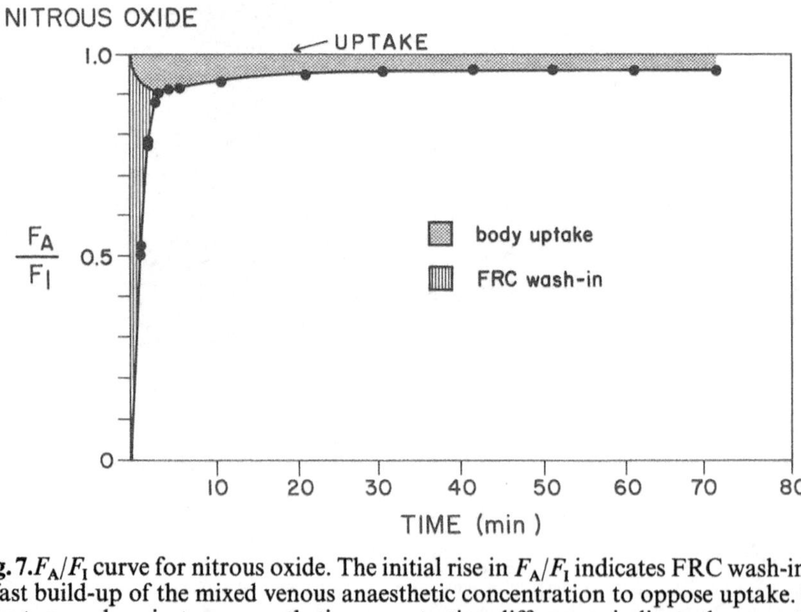

Fig. 7. F_A/F_I curve for nitrous oxide. The initial rise in F_A/F_I indicates FRC wash-in and not a fast build-up of the mixed venous anaesthetic concentration to oppose uptake. Since inspiratory and expiratory anaesthetic concentration differences indicate the anaesthetic uptake during constant-volume ventilation, the rate of true body uptake should be represented by the *shaded area*, which shows very limited change over 1 h. The rate of uptake is best expressed by the values above the F_A/F_I curve and not by the F_A/F_I curve itself. The initial lower rate of uptake can be explained by the fact that the inspired concentration of nitrous oxide cannot reach a peak at the alveolar level because nitrous oxide is diluted by the gases pre-existing in the FRC

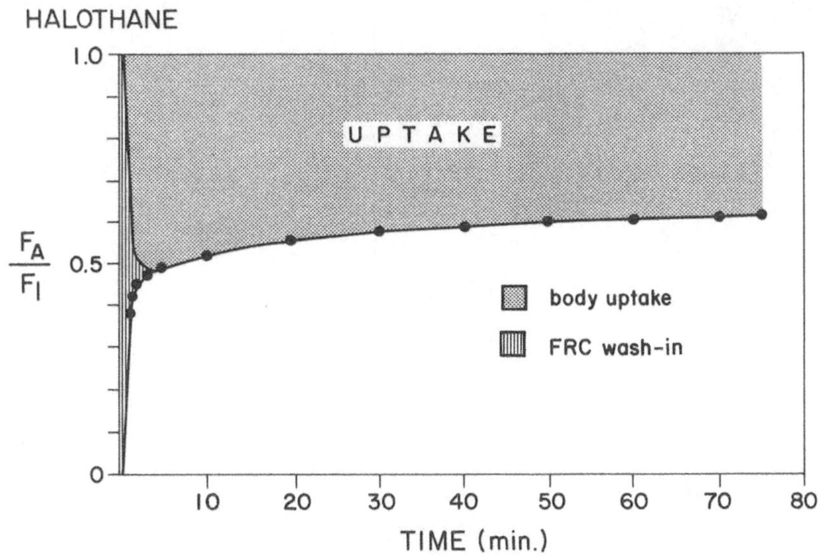

Fig. 8. F_A/F_I curve for halothane. The initial fast rise in F_A/F_I indicates FRC wash-in and not a fast build-up of the mixed venous anaesthetic concentration to oppose uptake (decreased partial pressure differences across the alveolar membrane). The true body uptake is represented by the *shaded* area, which shows a very limited change in the rate of uptake over 1 h. This diagram also demonstrates that, as inspired concentration increases, the rate of uptake increases. Thus, the rate of uptake can be approximated by the expression: inspiratory concentration × fraction of uptake × alveolar ventilation

centration and inspiratory concentration over time. Eger [8] has employed this relationship to demonstrate the rate of uptake. However, the initial rapid rise of the F_A/F_I curve for nitrous oxide in Fig. 7 is not indicative of a large uptake of nitrous oxide, but represents the FRC wash-in, as described above. In other words, because of the initial limited uptake of nitrous oxide, the alveolar concentration will quickly rise towards the inspired concentration (F_A/F_I). Since uptake of anaesthetics can be measured as the difference between inspired and expired concentration, we conclude that the rate of uptake is best represented not by the F_A/F_I curve, but by the region above the curve, i.e. the difference between F_A/F_I and the curve. The fractional N_2O uptake at a given time can be expressed as:

$$\text{Fraction of uptake} = 1 - F_A/F_I.$$

The same principle can be applied to other inhalation anaesthetics; the curve for halothane is shown in Fig. 8 and that for enflurane (Ethrane) in Fig. 9. The isoflurane (forane) curve is very similar to that for ethrane because of the similarity in their solubility coefficients. The fraction of uptake for several anaesthetic gases is given in Table 1. As mentioned before, the fact that the fraction of uptake for each of the gases changes very little with time indicates that the uptake of an anaesthetic can be considered to be nearly constant at a given inspired concentration over 1 h (with the assumption of constant cardiac output and constant alveolar ventilation).

As demonstrated by Eger, the F_A/F_I curves vary with ventilation and cardiac output. Much misleading information has been published on this variation in the

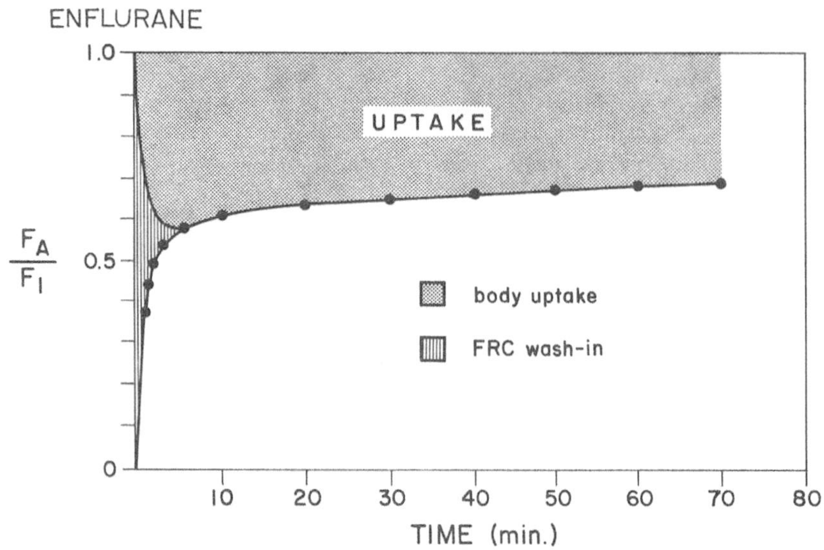

Fig. 9. F_A/F_I curve for enflurane. This again demonstrates the near-constancy of the rate of uptake over 1 h

Table 1. Fraction of uptake

Agent	Initial	After 60 min	After 120 min
N_2O	0.13	0.07	0.05
Halothane	0.50	0.40	0.35
Enflurane	0.40	0.35	0.30
Isoflurane	0.40	0.35	0.30
Methoxyflurane	0.80	0.75	0.70

Fraction of uptake $= [1 - F_A/F_I]$ (after FRC wash-in)

past because too much emphasis was placed on the value of the alveolar concentration. During shock or when the cardiac output is low, the alveolar concentration rises towards the inspired concentration faster than is the case under normal cardiac output conditions. This may reflect not an increase in the depth of anaesthesia, but a reduction in the fraction of uptake at a given concentration – an indication that anaesthetic uptake is lower. Ventilation also influences the shape of the F_A/F_I curve. A higher ventilation rate results in a higher F_A/F_I curve and lower ventilation gives a lower curve. Since the rate of uptake of anaesthetic after FRC wash-in can be expressed or estimated as: rate of uptake = inspired concentration × fraction of uptake × alveolar ventilation, altering the rate of ventilation should have a very limited influence on uptake except during the initial wash-in period (if the alveolar ventilation increases, the fraction of uptake decreases).

Monitoring During Closed-Circuit Anaesthesia. With these new concepts of uptake of inhalation anaesthetics in mind, we developed a very simple, practical, but safe method of closed-circuit anaesthesia for clinical use.

This new method does not deviate very much from the current practice of using a semiclosed system in terms of inspiratory concentration. The approximate amount of anaesthetic vapour needed to maintain a similar inspiratory concentration can be calculated with the use of the formula given above for the rate of uptake. After the initial wash-in period, when the system is closed, one can apply a very simple physics principle – the lower the flow, the longer the time constant. At its extreme, the circuit condition becomes a closed system, and the discrepancy between supply and demand volume becomes extremely small. With the small volume of fresh gas compared with the large circuit volume which we use during closed-circuit anaesthesia, the circuit volume will act as a giant buffer system. Unless there is a continuous supply of excessive amounts of anaesthetic into the circuit, it is difficult to change the existing circuit concentration and to have the inspired concentration reach an undesirable level.

Thus, at the alveolar membrane, the inspiratory-concentration-dependent uptake will function as a self-contained limited-feedback system. This eliminates the need for sophisticated equipment for continuous monitoring in the conduct of closed-circuit anaesthesia.

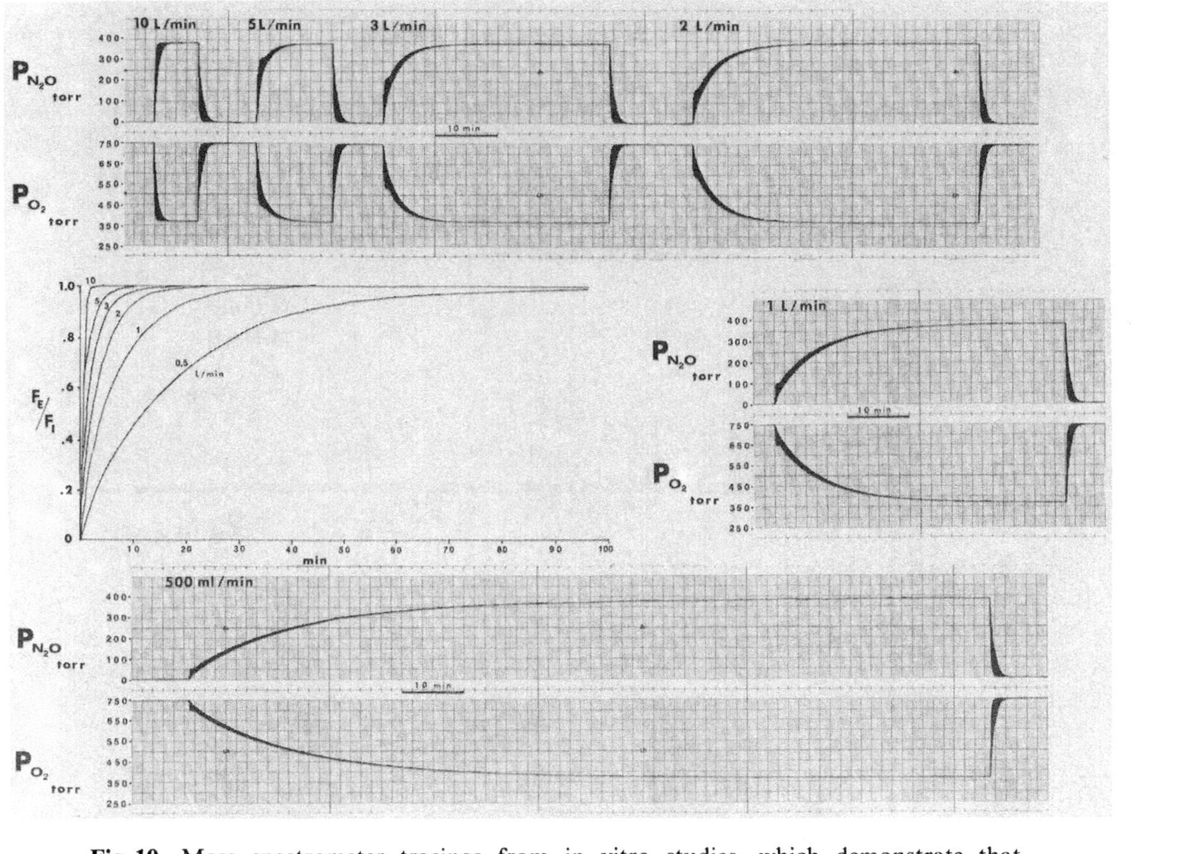

Fig. 10. Mass spectrometer tracings from in vitro studies, which demonstrate that equilibration of 50% nitrous oxide after wash-in into FRC and circuit anaesthetic is a function of the rate of fresh-gas flow. The higher the fresh-gas flow, the more rapidly one achieves equilibration, which is indicated in the *middle left panel* as $F_E/F_I = 1.0$. The curves also indicate that, once equilibration is reached, it is difficult to change the concentration by using a fresh-gas flow

After a brief period of FRC and circuit wash-in with a high fresh-gas flow (Fig. 10), one can apply a simple and practical method of closed-circuit anaesthesia based on three principles:

1. Near-constant uptake of anaesthetic during 1 h after initial FRC wash-in with a given anaesthetic concentration (at a step function of 1 h). This eliminates the necessity of following the complicated power function curve in supplying anaesthetic vapor.
2. Uptake depends on inspired anaesthetic concentration; when the supply of anaesthetic vapour exceeds the demand, then inspiratory concentration rises; uptake then increases, and this results in bringing down the inspired concentration towards the original level.
3. The large circuit volume and FRC serve as a buffer.

Preparatory Procedures and Equipment

Anaesthetic Machine Requirements

Rotameters for O_2 and N_2O Must be Accurate at low Flows (0- to 1-liter/min Type)

Absolute accuracy of the flowmeter at low flow rate is desirable, but is not a necessary criterion in the clinical setup, especially if 100% oxygen is used with potent inhalation anaesthetics or high-dose narcotics. When the total volume of the gas

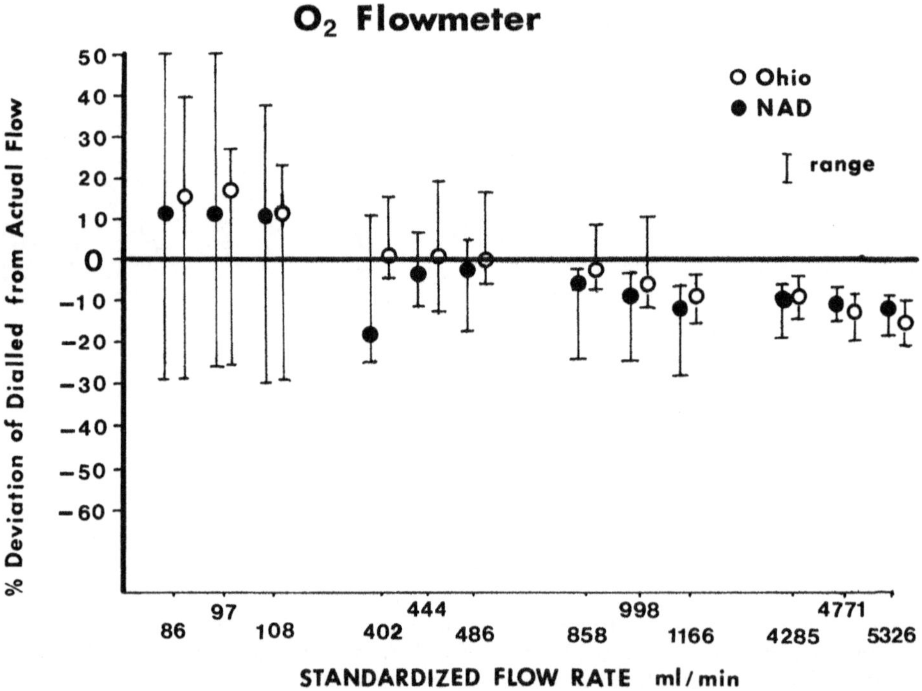

Fig. 11. Oxygen flowmeter accuracy as evaluated in 22 different anaesthesia machines. Higher actual flow than the dialled flow and large deviation of dialled flow and actual flows were demonstrated at lower flow rates

supply matches the total gas volume consumed by the patient, we achieve the condition of a closed system. When a high concentration and a high volume of nitrous oxide are going to be used clinically, the relationship of flow rates between nitrous oxide and oxygen becomes quite important. As shown in Figs. 11 and 12, we examined the anaesthetic machines in our hospital and found a very wide variation in flowmeter accuracy from machine to machine. When we compared the

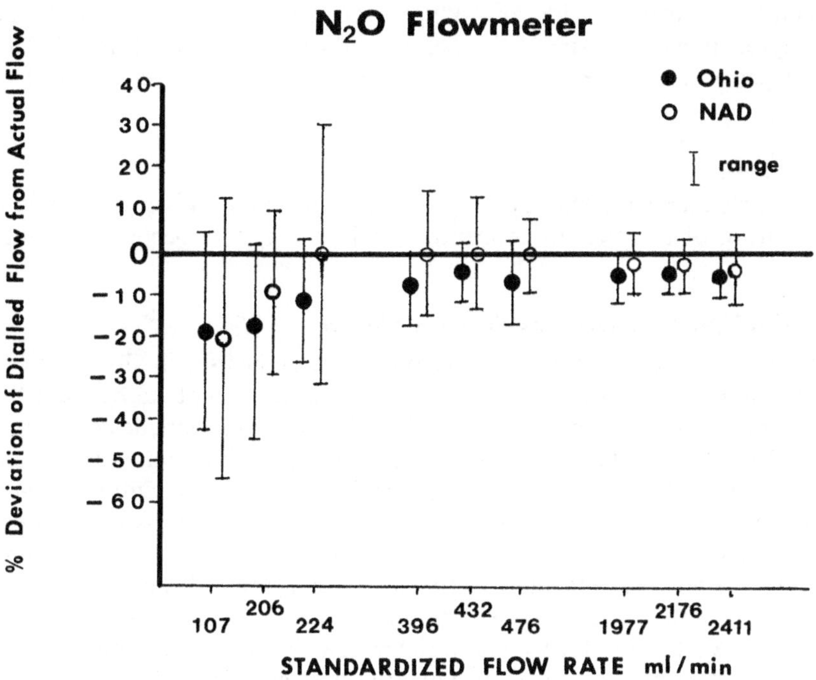

Fig. 12. Nitrous oxide flowmeter accuracy, as evaluated in 22 different anaesthesia machines by means of the bubble meter technique. Lower actual flows than dialled flow and very large deviations of dialled flow from actual flows were demonstrated at lower flow rates

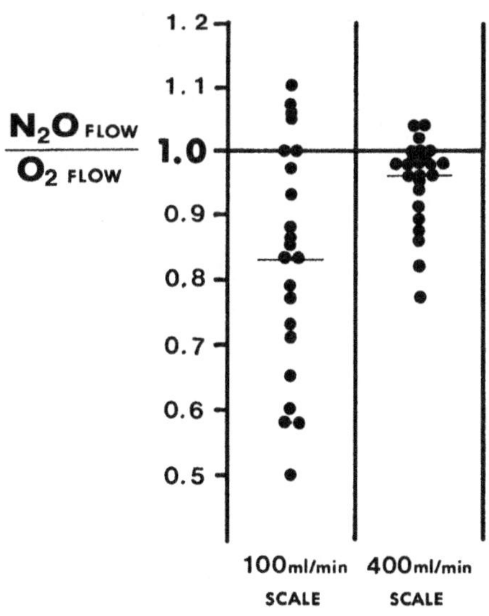

Fig. 13. Actual flow rates of nitrous oxide and oxygen were compared at 100 ml/min and 400 ml/min dial setting on each anaesthesia machine tested. Wide scatter between nitrous oxide and oxygen flow was demonstrated at both dialled flow rates. The low N_2O/O_2 ratios at 100 ml/min dial scale indicate lower actual nitrous oxide flow than actual oxygen flow

nitrous oxide and oxygen flowmeters (Fig. 13) at a similar dialled flow rate, we found that the nitrous oxide flowmeter registered a higher value than the actual flow, which seems to indicate the built-in safety factor in the manufacture of flowmeters. Therefore, we recommend checking the ratio of flow between nitrous oxide and oxygen on each anaesthetic machine intended for use with the closed-circuit technique. This can be done simply with an oxygen analyzer. The calibrated oxygen analyzer is attached to the outlet of the fresh-gas flow for 15 min, with the flowmeters for nitrous oxide and oxygen set at the same flow rate. If the oxygen analyzer shows more than 50% oxygen at the end of 15 min, this indicates that the oxygen flow is higher than the nitrous oxide flow at the registered flow rate.

Oxygen Analyzer

This is preferably located in the expiratory arm of the circuit. If nitrous oxide is used, monitoring of the oxygen concentration in the system becomes mandatory.

Ventilator with Upward Bellows, Such as Air Shields

It is recommended that ventilator-controlled respiration be used in all closed-circuit anaesthesia cases. This provides an easy estimation of uptake because the constant alveolar ventilation provides stability of inspired anaesthetic concentration at the alveolar level; hence, the anaesthesia uptake will remain nearly constant on a breath-by-breath basis. It is also recommended that a ventilator with upward bellows be used. When a downward bellows ventilator is used in closed-circuit anaesthesia, it is difficult to observe the volume equilibration at the end of expiration or a volume deficiency at the end of expiration. When the volume supply falls short of the patient's consumption, this results in creation of negative pressure in the circuit due to the weight of the bellows, and volume compensation from the atmosphere may occur. Consequently, nitrogen may accumulate continuously in the circuit as demonstrated in Fig. 14.

Vaporizers

Many different methods can be utilized to supply anaesthetic agents to the circle system during closed-circuit anaesthesia. In terms of use of flow-through Tek-type vaporizers, our measurements demonstrate that available vaporizers, except for the Fluotec Mark II, will provide accurate vapour output at a flow of 100 ml/min. This type of vaporizer can therefore be utilized for closed-circuit anaesthesia with reasonable accuracy and convenience [9]. This type of vaporizer seldom produces excessively higher vapour output than dialled, but it is recommended that the vaporizer be checked with a mass spectrometer, gas chromatograph or an eye movement measuring apparatus (EMMA) type of device to ensure the adequacy of its performance. Current flow-through Tek vaporizers have a maximum output limit of 5% for halothane vaporizers, 7% for enflurane vaporizers and 5% for isoflurane vaporizers. This is because the anaesthetic vapour mass output relies upon total gas flow through the vaporizer; hence, when 100% oxygen is chosen as the carrier gas, it may not be possible to deliver sufficient anaesthetic vapour into the circle system during clinical anaesthesia. For example, a 2% enflurane inspired concentration is required in order to maintain anaesthesia if 100% oxygen was used with the semiclosed system. A 2% inspired enflurane concentration means an enflurane uptake of 32 ml/min for the 1st h of anaesthesia (2% × 0.4 × 4000 = 32 ml/min). With a total fresh-gas flow of 200–250 ml/min and a maximum dial setting of 7%, an enflurane Tek vaporizer provides only 14–17.5 ml/min ethrane, which is far short of the requirement of 32 ml/min. When nitrous oxide is used with oxygen, the total gas flow will be increased to 400–450 ml/min, which provides an enflurane vapour output of 28–31.5 ml/min at the maximum dial setting of 7%. This merely matches the vapour requirement in order to maintain a reasonable depth of enflurane anaesthesia with a closed circuit.

In contrast to this limitation, side-arm Vernitrol or copper-kettle-type vaporizers are able to provide a wide range of vapour outputs into the circle system by having available separate metered flows. A drawback of this type of vaporizer is the requirement of a flowmeter that is very accurate at low flow rates.

Direct injection of liquid anaesthetic into the system, as advocated by Lowe [10], is another alternative for placing anaesthetics into the circle system. This approach uses the physical property of liquid anaesthetics, is economical and requires no special vaporizing equipment; also, it is not necessary to depend on the accuracy of the flowmeter at a low flow rate. Most of the potent inhalation an-

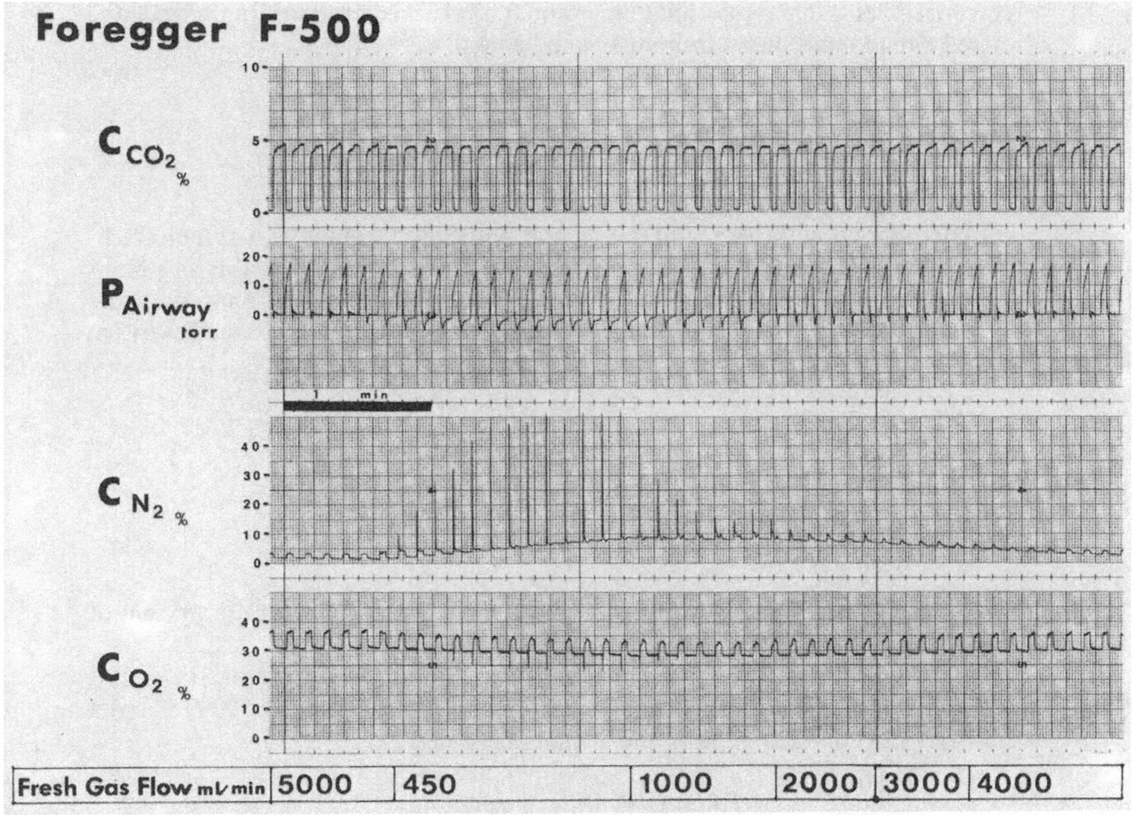

Fig. 14. Significant increase of nitrogen concentration and simultaneous demonstration of negative pressure during expiration in the circuit when fresh-gas flow was reduced from 5000 ml/min on a patient ventilated with a downward bellows ventilator

aesthetics will provide approximately 200 ml anaesthetic vapor/ml anaestic liquid. This, compared with the usual maintenance dose of 10–20 ml/min anaesthetic vapor, indicates that the anaesthetic liquid should be added to the circle system in a small aliquot in order to prevent overdosage or the bolus effect. When this approach is chosen, the anaesthetic liquid should be added to the expiratory arm of the circle system to provide the maximum vaporization effect. Care must be taken to guard against injection of an excess of liquid anaesthetic, by syringe, into the circle system.

Preliminary Checkout

1. At least once before use in a low-flow or closed-circuit system, verify the accuracy of the rotameters with a flowmeter verification device.
2. Each day, check the oxygen analyzer against room air and pure oxygen.
3. For each case, check the circuit for leaks by attaching a 3-litre bag at the ETT connection and, with a full circuit, run a fresh-gas flow of 100 ml/min. If the ventilator bellows do not fall over a period of several minutes, then there is no more than a minimal leak in the circuit.
4. Check the soda lime before each case.

Effective absorption of CO_2 is an essential factor in the practice of closed-circuit anaesthesia. Therefore soda lime should be checked every morning when the closed-circuit anaesthesia technique is to be used.

Procedure of Anaesthesia with N_2O

1. Preferably use preoxygenation before induction.
2. After induction, just as with the regular semiclosed technique, use high fresh-gas flows (5000 ml/min) for approximately 6 min (3 time constants as a minimum). This is done to eliminate nitrogen and equilibrate the circuit to the desired anaesthetic concentration. The time constant formula is usually written as:

$$\frac{\text{circuit volume} + \text{FRC}}{\text{fresh gas flow}} = 1 \text{ time constant.}$$

The actual formula should be:

$$\frac{\text{circuit volume} + \text{FRC}}{\text{fresh gas flow} - \text{uptake}} = 1 \text{ time constant.}$$

However, since the rate of uptake is quite small compared with the amount of fresh-gas flow and the circuit volume, it can be neglected.

For a typical anaesthesia machine with an Ohio absorber system, the circuit volume is 6000 ml. With this value, an estimated FRC volume of 3000 ml and a fresh-gas flow of 5000 ml/min, the formula becomes:

$$\frac{6000 + 3000}{5000} = 1.8 \text{ min} = 1 \text{ time constant.}$$

Thus, 6 min represents a little more than 3 time constants for the system. One time constant will achieve 63% equilibration. Therefore, 3 time constants are required to achieve 95% equilibration of the supplied anaesthetic concentration in the anaesthetic circuit and lungs.

3. After 6 min of high flow, close the system with 250 ml/min O_2 and 200 ml/min N_2O. If a completely closed system is wanted, then watch the bellows of the ventilator, adjusting the total gas flow in order just to prevent the bellows from touching the top, but *never set the N_2O flow higher than the O_2 flow*. The flow seldom requires adjustment over a 1-h period. For the 2nd h, the N_2O flow can be cut to two-thirds or one-half of the original flow without any change in the O_2 flow. Beginning with the 3rd h, the N_2O flow can be diminished to one-half or one-third of the original low-flow level, or simply shut off, with O_2 used alone to maintain the circuit volume. If the N_2O supply is shut off, one should use a completely closed circuit in order to prevent too rapid a washout of the N_2O.
4. For potent inhalation anaesthetics: First, the uptake of the inhalation anaesthetic during maintenance should be calculated. For example, when the semiclosed system technique is used with halothane, induction is usually achieved with 2%–2.5% halothane for 5–10 min; this is then decreased to 1% and maintained at this concentration unless untoward haemodynamic changes are encountered. With the closed-circuit system, during the first 6 min of high-flow wash-in, 2% halothane can still be used; however, when the circuit is closed, only the amount of anaesthetic which would be taken up during maintenance should be supplied (equivalent to uptake from a 1% inspired concentration with the semiclosed technique). The rate of uptake can be calculated as: inspired concentration × fraction of uptake × alveolar ventilation = rate of uptake, where inspired concentration (1%) = 0.01, fraction of uptake for halothane = 0.5 and alveolar ventilation = 3000; or 0.01 × 0.5 × 3000 ml/min = 15 ml/min.

The stated alveolar ventilation should not be mixed with the minute ventilation or minute volume, which is always noticeable during anaesthesia. The minute ventilatory volume, as calculated from the tidal volume and rate of ventilation, consists of alveolar and anatomical dead space other than alveolar ventilation; it also includes the compressed circuit volume and expandable gas volume from the positive-pressure ventilation used. This, in fact, increases the V_d/V_t ratio to more than 0.3, frequently reaching 0.5 or more during closed-circuit anaesthesia.

If the arterial blood gases are measured during anaesthesia, this provides not only blood gas data, but also an easy method for calculation of alveolar ventilatory volume from the alveolar equation:

$$FCO_2 = \frac{CO_2\text{ production}}{\text{alveolar ventilation}} = \frac{CO_2\text{ production}}{(V_t - V_d)\times\text{rate}} = \frac{O_2\text{ consumption}\times 0.8}{(V_t - V_d)\times\text{rate}}.$$

For example, if $pCO_2 = 35$ torr, $TV = 800$ ml, rate $= 10$/min and O_2 consumption $= 250$ ml/min, then CO_2 production will be $250 \times 0.8 = 200$ ml/min and FCO_2 will be $\frac{35}{710}$; so V_d will be

$$V_d = \frac{(350\times 800) - (710\times 200)}{35\times 10} = 394{,}3\text{ ml.}$$

Thus $V_d/V_t = 0.49$, and the alveolar ventilation volume will be

$$VA = (V_t - V_d) \times R = (300 - 394.3) \times 10 = 4057 \text{ ml/min}.$$

With machines having a calibrated variable-bypass flowover vaporizer, such as the Ohio, Dräger, Fluotec Mark III, or Fluomatic, the vaporizer dial setting for 15 ml/min halothane is calculated as follows:

$$\text{dial setting (\%)} = \frac{\text{uptake of anaesthetic vapour (ml/min)}}{\text{total fresh-gas flow (ml/min)}}$$

so that, for a fresh-gas flow of 500 ml/min, dial setting $= \frac{15}{500} \times 100 = 3\%$.

For side-arm Vernitrol or copper kettle-type vaporizers, the amount of anaesthetic vapour delivered will be one-half of the vaporizer flow setting for halothane and about one-third of the vaporizer flow setting for either enflurane or forane. Thus, a vaporizer flow of 30 ml/min will provide 10 ml/min enflurane vapour or 15 ml/min either halothane or forane vapour.

During 1 h of closed-circuit anaesthesia with a constant supply of halothane vapour, the inspiratory halothane concentration does not change significantly. This is because the fraction of uptake does not change significantly over time (after wash-in, uptake is nearly constant) and because the circuit volume is very large compared with the total fresh-gas flow with a closed circuit. With the dependence of uptake upon inspiratory concentration, the circuit thus serves as a limited-feedback, self-regulatory system, minimizing the risk of raising the circuit concentration to significantly higher levels.

For enflurane, a patient is normally anaesthetized with 3%–4% of the agent for about 10 min, then maintained at 2% (equivalent to 1.3 MAC) with the semiclosed technique. For closed-circuit anaesthesia, the uptake at a 2% inspired concentration is first calculated:

$$0.02 \times 0.4 \times 3000 \text{ ml/min} = 24 \text{ ml/min}.$$

Therefore, as in the semiclosed technique, use 3%–4% for wash-in (6 min with a fresh-gas flow of 5000 ml/min or 9 min with a fresh-gas flow of 3000 ml/min), then close the circuit. If only 450 ml/min fresh-gas flow is required after the circuit is closed, the dial setting for the enflurane vaporizer is

$$\frac{24}{450} \times 100\% = 5.3\% .$$

The fraction of uptake shown in Table 1 is derived from data on patients with normal cardiac output and normal ventilation. Remember that, in cases of low cardiac output, the fraction of uptake will be diminished significantly (F_A will rise faster than normal, indicating that $1 - F_A/F_I$ approaches 0). Ventilation will affect F_A/F_I, but this effect does not have significant impact on the rate of uptake since increase in ventilation results in higher placement of F_A/F_I curve, which is indicative of the reduction in fraction of uptake ($T - F_A/F_I$), so that the rate of uptake will not be considerably altered with the ventilatory change.

Rate of uptake = (inspired concentration) × (fraction of uptake) × (alveolar ventilation).

5. If any problem arises, simply change back to high flow for a few minutes.

6. It is recommended that ventilator-controlled respiration be used in all closed-circuit cases. This provides easy estimation of uptake because the alveolar ventilation is held constant; and, with the stability of the inspired anaesthetic concentration, uptake will remain nearly constant breath by breath.
7. Use of the Fluotec Mark II vaporizer in closed-circuit anaesthesia should be avoided because this vaporizer fails to provide predictable output concentration when flow is reduced to less than 2000 ml/min.

References

1. Lin CY, Mostert JW (1977) Inspired oxygen and nitrous oxide concentration in essentially closed circuits. Anesthetist 26:514–517
2. Lin CY, Mostert JW, Benson DW (1980) Closed circle systems. A new direction in the practice of anesthesia. Acta Anaesthesiol Scand 24:354–361
3. Lin CY (1982) Nitrous oxide uptake in adults (abstract). Anesthesiology 57:S372
4. Severinghaus JW (1954) Rate of uptake of nitrous oxide in man. J Clin Invest 33:1183–1189
5. Lowe HJ (1981) The anesthetic continuum. In: Aldrete JA, Lowe HJ, Virtue RW (eds) Low flow and closed system anesthesia. Grune and Stratton, New York, pp 11–37
6. Mapleson WW (1973) Circulation-time models of the uptake of inhalation anaesthetics and data for quantifying them. Br J Anaesth 45:319–334
7. Pipper J (1981) Blood-gas equilibration in lungs and pulmonary diffusion capacity. Prog Resp Res 16:115–125
8. Eger EI (1974) Anesthesia uptake and action. Williams and Wilkins, Baltimore
9. Lin CY (1980) Assessment of vaporizer performance with reference to low-flow and closed-circuit anesthesia. Anesth Analg 59:359–366
10. Lowe HJ (1972) Dose regulated penthrane anesthesia. North Chicago Abbott Laboratories, Chicago

Closed-Circuit Anaesthesia for Paediatric Patients

C.-Y. Lin

Although closed-circuit anaesthesia has several distinct advantages, such as conservation of heat, maintenance of airway humidity and reduction of anaesthetic gas pollution in the operating room, anaesthesia with an adult circle system for paediatric cases has been considered unsafe and impractical in the past because of problems of dead space, compliance and airway resistance. This belief stems mainly from the choice of the circle system for paediatric anaesthesia. In the past, elimination of apparatus dead space and elimination of minimal resistance to respiration were the two most important factors considered in the selection of anaesthesia apparatus for the paediatric patient [1]. This is certainly correct when general anaesthesia is administered with spontaneous respiration, but it becomes a minor consideration in the selection of anaesthesia apparatus for the paediatric patient under general anaesthesia with controlled or assisted ventilation.

With increasing complexity of surgical procedures, maintenance of body heat and humidity of airway gases became the focus of attention in recent years with regard to the selection of anaesthetic apparatus for paediatric patients undergoing extensive surgery. An add-on humidifier seems an excellent solution to the problem of maintenance of humidity for high-flow or non-rebreathing-type systems requiring a high fresh-gas flow; but this is not without inconvenience or complexity. In contrast, a closed circuit provides airway humidity and better maintenance of heat, with rebreathing of the expired gases and minimal use of dry, cold fresh gases. In other words, the gases inhaled from the closed-circuit system consist mainly of previously exhaled warm gas containing water vapour near saturation.

Since the introduction and practice of a simple method of closed-circuit anaesthesia based on new concepts of uptake of inhalation anaesthetics [2], this method has been extended to paediatric cases in which the time of anaesthesia is expected to be long. It has proved to be as safe and simple in children as in adults.

Equipment

A regular Ohio circuit system (Ohio 2000) with double-canister and Air-Shields ventilator is used. For patients weighing less than 25 kg, the corrugated rubber tubing usually placed between the outlet and inlet is replaced by 200 cm of 3/8-inch Tygon tubing, or with Rüsch tubing, because this reduces the compliance of the system. The compliance loss after modification of this system is 4 ml/cm H_2O

airway pressure. Ventilation is maintained at 10 ml/kg for the basal tidal volume, and the rate is determined from Radford's nomogram [3].

Eger [4] demonstrated that a different arrangement of various components of a circle system, inlet port, inlet valve, outlet valve and exhaust valve, can influence the performance of the system considerably; but, as demonstrated by Schoonbee and Conway [5], this only applies to the condition of high fresh-gas flow. With a closed-circuit system, a very small portion of the tidal volume is composed of fresh gas, and the majority of the tidal volume consists of exhaled gas; thus, little change has resulted from a different arrangement of various components of the circle system. Gases within the circle system (approximately 5000 ml) will tend to be uniformly mixed.

The large-circle system volume influences the time required for initial priming of the circuit with the desired anaesthetic gas concentration, but it also provides a tremendous buffering capacity for any change in the gas composition in the circuit. The lower the flow, the longer the time constant. Thus, the lower the flow of fresh gas, the longer it takes for a change in fresh-gas concentration and a comparable change in the inspiratory concentration. During closed-circuit anaesthesia, the fresh-gas supply is very low; even with an excess supply of potent inhalation-anaesthetic gases, a very long time is needed for these gases to reach a dangerously high level in the circuit. As mentioned in another chapter, uptake of anaesthetics at the level of the alveolar membrane is determined mainly by the partial pressure gradient between the outside and inside of the membrane. An excess supply of anaesthetics results in an increase in the inspired concentration; this may enhance the uptake and, hence, results in reduction of the expired anaesthetic gas concentration which brings the anaesthetic concentration in the circuit towards the original level.

The Ohio 2000 anaesthetic machine provides both high and low (0- to 700-ml/min full-scale) flowmeters. These were tested with a verification device before the machine was used for closed-circuit anaesthesia. We also determined the flow ratio between oxygen and nitrous oxide for each machine with an oxygen analyzer. The significance of this ratio determination is discussed in another chapter.

Practical Considerations

Ventilation

Usually, an airway pressure of 20 cm H_2O at a reasonable inspiratory flow rate will provide a reasonable tidal volume, unless the child has a very low-compliance lung. In order to ensure adequate ventilation, effective thoracic cage movement should be observed clinically, and the actual tidal volume (10 ml/kg) should always be calculated from a simple formula which takes into account the volume loss resulting from the compliance of the circle system (in our case, 4 ml loss per cm H_2O of airway pressure).

From our mass spectrometry observations, we confirmed that expired CO_2 is completely absorbed by a single path of soda lime canisters and that CO_2 is therefore not contained in the recirculated inspiratory gases. Despite this, our initial clinical trial of closed-circuit anaesthesia in paediatric patients, with 10 ml/kg tidal volume and a respiratory rate obtained from Radford's nomogram, demonstrated a slight increase in arterial pCO_2. Although this slight increase can be corrected by a 10%–15% increase in the ventilatory rate, it indicates two possibilities: either miscalculation of the ventilatory volume and rate or an increase in the respiratory dead space due to the low fresh-gas flow.

Circle System

As mentioned before, our circle system has a volume of approximately 5000 ml. Once this volume is primed with the desired concentration of anaesthetic gases (because the anaesthetic uptake and the anaesthetic gas supply are quite small compared with the circuit volume), a very long time is required for a change in concentration from the initial level. In other words, the circuit volume serves as a buffer and safeguard in preventing potentially dangerous changes in gas composition in the circuit during closed-circuit anaesthesia.

During induction, this large, non-collapsible volume of the circuit certainly poses an obstacle to providing closed-circuit anaesthesia starting from time zero, especially when high concentrations of nitrous oxide are used. Despite meticulous attention, priming of the circuit with nitrous oxide is impossible without allowing some of the nitrous oxide-oxygen gas mixture to escape from the circuit. Barton [6] achieved priming by complete flushing and suctioning of the circuit system prior to its attachment to the patient, but this is not only a complicated and cumbersome procedure, but also neglects the patient's FRC.

Lowe [7] advocates priming with nitrous oxide according to a power function of time by turning on a high flow of nitrous oxide for only a few minutes, until a desired oxygen concentration in the circuit is reached. This procedure is complicated and diverts the anaesthesiologist's attention completely from the patient. Also, one cannot avoid the escape of administered nitrous oxide from the circuit during the initial FRC wash-in period.

This is the main reason why we recommend the use of high fresh-gas flows of anaesthetic at the desired concentration during the initial period, similar to the practice with the semiclosed system. This high fresh-gas flow for a short period provides equilibration of the circuit to the delivered and desired anaesthetic concentration; it also eliminates almost all of the nitrogen from the circuit and FRC. In our experience with several thousand cases of closed-circuit anaesthesia monitored with a mass spectrometer in the past 10 years at the University of Chicago, we seldom observed an accumulation of nitrogen in the circuit which exceeded the level of 35 torr.

Anaesthetic Requirements

Nitrous Oxide

As mentioned and explained in another chapter, the rate of true body uptake of nitrous oxide should be considered as being near-constant for a given concentration, and one should not relate it to the complicated power function. After initial wash-in of the anaesthetic gas mixture into the patient FRC and the circuit, the anaesthetic concentration in the circuit and FRC soon reaches an equilibrium with the delivered anaesthetic concentration. The circle system then can be closed and maintained with a very limited supply of nitrous oxide and oxygen. During closed-circuit anaesthesia, most of the volume which the patient breathes comes from the gaseous mixture in the circuit, and a very limited volume is contributed from the fresh-gas flow. This is quite contrary to the situation in a non-rebreathing or semiclosed system, where the volume patient breath is almost exclusively related to the fresh gas. When the circle system is closed, with a continuous supply of an approximated volume of nitrous oxide and oxygen, the circuit concentration of nitrous oxide or oxygen seldom deviates from the original level over a long time because of the buffering effect of the large circuit volume as compared with the rather small volume of fresh gas supplied during closed-circuit anaesthesia. This buffering effect is further enhanced by the fact that the anaesthetic uptake is mainly controlled by the inspired concentration at the alveolar membrane: The inspired concentration increases when the supply of anaesthetic vapor exceeds the demand or the uptake; this causes uptake to rise and brings the anaesthetic concentration in the circuit towards the original level.

Although this concentration effect on uptake and the buffering effect of the large circuit volume provide limited self-feedback control in maintaining a near-constant nitrous oxide concentration in the circuit during closed-circuit anaesthesia, monitoring of the oxygen concentration in the system is mandatory from the medicolegal standpoint.

Supply of nitrous oxide requires readjustment only every hour following initial wash-in despite the fact that the rate of uptake is not constant but, because of the buffering effect of large circuit volume and near-constant uptake of inhalation anaesthetics at a given anaesthetic concentration, requires few adjustments during closed-circuit anaesthesia. As shown in Figs. 1 and 2, with a fixed-volume supply of nitrous oxide and oxygen over 50 min during closed-circuit anaesthesia, there is only an average 5% deviation of end-expiratory oxygen concentration from the original oxygen concentration at the end of the initial high-flow wash-in period.

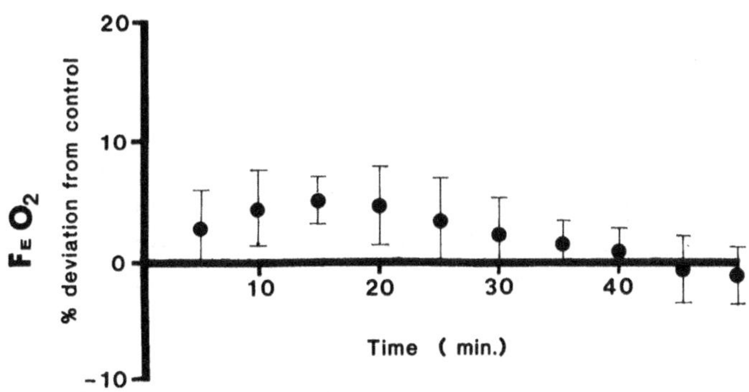

Fig. 1. An average 5% deviation of end-expiratory oxygen concentration from the original oxygen concentration at the end of the initial high-flow wash-in period occurred during closed-circuit anaesthesia. This deviation reached its peak 15 min after initiation of closed-circuit anaesthesia and gradually returned to the original level at 43 min. This indicates that a fixed-volume supply of nitrous oxide and oxygen over 50 min did not match the exact uptake requirement of the patient; but the approximation of uptake is close enough for 1 h duration. An initial slightly higher uptake of nitrous oxide produces an increase in F_EO_2

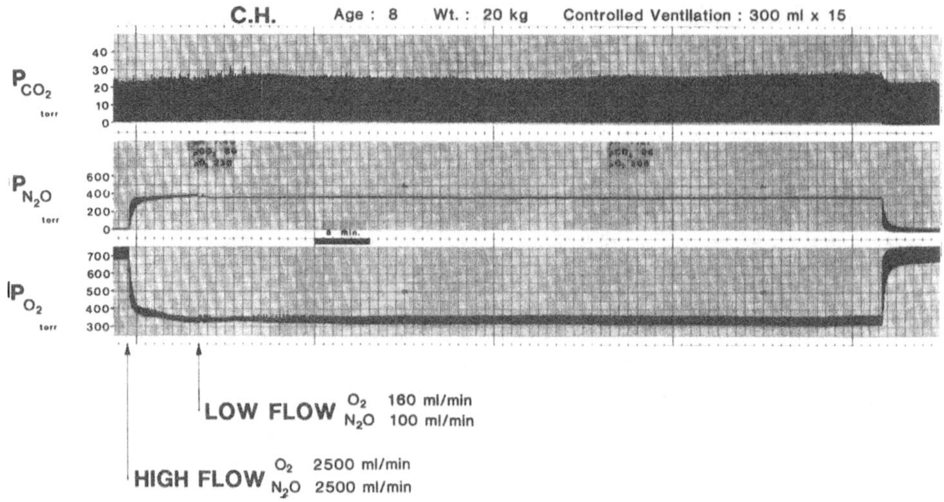

Fig. 2. The tracings show the steady uptake of anaesthetic (nitrous oxide) in an 8-year-old boy. During 70 min, the anaesthetic gas flow was changed only once. At the beginning, a high flow was used to equilibrate the circuit, including the FRC, with an N_2O-O_2 mixture of 2500–2500 ml/min for 6 min; then the system was closed with 160 ml/min O_2 and 100 ml/min N_2O. There was a slight rise in pO_2, which reached its peak 5 min after initiation of closed-circuit anaesthesia, then gradually declined to 10 torr, below the pO_2 value at the beginning of closed-circuit anaesthesia. The maximum deviation of 30 torr in the end-expiratory pO_2 with a steady supply of fresh-gas mixture indicates a near-constant uptake of nitrous oxide. The initial rise in pO_2 indicates that a steady supply of 100 ml/min nitrous oxide during the initial phase of closed-circuit anaesthesia fell short of the patient's nitrous oxide uptake; but with declining nitrous oxide uptake, the oxygen tension gradually declined to a level slightly below the initial one

This indicates that a fixed-volume supply of nitrous oxide and oxygen over 1 h did not match the exact uptake requirement of the patient; but the approximation of uptake is close enough for 1 h duration.

Potent Inhalation Anaesthetics

Similar to the rate of uptake of nitrous oxide, the rate of uptake of potent inhalation anaesthetics can also be considered as being near-constant at a given concentration after the initial FRC wash-in period. This concept not only provides easy calculation of the rate of uptake on the basis of the inspired concentration and the alveolar ventilation, but also provides easy practice of closed-circuit anaesthesia, since there is no need to change the rate of anaesthetic supply for 1 h.

It is true that, during clinical anaesthesia, the anaesthetic dose delivered depends heavily on the haemodynamic response of the patient, and that the dose must be regulated accordingly. During closed-circuit anaesthesia, there is no exception to this rule, and we can adjust the dose according to the patient's response. For example, a healthy boy weighing 20 kg was anaesthetized with halothane and maintained with 1.25% inspired halothane concentration for 15 min. His blood pressure dropped to 80 torr and seemed to have tendency to decrease further. With a semiclosed system, the response of most anaesthetists will be a reduction of the inspired anaesthetic concentration to 0.75% or less. Uptake of halothane vapour at 1.25% inspired halothane concentration will be 0.0125 × 0.5 × 1500 = 9.4 ml/min, and at 0.75% inspired concentration it will be 0.0075 × 0.5 × 1500 = 5.6 ml/min. Thus, if a 1.25% inspired halothane concentration was maintained before the change in blood pressure, we can reduce the halothane vapour from 9.4 ml/min to 5.6 ml/min or lower.

The difference in time for the change should also be considered during closed-circuit anaesthesia. The above change in the supply of halothane vapour from 9.4 ml/min to 5.6 ml/min, and thus the change in inspired concentration from 1.25% to 0.75%, may require quite a long time during closed-circuit anaesthesia because large circuit volume serves as a buffer. Therefore, if a very rapid change in the inspired concentration is required or desired, one should consider switching to a semiclosed system with a high fresh-gas flow for a short period. Alternatively, one can maintain the system closed, but shut off the supply of potent inhalation anaesthetic, in this case, halothane.

Normally, the anaesthetic vapour requirement can be calculated as desired inspired anaesthetic concentration × fraction of uptake × alveolar ventilation. The fraction of uptake does not change significantly with time, as explained above. This, associated with the large buffering capacity of the circle system and the inspired-concentration-dependent uptake, means that the vapour supply may require adjustment only once every hour. This simplifies the practice of closed-circuit anaesthesia significantly.

Application of Closed-Circuit Anaesthesia to Paediatric Patients

Induction of Anaesthesia

Anaesthesia is usually induced with thiopental sodium, up to 4 mg/kg; this is followed by a non-depolarizing muscle relaxant, orotracheal intubation and ventilation with a nitrous oxide-oxygen mixture at 2:1, or 3:2, patients in the older paediatric age group.

For younger paediatric patients, inhalation induction or intramuscular ketamine at a dose of 10 mg/kg may be used until consciousness is lost. An intravenous route can be established thereafter, and intravenous administration of a non-depolarizing muscle relaxant can facilitate intubation.

Maintenance of Anaesthesia

Following intubation, our simple, practical method of closed-circuit anaesthesia begins with a high fresh-gas flow of a nitrous oxide-oxygen mixture with or without a potent inhalation anaesthetic. This does not differ from the procedure with a conventional semiclosed system. For a 10-kg patient, we commonly use 3000 ml/min nitrous oxide and 2000 ml/min oxygen and 1% of halothane. Ventilation is controlled, with a tidal volume of 10 ml/kg and a rate of 18/min. After 5 min, the high fresh-gas flow is reduced; the nitrous oxide flow is now 150 ml/min and the oxygen flow 200 ml/min. In contrast to the reduction in fresh-gas flow, the vaporizer setting for halothane is increased to 1.5%. At the 1.5% dial setting with a total fresh-gas flow of 350 ml/min, a flow-through vaporizer will pick up and deliver to the circle system approximately 5.1 ml/min halothane vapour. If the existing halothane concentration of 1% is maintained in the circuit, the patient will continue taking up the halothane vapour at the rate of $0.01 \times 0.5 \times 1000 = 5$ ml/min.

(A 10-kg patient will have 60 ml/min oxygen consumption and 50 ml/min CO_2 production. If a pCO_2 of 35 torr is maintained by controlled ventilation, this indicates an alveolar ventilation of $50 \times 710/35$ – about 1000 ml/min.)

If the time or the conditions allow it, one can further provide fine tuning of the rate of fresh-gas flow in order to achieve a state of total closed-circuit anaesthesia. When the bellows continuously reach the top of the ventilator, this indicates that the fresh-gas flow must be reduced.

We recommend total closed-circuit rather than low-flow anaesthesia for paediatric patients since closed circuit will provide limited self-feedback in keeping the inspiratory concentration constant.

In the case of younger patients for whom a non-cuff endotracheal tube is used, the fresh-gas requirement for closed-circuit anaesthesia is unpredictable and requires a much higher volume per body weight because gas leakage occurs around the non-cuffed tube during positive-pressure ventilation. This was clearly demonstrated in a study which we performed (Fig. 3).

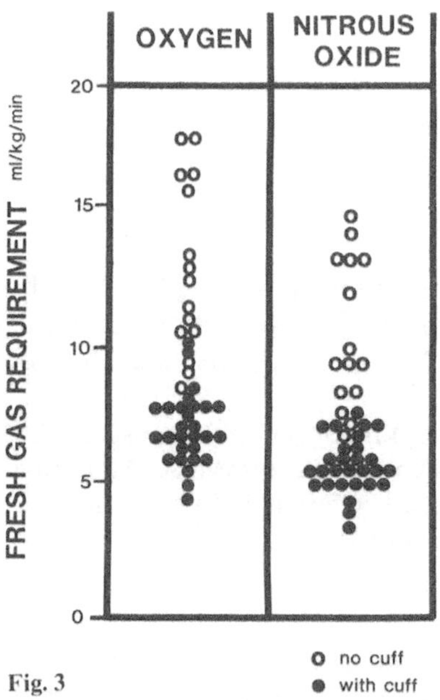

Fig. 3

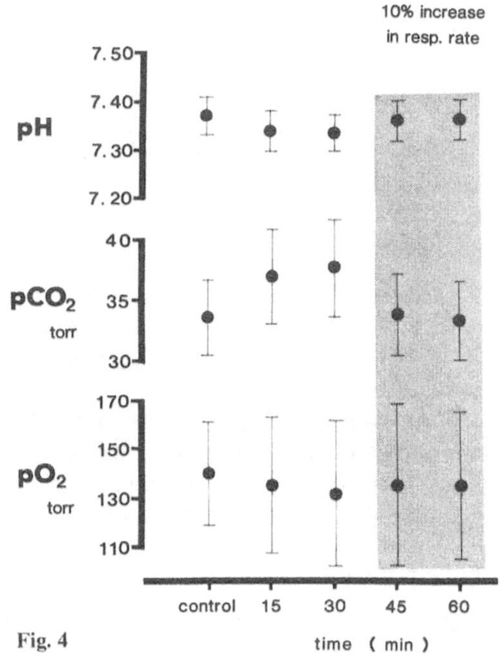

Fig. 4

Fig. 3. When closed-circuit anaesthesia was administered to paediatric patients with a cuffed endotracheal tube in place, the fresh-gas requirement tended to cluster at 6–7 ml per Kilogram per minute area for oxygen and 5 ml per kilogram per minute for nitrous oxide. Patients under 4 years of age, for whom a non-cuffed endotracheal tube was used, demonstrated an unpredictably large fresh-gas requirement for maintenance of the circuit volume because of gas leakage around the endotracheal tube

Fig. 4. Blood gas changes in paediatric patients during closed-circuit anaesthesia. A slight increase in pCO_2 was observed soon after initiation of closed-circuit anaesthesia when the patients were ventilated at 10 ml/kg tidal volume at a ventilatory rate determined from the Radford nomogram. This increase in pCO_2 can easily be corrected with a 10%–15% increase in the ventilatory rate

If one chooses not to use nitrous oxide, one can start the closed-circuit anaesthesia without the initial period of high fresh-gas flow, but the use of a circulator such as the Revel type in the circuit is recommended in order to eliminate the hazardous bolus effect associated with the initial dose. Use of vaporizers other than a calibrated flow-through Tek vaporizer should be considered. With an oxygen fresh-gas flow of less than 200 ml/min at a maximum halothane dial setting of 5%, at most 10 ml/min halothane vapour can be delivered to the circuit. This indicates that almost 6 min are required to reach a 1% halothane concentration in the circuit if uptake during this period is disregarded.

As shown in our study (Fig. 4), during closed-circuit anaesthesia there was a tendency towards an increase in pCO_2, which may result from an increase in dead-space respiration. This increase in pCO_2 can easily be corrected with a 10% –15% increase in the ventilatory rate.

Emergence from Anaesthesia

In the case of abdominal surgery, a non-depolarizing muscle relaxant and halothane are used for anaesthesia. As soon as the abdominal fascia is closed, one can reverse the muscle relaxant with the proper dose of a reversal agent. Then the halothane supply is turned off and the rate of ventilation is lowered to a minimal rate in order to accumulate CO_2 in the body. If nitrous oxide was used, continue with it. Spontaneous respiration will soon return. Since the circuit is still closed, one can observe the return of spontaneous respiration, registered as tidal volume on the ventimeter, and the progress of recovery. This condition also provides coasting of the halothane concentration in the blood. Although halothane uptake continues, the blood level will drop gradually due to redistribution and continuous uptake by the poorly perfused organs. When complete closure of the skin is accomplished, the circuit should be opened with a high flow of oxygen, but use of the ventilator should continue until ready for extubation.

In the case of balanced anaesthesia and with no potent inhalation anaesthetic used, the muscle relaxant should be reversed at the end of surgery avoiding unnecessary movement.

In conclusion, we apply the practice of a simple method of closed-circuit anaesthesia in paediatric patients based on our new concept of uptake of inhalation anaesthetics and use of a regular adult circuit with limited modifications. This has proved to be as safe and simple in children as in adults.

References

1. Adriani J, Griggs T (1953) Rebreathing in pediatric anesthesia: recommendations and descriptions of improvement in apparatus. Anesthesiology 14:337–347
2. Lin CY, Mostert JW, Benson DW (1980) Closed circle systems. A new direction in the practice of anesthesia. Acta Anaesthesiol Scand 24:354–361
3. Radford EP (1955) Ventilation standards for use in artificial respiration. J Appl Physiol 7:451
4. Eger II EI, Ethans CT (1968) The effect of inflow, overflow and valve placement on economy of the circle system. Anesthesiology 29:93–100
5. Schoonbee CG, Conway CM (1981) Factors affecting carbon dioxide homeostasis during controlled ventilation with circle systems. Br J Anaesth 53:471–477
6. Barton F, Nunn JF (1975) Totally closed circuit nitrous oxide-oxygen anaesthesia. Br J Anaesth 47:350–357
7. Lowe HJ, Ernst EA (1981) The quantitative practice of anesthesia: use of closed circuit. Williams and Wilkins, Baltimore

Integrated Monitoring of Closed-Circuit Anaesthesia

M. Paloheimo

A closed circuit is a sophisticated version of a semiclosed anaesthesia system; the overflow valve is closed, all possible leaks (including the endotracheal cuff) are minimized, and composition and mass flow of fresh gas are adjusted to maintain desired fractions of gases as well as to keep the circuit volume within acceptable limits. Supplementation of anaesthetics and oxygen must meet individual demands, which vary with time and the stage or degree of surgery.

There are two ways to manage an anaesthetic in the closed milieu:

1. The square root of time model

The use of known facts about organ blood flows, organ volumes and tissue anaesthetic solubilities allows for the application of a schematic delivery system to reach and maintain desired arterial molar concentrations of anaesthetic agents [1]. Mathematical prediction of the anaesthetic doses as a function of time, however, does not take individual requirements into account. Monitoring of at least the inspiratory oxygen concentration is considered as mandatory [2].

2. The feedback model

On-line monitoring of the anaesthetic agent concentrations makes possible injection or intermittent(/continuous) infusion of incremental supplementary doses according to the measured alveolar level of the agent. Simultaneous measurement of oxygen and carbon dioxide concentrations offers full control of the gas exchange. According to available methods and their sensitivity one can draw conclusions about the anaesthesia system, the patient's metabolic state and the adequacy of the whole anaesthesia.

Integrated monitoring of closed-circuit anaesthesias may be accomplished at three levels:

Monitoring Approach. Breath-by-breath monitoring of carbon dioxide and anaesthetic agent concentrations in the inspiratory and expiratory gas is possible with the existing infrared measuring techniques [3]. Response times (time from 10% to 90% of full scale) in the commercially available gas monitors can follow gas concentrations accurately up to 35 breaths/min. Separate alveolar samples may be obtained from children by occasional extended expirations. Oxygen electrodes can be placed into the circuit or into the sampling flow of CO_2 monitors. Polarographic oxygen cells float between the inspired and expired concentrations, measured by the inspired/expired time ratio. In the near future we may expect to obtain fast oxygen monitors which give "oxygrams" resembling reverse capnograms. Measurement of nitrous oxide in routine clinical practice is also not far away. The real necessity of using nitrous oxide is a matter of dispute; air enriched with oxygen certainly makes things easier in the closed circuit.

Adjustable, sensitive alarms aid the smooth control of the system. This approach is applicable to any existing low-flow anaesthesia system.

Feedback Control Approach. The features above may be used to suggest to the anaesthesiologist what corrective or effective measures should be made to reach a desired state. A further step in this concept is feedback to an anaesthesic agent and O_2/N_2O administrator, Intermittent Positive Pressure Ventilation device and the patient record.

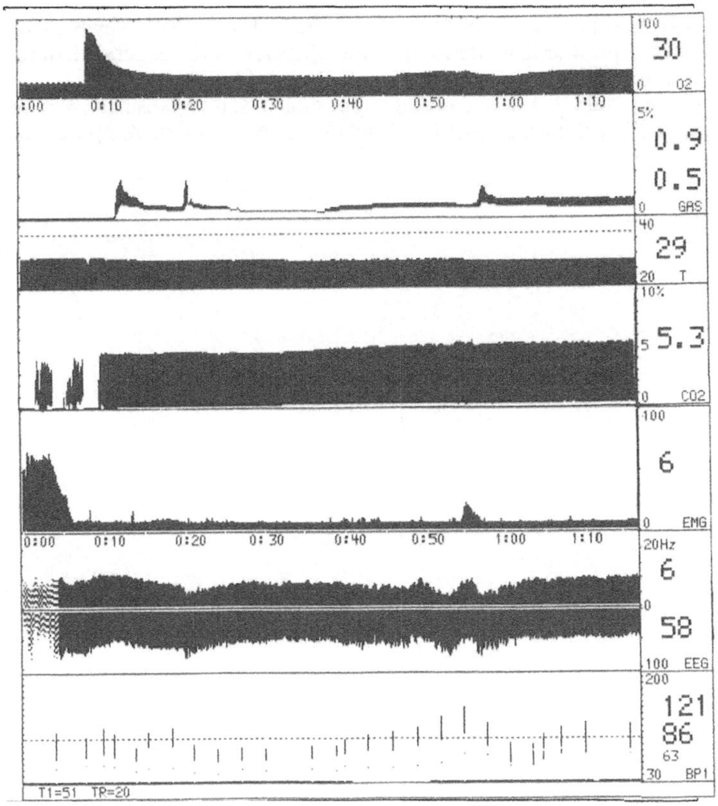

Fig. 1. A printed record of an anaesthetic starting with the circuit semiclosed (induction with thiopentone, intubation in succinyl choline relaxation); fresh gas (*FG*) = 5 litres/min until 8 min, where FG = 1.5 litres/min. The circuit was closed at 12 min and two injections of unit doses of enflurane were administered. The patient's blood pressure dropped and the plans had to be changed. The operation started at around 35 min, when the circuit was made semiclosed, FG = 1.5 litres/min, and the vapirozer was used for enflurane administration. At 45 min FIO_2 was increased to 35%. At 55 min the patient showed some responsiveness and the vaporizer was turned on at 5% for 50 s in order to deepen the anaesthesia; blood pressure levels dropped. The tracings are, starting from top: oxygen, anaesthetic agent, airway temperature, carbon dioxide, frontalis EMG, mean EEG frequency, mean EEG amplitude and blood pressure; they are derived from Datex OT-102, NorMac, Normocap, ABM and Dynamap and are recorded with a video printer

Constant Volume Approach. A method for maintaining a constant volume in the system added to the previous features enables complete control of the patient/circuit system and provides the user with information of gas turnover and metabolic parameters. This topic is covered elsewhere in this volume.

Through integration of informative patient parameters such as blood pressure, heart rate, frontalis muscle EMG activity and compressed EEG trends on a common time scale it seems to be possible to conduct very low flow and closed circuit anaesthesia more individually and, certainly, more safely (Fig. 1).

References

1. Lowe HJ, Ernst EA (1981) The quantitative practice of anesthesia. Use of closed circuit. Williams and Wilkins, Baltimore
2. Kofke WA, Latta WB (1982) Closed circuit anesthesia. In: Lebowitz PW, Newberg LA, Gillette MT (eds) Clinical anesthesia procedures of the Massachusetts General Hospital. Little, Brown, Boston, pp 464–476
3. Sykes MK, Vickers MD, Hull CJ (1981) Gas and vapur analysis. In: Sykes MK, Vickens MD (eds) Principles of clinical measurement. Blackwell Scientific, Oxford, pp 220–241

Monitors in Closed-Circuit Anaesthesia

M. Yamashita, H. Ishihara, and T. Oyama

Introduction

Monitoring of the central nervous or cardiovascular system during closed-circuit anaesthesia is no different from that in high-flow system anaesthesia. However, during closed-circuit anaesthesia, monitoring of oxygen, carbon dioxide and halothane concentrations in the circuit is an essential and integral part of the practice of this system.

Principles of measurements of oxygen, carbon dioxide and halothane are discussed briefly in this paper.

Oxygen and carbon dioxide concentrations can be measured simultaneously by relatively simple instruments such as the Datex Normocap or Clinical Gas Monitor (NEC San-ei). These instruments use the polarographic electrode method and the infrared absorption method for the analysis of O_2 and CO_2, respectively.

Halothane concentration can be measured by simple equipment using the physiochemical method (Narkotest) or with more complicated equipment using the ultraviolet absorption method (Penlon Halothane Meter). All these concentrations can be measured simultaneously by a more sophisticated machine, i.e. the gas mass spectrometer.

Oxygen Analyzer

The O_2 analyzer should be placed on the expiratory limb, the site where the lowest concentration of oxygen might be anticipated (Fig. 1); the O_2 concentration

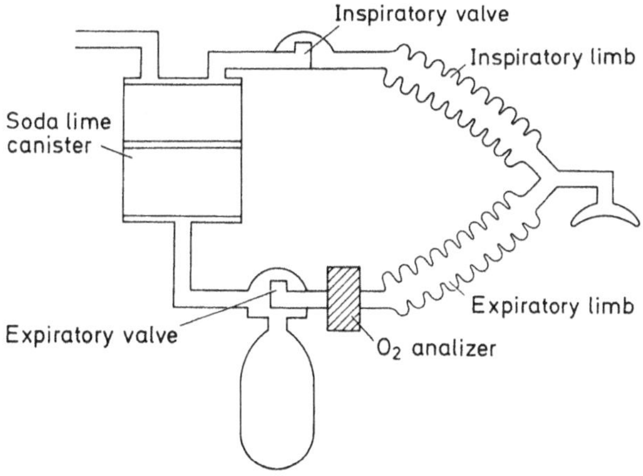

Fig. 1. Placement of the O_2 analyzer on the expiratory limb

Table 1. Characteristics of the O_2 analyzer

	Paramagnetic method	Oxygen electrode method			Gass mass spectrometric method
		Galvanic oxygen analyzer	Solid electrolyte fuel cell analyzer	Polarographic fuel cell analyzer	
Interfered with anaesthetic vapour	No	No	Yes	Minimum	No
Response time	Slow	Rapid	Rapid	Rapid	Rapid

should be kept above 25%–30%. The characteristics of different O_2 analyzers are summoned up in Table 1.

Paramagnetic Method

1. Principle
   a) Paramagnetic property of oxygen molecules.
   b) Oxygen molecules experience a force in a magnetic field proportional to the oxygen partial pressure (at constant temperature).
2. Advantages of this method: it is inexpensive and accurate in the presence of anaesthetic gas.
3. Disadvantages: it responds slowly and not quickly enough to monitor the breath-by-breath changes. Samples have to be taken from the system, and the samples have to be dried through a filter.
4. Model: Servomex Controls Ltd, type OA150

Oxygen Electrode Methods

These methods are based on the ability of oxygen to accept an electron.

Galvanic Oxygen Analyzer

1. Principle
   An electrical current generated between the electrochemical reduction of the oxygen on the catalytic electrode (cathode) and the corresponding oxidation on the lead counter electrode (anode) is proportional to the oxygen partial pressure.
2. Advantages of this method: It does not need external power, is unaffected by humidity and anaesthetic vapours, no warm up time is required and it is durable. Its sensors are disposable and inexpensive and it requires simple calibration.
3. Disadvantages of this method: Response time increases with the age of the sensor and it depends on the supply of replacement electrode.
4. Models: Mini OX M25 RAD Medical Oxygen Monitor (Catalyst Research Corporation).

Its specifications are as follows:
a) Cell life is 1 year and response time is 6 s for 90% change
b) Accuracy is to within ±0.1% of full scale
c) Cell linearity is to within ±0.1% of full scale
d) Display linearity is to within ±0.1% of full scale
e) long-term stability is to within ±1% of the initial value in 8 h
f) Warm-up time is not required

5. Interferent gas and vapors:

Interferent	Volume % dry	Interference equivalent of percentage O_2
CO_2	12%	<0.1%
Enflurane	4%	<0.5%
Halothane	5%	<0.9%
N_2O	80%	<0.5%

Solid Electrolyte Fuel Cells Analyzer

1. Principle
This is a Westinghouse oxygen monitor, which uses two solid/half solid cells: platinum/zirconium oxide/platinum.
The zirconium oxide is permeable to the reduced oxygen when heated, and the concentration of oxygen at each platinum/zirconium oxide interface determines the half-cell voltage according to the Nernest equation. [1]
2. Advantages: it is highly accurate and the response is rapid.
3. Disadvantage: it requires heating the zirconium oxide to 850 °C, and the agents combustible when heated, such as halothane, cause interference.

Polarographic Electrode Oxygen Analyzer

1. Principle
It based on the polarizing voltage between a cathode and a silver anode in an electrolyte solution. At any particular voltage, the current produced varies in parallel with the oxygen tension.
2. Advantages: the response is fast, and it is accurate under the condition of high humidities. It is unaffected by CO_2 and N_2O. It receives the minimum effects by positive pressure.
3. Disadvantages: it is battery powered and regular changes of membrane (once a year) and electrolyte (four times a year) are needed.
4. Models:
a) Ohio model 401, 201: this has an accuracy of ±1% O_2 and its response time is 97% of the O_2 within 20 s.
b) Datex Normocap O_2 monitor [2] this has a linearity error of less than 2% of the full scale; drift versus time is less than 1% of the reading/8 h. Drift versus temperature is less than 1% of the reading/°C. The response time is 20 s to 97% of the final reading. Membrane life is 1 year, the electrode life is 3 years and the electrolyte life is 3–5 months.

[1] The Nernest equation for the cell: $V = 55 \log Pr/10Ps$, where V = the voltage developed by the cell, Pr = the pO_2 of the reference gas (usually air) and Ps = the pO_2 of the sample gas.

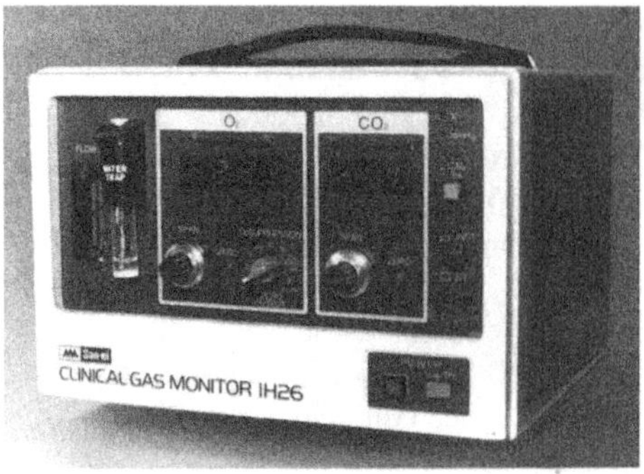

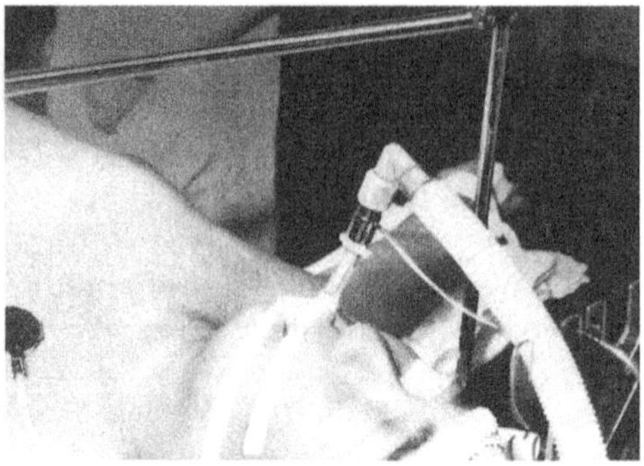

Fig. 2. Clinical gas monitor (NEC San-ei)
Fig. 3. Placement of the sampling tip between the endotracheal tube and the angle piece

c) Clinical Gas Monitor IH26 (NEC San-ei)[2] (Fig. 2): this has a linearity of ±1.5% of the full scale. Its response time is 90% step change in 200 ms and it has a stability of ±2% of the full scale/8 h. Anaesthetic gas interference by N_2O is less than 3% of the full scale against 70% N_2O. That of fluothane is less than 1% of the full scale against 3% fluothane.

Gas Mass Spectrometric Method

Oxygen monitoring by the gas mass spectrometric method is discussed in a special chapter below.

Carbon Dioxide Monitor

The sampling tip is connected between the angle piece and the endotracheal tube (Fig. 3). And end-tidal CO_2 is usually kept between 4% and 5%.

Infrared CO_2 Analyzer

1. Principle
   Most gases and vapours, including carbon dioxide, have characteristic absorption bands in the infrared region of the spectrum. The infrared CO_2 analyzers used in anaesthesia are equipped with cells containing N_2 to eliminate the interference from N_2O in the sample.
2. Advantages: It is accurate and the response time is fast.
3. Disadvantage: Samples have to be drawn from the respiratory system and it needs warming-up time.
4. Models:
   a) Datex Normocap CO_2 Meter: This has a measurement range of 0%–10% (CO_2 volume percentage). Zero point drift is ≦0.02% CO_2/°C; gain drift is ≦0.02% CO_2/°C; linearity error is ≦2% of the full scale, the compen-

[2] These instruments measure O_2 and CO_2 concentrations simultaneously. Therefore, the sampling tips are placed between the angle piece and the endotracheal tube (Fig. 3).

sation accuracy error of N_2O is $\leq 0.2\%$ for a gas mixture of 70% N_2O, 25% O_2 and 5% CO_2. Sampling flow rate is 150 ml/min or 50 ml/min. Warming-up time is less than 3 min.

b) Engstrom Eliza CO_2 Analyzer: This has a measurement range of pCO_2 0–75 mmHg or FCO_2 0%–10%. Accuracy is $\pm 0.1\%$ CO_2 + 2% of the reading after a warm-up time of 30 min. Response time is 100 ms at 100 ml/min. Sampling flow rate is 100 ml/min.

c) Clinical Gas Monitor 1H26 (NEC San-ei): This has a measurement range of 0%–10% or 0–76 mmHg. Linearity is $\pm 1.5\%$ of the full scale. Sampling flow rate is 20 ml/min (standard), adjustable from 10 to 40 ml/min. Response time is 90% step change in 200 ms. Stability is $\pm 2\%$ of the full scale/8 h. Warm-up time is approximately 5 min with preheat or approximately 30 min with the preheat off. Anaesthetic gas interference is $<3\%$ of the full scale against 70% N_2 and is $<1\%$ of the full scale against 3% fluothane.

Gas Mass Spectrometric Method

Oxygen monitoring by the gas mass spectrometric method will be discussed in the section "Gas Mass Spectrometer".

Halothane Analyzer

Ultraviolet Halothane Meter

1. Principle
   Halothane absorbs ultraviolet light with a peak absorption in the region of 200 nanometers.
2. Advantages: It is reasonably accurate and has a rapid response time.
3. Disadvantages: Preheating time is needed. Samples have to be drawn from the system, usually a normal flow rate of 50 ml/min.
4. Model
   Penlon Halothane Monitor

Physiochemical Method (Dräger Narkotest)

1. Principle
   The principle of this method is relaxation of elasticity of silicon rubber bands in the presence of halothane vapour (Fig. 4).
2. Advantages: It is a simple instrument and is reasonably accurate. It does not need an electrical source and preheating is not required.
3. Disadvantages: Its response is slow, and it is influenced in the presence of N_2O. Furthermore, it is not specific for halothane.
4. Model
   Dräger Narkotest: This is a useful instrument for the measurement of halothane vapour concentration up to 3%. Accuracy is $\pm 0.15\%$ over 0%–3% of halothane.

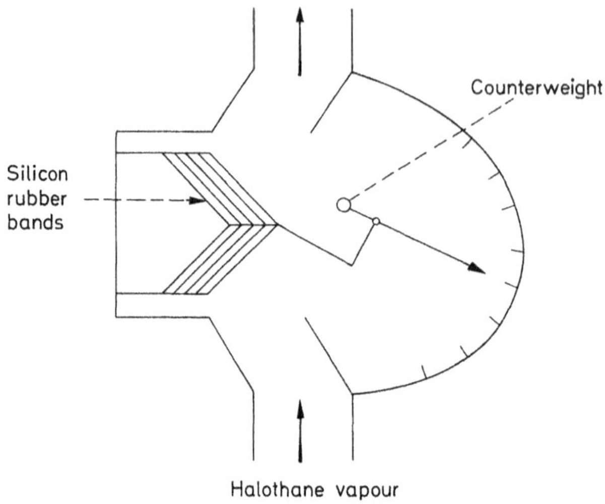

Fig. 4. Measurement of halothane by means of silicon rubber bands (Dräger Narkotest)

Gas Mass Spectrometer

Monitoring of halothane concentration by the gas mass spectrometer is discussed in the next section.

Gas Mass Spectrometer

The mass spectrometer measures the composition of inspired and expired gases. Oxygen, carbon dioxide, nitrogen and anaesthetic gases including halothane and nitrous oxide can be measured on a simultaneous and essentially instaneous breath-to-breath basis. It is presently the most advanced method of measuring gas

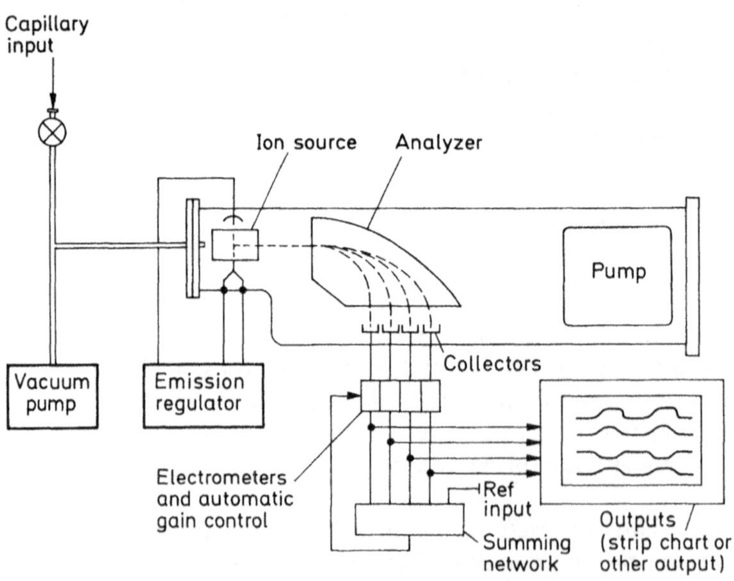

Fig. 5. Block diagram of the Perkin-Elmer medical mass spectrometer

concentration. By simplifying its operation and designing it specifically for respiratory gas analysis, it has been used in the pulmonary function laboratory.

Response time is 100 ms or less from 0 to 90%, and the sample gas flow to the inlet is relatively small (1 ml/s). Therefore, the mass spectrometer provides reasonable measurement of respiratory gases during closed-circuit anaesthesia accurately and easily.

Gas concentrations are displayed on a selectable digital display located on the front of the instrument. Readings are either "per cent" or "mmHg".

Principle of Operation of the Medical Mass Spectrometer. At a point along the capillary where the pressure has been reduced, a small proportion of the sample is admitted to the analyzer where it is ionized at a reduced pressure by an electron beam. These ions are focused into a beam by an electrostatic lens, then pass through a magnetic field. Each ion has a characteristic mass and carries an electric charge, or mass-to-charge ratio, with heavier ions following larger radii. Ion collectors are placed at appropriate locations to collect specific ions. Each ion current is amplified to a level convenient for use with conventional meters or recording devices. An ion vacuum pump maintains internal parts of the mass spectrometer at appropriate pressures, and suitable power supplies are provided (Fig. 5).

O_2 Consumption ($\dot{V}O_2$) and CO_2 Production ($\dot{V}CO_2$)

The $\dot{V}O_2$ and $\dot{V}CO_2$ are usually calculated as follows:

$$\dot{V}O_2 = \int_0^t \dot{V}_I F_{IO_2} dt - \int_0^t \dot{V}_E F_{EO_2} dt$$

$$\dot{V}CO_2 = \int_0^t F_{ECO_2} \cdot \dot{V}_E dt \,,$$

where $\dot{V}_I$ = inspired volume, $\dot{V}_E$ = expired volume, F_{IO_2} = fraction of inspired oxygen, F_{EO_2} = fraction of expired oxygen and F_ECO_2 = fraction of expired carbon dioxide.

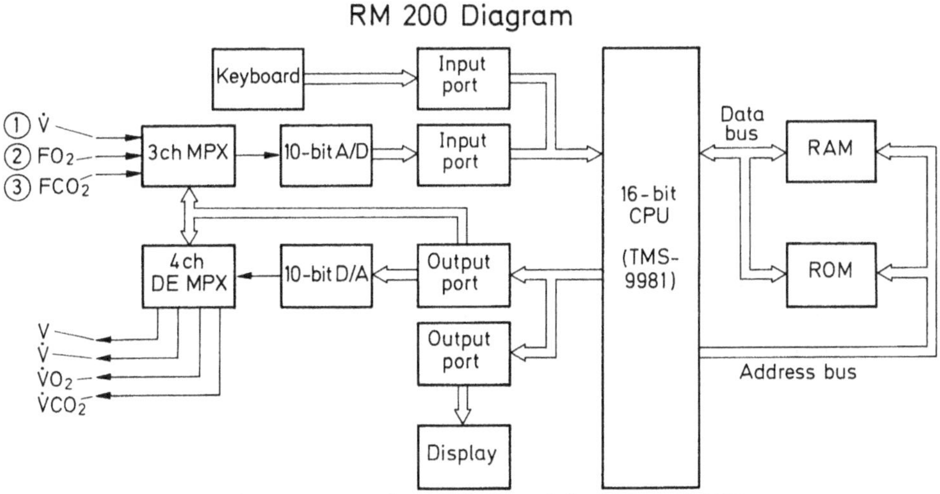

Fig. 6. Diagram of a microcomputer for calulation of the $\dot{V}O_2$ and $\dot{V}CO_2$

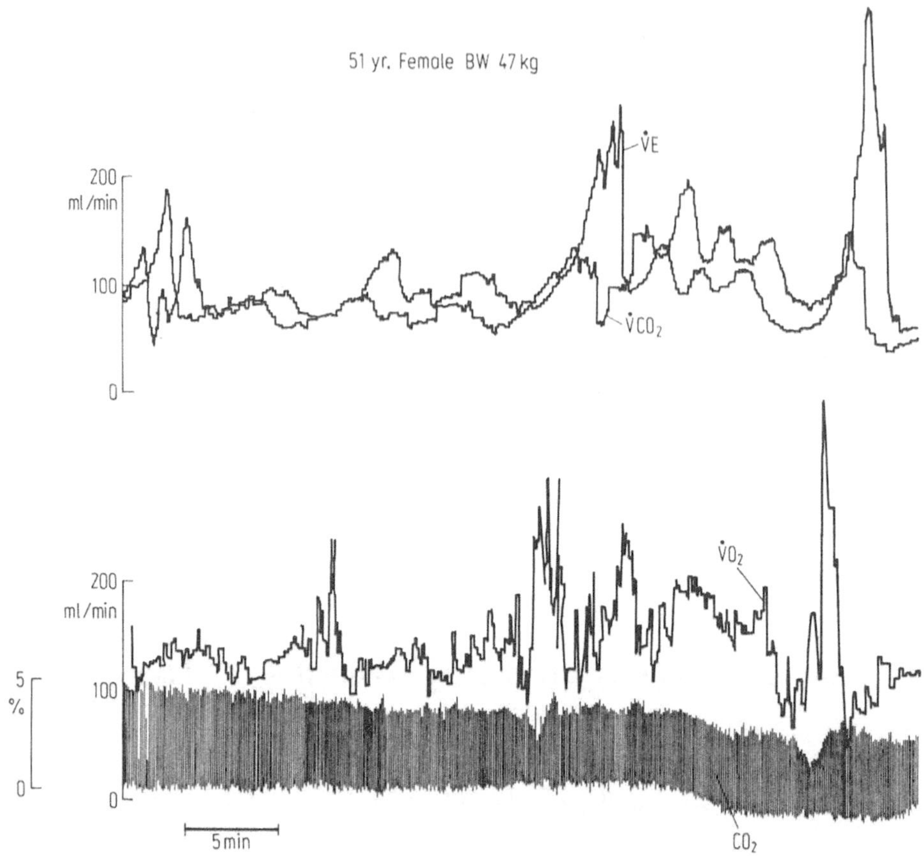

Fig. 7. Measurement of $\dot{V}O_2$ and $\dot{V}CO_2$ during closed-circuit anaesthesia

Both a mass spectrometer and a compact flowmeter with quick response are required to measure $\dot{V}O_2$ and $\dot{V}CO_2$. The hot-wire flowmeter is a hot-wire anemometer of a constant-temperature type (Respiromonitor, RM-100, Minato Medical Science). It is designed as a respiratory monitor in anaesthesia and intensive care.

Breath-by-breath integration of respiratory flow is achieved and $\dot{V}_I$ and $\dot{V}_E$ are calculated.

In order to compute $\dot{V}O_2$ and $\dot{V}CO_2$ a microcomputer is also needed. Output data from a hot-wire flowmeter and a mass spectrometer are entered in to a 16-bit microcomputer (Fig. 6).

A delay is introduced in the output of the flowmeter to compensate for the pneumatic delay introduced by the capillary at the mass spectrometer inlet. This delay is usually 250 ms for a 2-m sample line. The flowmeter output should be delayed in time to coincide with the output from the mass spectrometer. The lag time and time constant of the hot-wire flowmeter are corrected intentionally using the keyboard of a 16-bit computer. Thus breath-by-breath integration of O_2 and CO_2 concentration is accomplished and $\dot{V}O_2$ and $\dot{V}CO_2$ is computed (Fig. 7).

References

1. Scurr C, Feldman S (ed) (1982) Scientific foundation of anaesthesia, 3rd edn. Heinemann, London
2. Gerson GR (1981) Monitoring during anaesthesia. Int Anesthesiol Clin 19:31–59
3. Diprose KV, Epstein HG, Redman LR (1980) An improved ultraviolet halothane meter. Br J Anaesth 52:115–1160
4. Duffin J (1976) Physics for anaesthetists. Thomas, Springfield, USA
5. Schreiber P (1972) Anaesthesia equipment. Performance, classification and safety. Springer, Berlin Heidelberg New York
6. Lowe HJ, Hagler K (1971) Clinical and laboratory evaluation of an expired anesthetic gas monitor (Narko-test). Anesthesiology 34:378–382
7. Operation Manuals of Normocap (Datex), Clinical Gas Monitor IH26 (NEC San-ei), Engstrom Eliza CO_2 analyzer, Mini OX M25RAD medical oxygen monitor (Catalyst Research Corp), and Ohio Oxygen monitor 401

Closed-Circuit Anaesthesia: Actual Inspired Gas Concentrations Measured by Mass Spectrometer

G. Rolly and L. Versichelen

The mass spectrometer is a sophisticated apparatus, which makes possible the qualitative and quantitative measurement of all respiratory gases present in the normal breathing gases or artificially introduced in the breathing circuit. The gases are identified and analysed according to the mass number, or more correctly according to their mass charge ratio. This occurs on a simultaneous and continuous breath to breath basis. It is the only method that provides complete insight into the gas exchange, and accordingly it is very useful in clinical anaesthesia, but especially for research purposes.

The apparatus we use is the Centronic mass spectrometer (Centronic House, Croydon, England), which is of the anaesthetic model type, with automatic stability control (ASC) and spectrum overlap eraser for anaesthetic gases [1] (Fig. 1). The respiratory gases are continuously sampled by means of a small-bore catheter, at a flow of 100 ml/min. The catheter is introduced through the Y-piece of the breathing circuit. The mass numbers at which the gases are analysed are shown in Table 1. The mass spectrometer output is connected to a Watanabe recorder, permitting full-scale deflection for each gas. At normal speed recording,

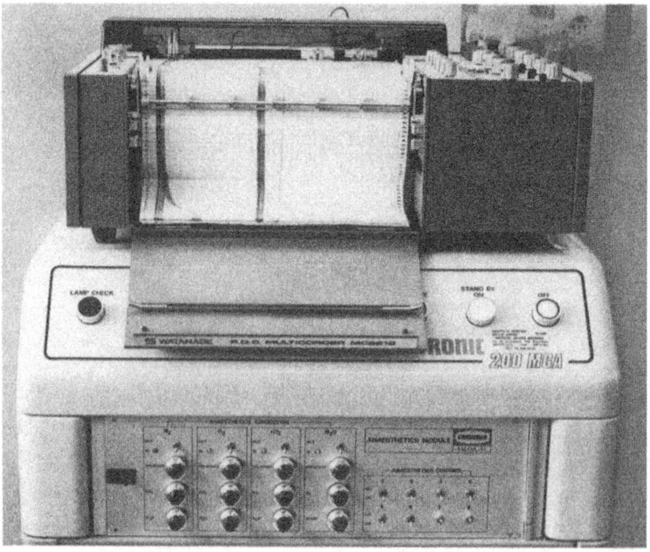

Fig. 1. Centronic mass spectrometer and Watanabe recorder

Table 1. Mass numbers used

He	4
N_2	28
N_2O	30
O_2	32
Arg	40
CO_2	44
Isoflurane	51
Enflurane	51
Halothane	116

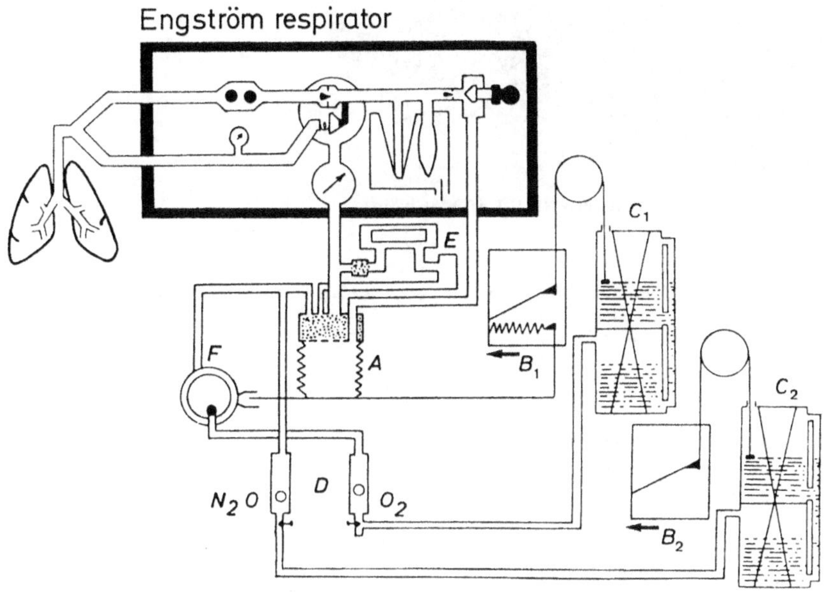

Fig. 2. EHN spirometer connected to an Engström respirator, for closed-circuit anaesthesia

breath to breath changes can be studied and at low-speed recording the curves give a good visual picture of the pharmacokinetics of inhalation anaesthetics.

We use the mass spectrometer for studies during open-circuit, semiclosed and closed-circuit anaesthesia. These last two applications will be discussed here.

In the first setup, an Engström 300 respirator is used in closed circuit. This apparatus has undergone some minor modifications to make it completely airtight; this is checked before each use. The Engström respirator is used in connection with an EHN spirometer [2] (Engström, Herzog and Norlander 1961) (Fig. 2). This last device enables the O_2 inflow in the system to be automatically adjusted, so to keep constant the volume of the apparatus-patient system. The O_2 concentration in the system is measured with a fuel cell and is kept constant by a variable inflow of N_2O during N_2O/O_2 anaesthesia. Liquid inhalation anaesthetic (isoflurane, enflurane or halothane) is injected in a special vaporizing chamber mounted in the circuit (Fig. 3). The copper home-made chamber has a capacity of ± 2 ml. A three-way stopcock permits injection by means of a small insulin syringe. Lowe's formula is used.

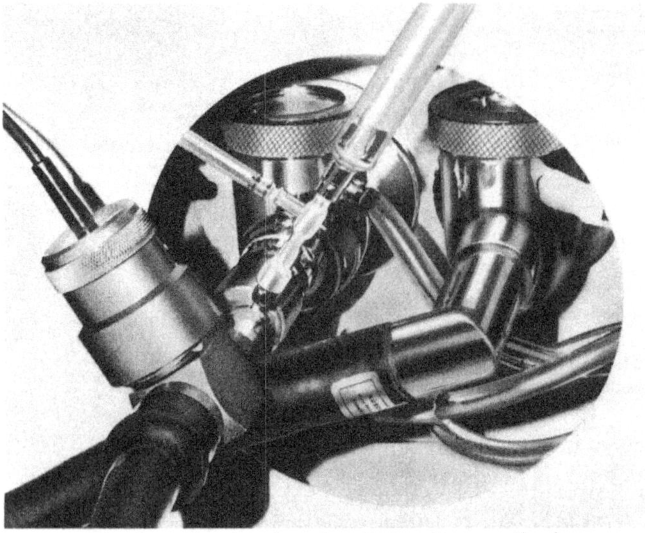

Fig. 3. Injection chamber for closed-circuit anaesthesia

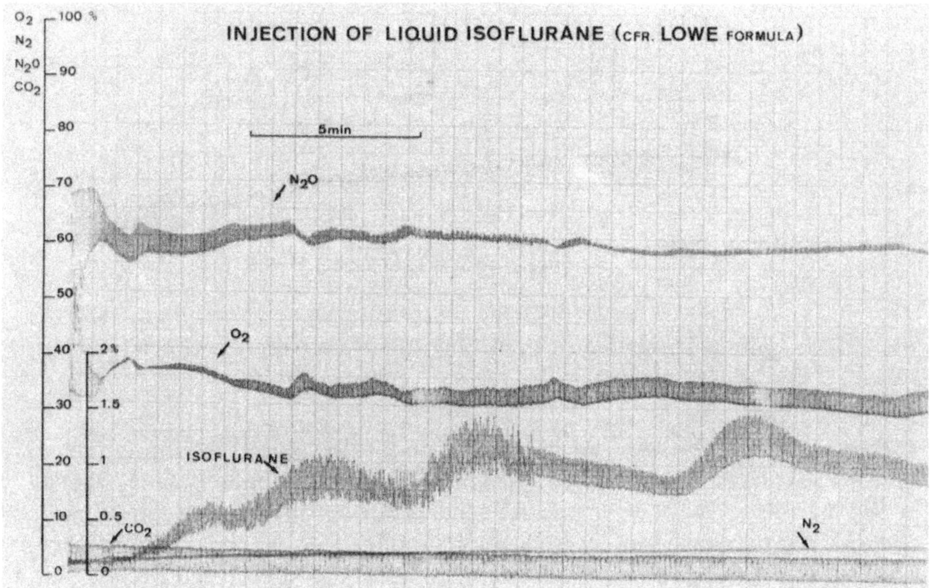

Fig. 4. Closed-circuit anaesthesia, with injection technique (controlled ventilation)

This technique is used in a selected group of adult patients anaesthetized for minor gynaecological procedures. Either isoflurane or halothane is used. Mostly it is possible by manual adjustment of the N_2O inflow to keep the O_2 and N_2O concentrations constant (Fig. 4). Nevertheless sometimes short-lasting major deviations from the aimed target are present, as only the normal rough assessments are immediately available to the anaesthetist, because the mass spectrometer is located outside the operating theatre (Fig. 5). After 20–30 min anaesthesia, the target concentrations are much easier to control carefully.

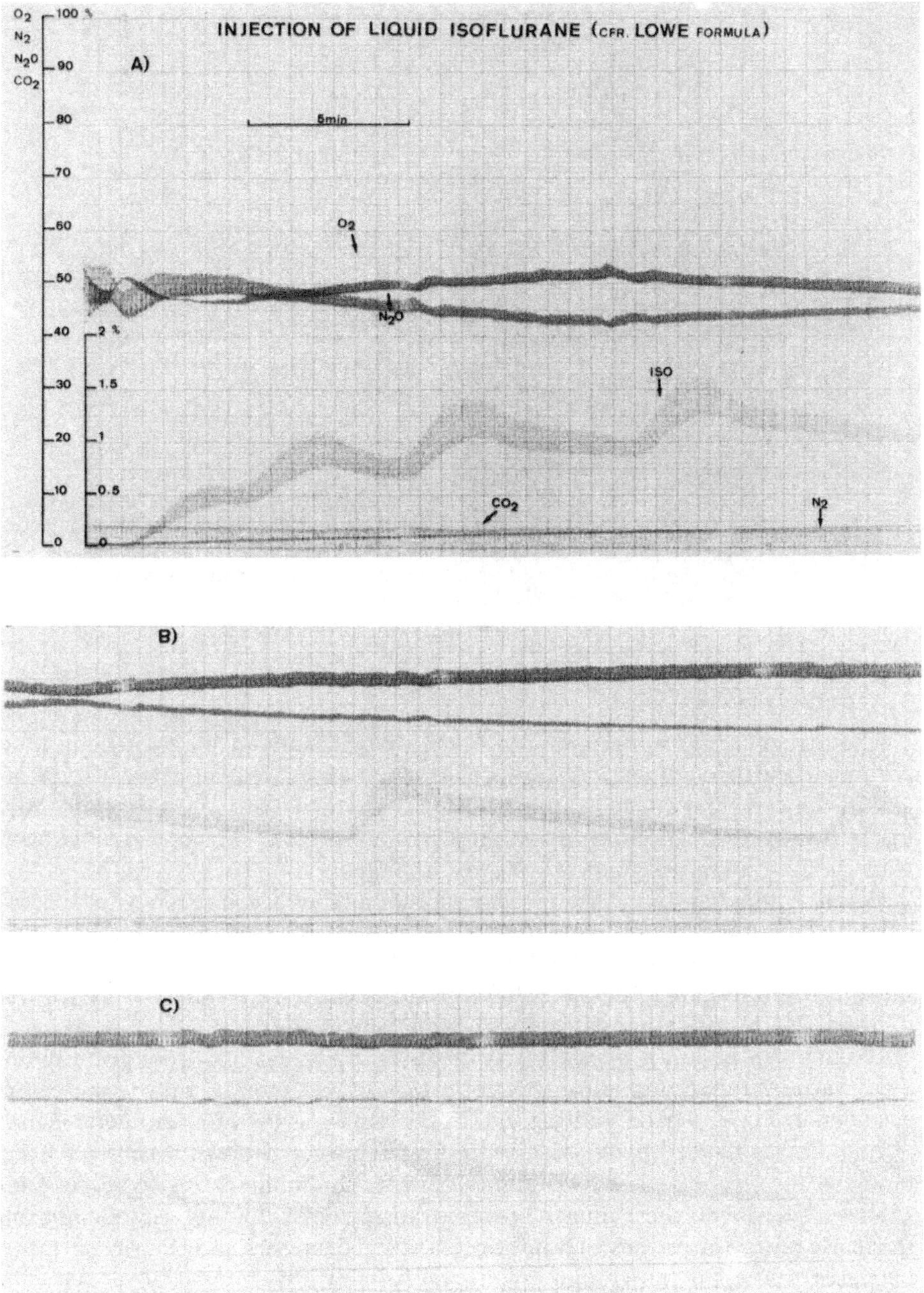

Fig. 5. Closed-circuit anaesthesia, with injection technique (controlled ventilation)

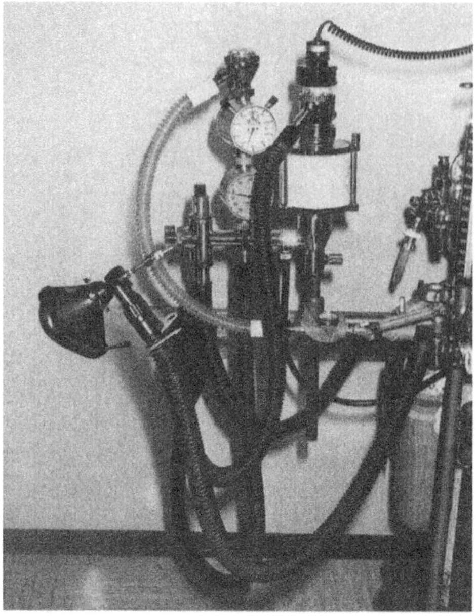

Fig. 6. Dräger circuit, with special injection chamber (sampling of respiratory gases for the mass spectrometer is done at the Y-piece)

The actual concentrations of isoflurane or halothane given by injection, according to the time sequence of Lowe, show a seesaw movement of the inspiratory and of the end-tidal concentrations during controlled ventilation. Initially large inspired to end-tidal concentration gradients are present. The end-tidal concentrations show a less pronounced stepwise change.

When liquid halothane is injected in the special home-made vaporization chamber, mounted in a Dräger circuit (Fig. 6), and only basal O_2 is fed to it, pronounced inspiratory end-tidal halothane gradients can be observed during spontaneous respiration (Fig. 7). After brief preoxygenation, a residual concentration of about 8% N_2 (together with some Argon) is present.

In clinical practice, it is usual first to start with a high gas flow given over a "tec" vaporizer and afterwards convert it to a low or minimal flow. An example is shown in Fig. 8, whereby initially 33% O_2 / 66% N_2O / 1% halothane is used at high flow, followed by a 750-ml/min flow (between the two arrows). At that moment, the actual inhaled halothane concentration immediately decreases from 1% to 0.5%, due to the diminished mass transport of halothane vapour. During that early part of anaesthesia, N_2O concentration decreases and O_2 concentration increases, due to the initial high uptake of N_2O.

Recently we had the chance to use the experimental apparatus Narcocon (Mijnhardt), developed for closed-circuit anaesthesia. In this device the O_2 concentration is kept constant at a desired, computer-programmed level, the balance being N_2O. Liquid inhalation anaesthetic is injected by syringe into the circuit (Fig. 9). N_2 concentration progressively rises despite 10 min denitrogenation, due to the continuous slow excretion of N_2. Small boluses of enflurane are injected so as to keep the end-tidal concentration at a minimum level of 0.75%, as measured with the Datex Normac apparatus.

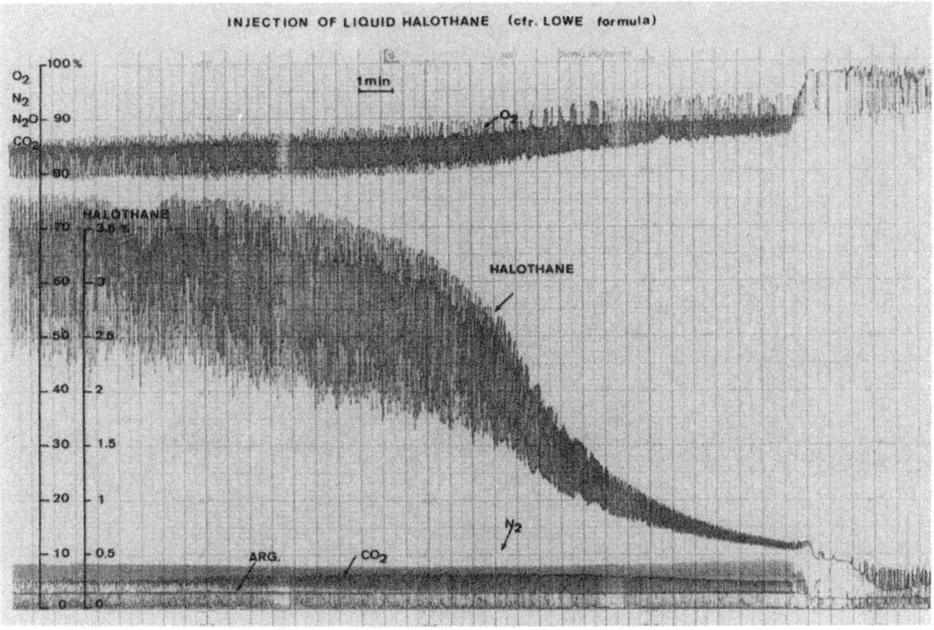

Fig. 7. Closed-circuit anaesthesia, with injection technique (spontaneous respiration)

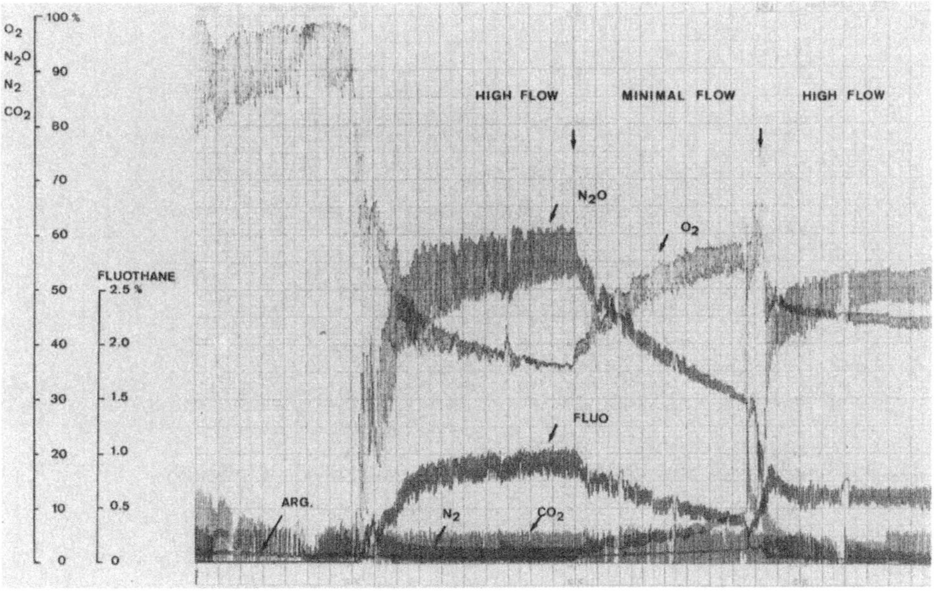

Fig. 8. Closed-circuit anaesthesia, with injection technique (spontaneous respiration)

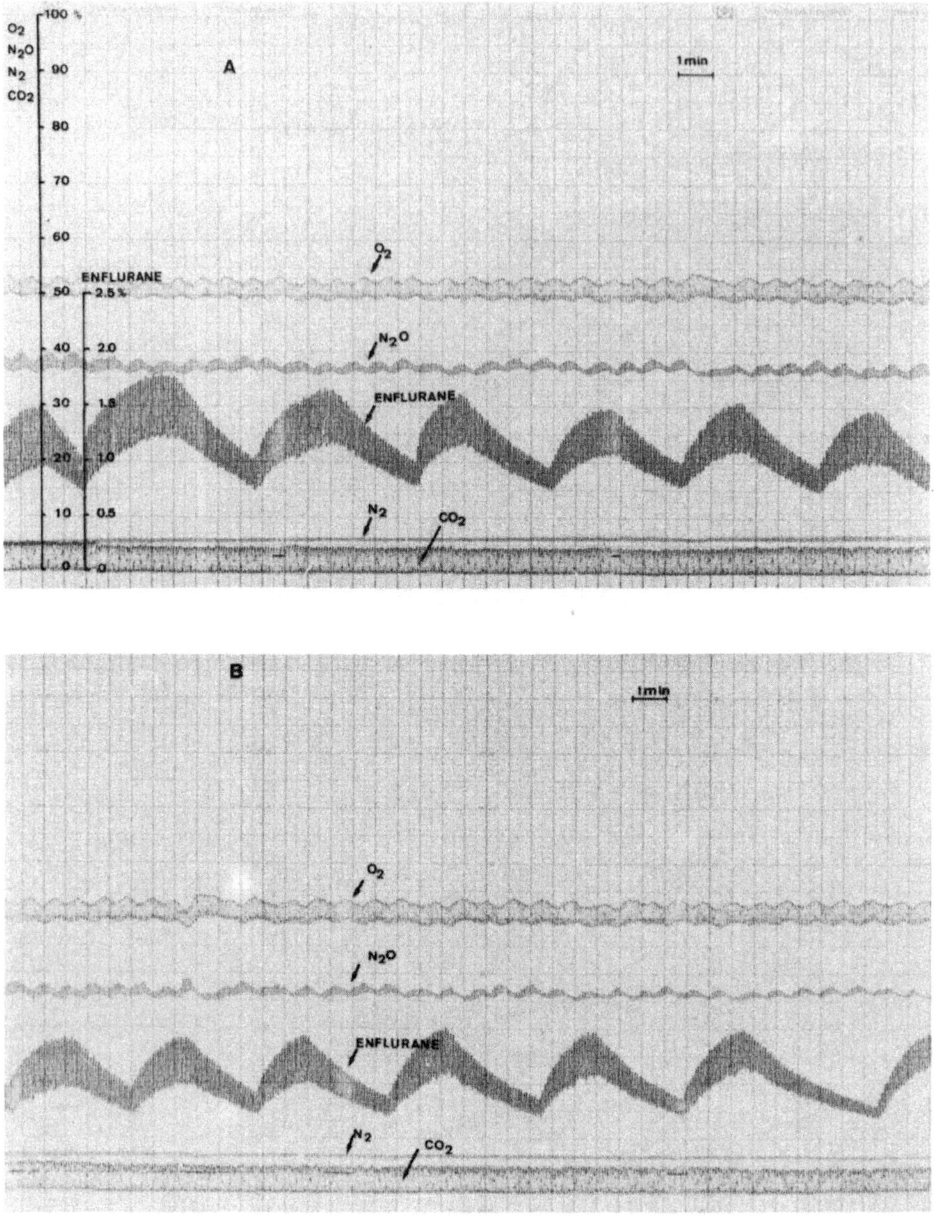

Fig. 9. Closed-circuit anaesthesia with Narcocon (controlled ventilation)

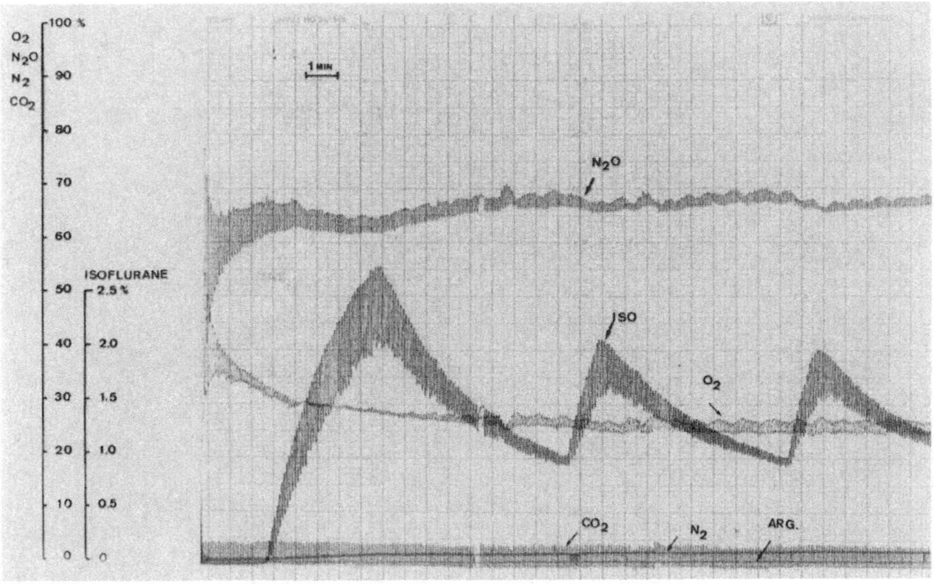

Fig. 10. Closed-circuit anaesthesia with Narcocon (controlled ventilation)

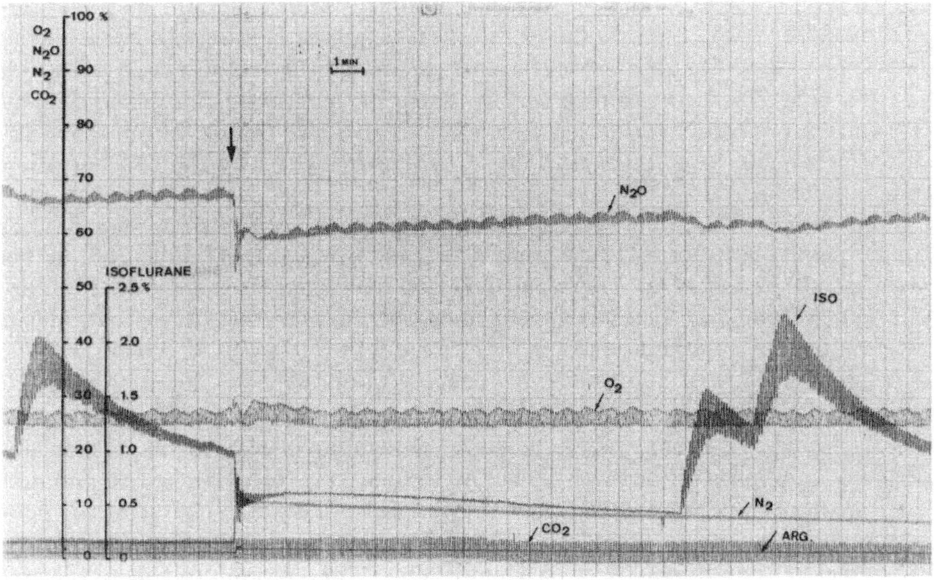

Fig. 11. Closed-circuit anaesthesia with Narcocon (artificial decrease of isoflurane concentration: *the arrow* indicates the point at which a charcoal cannister is temporarily opened)

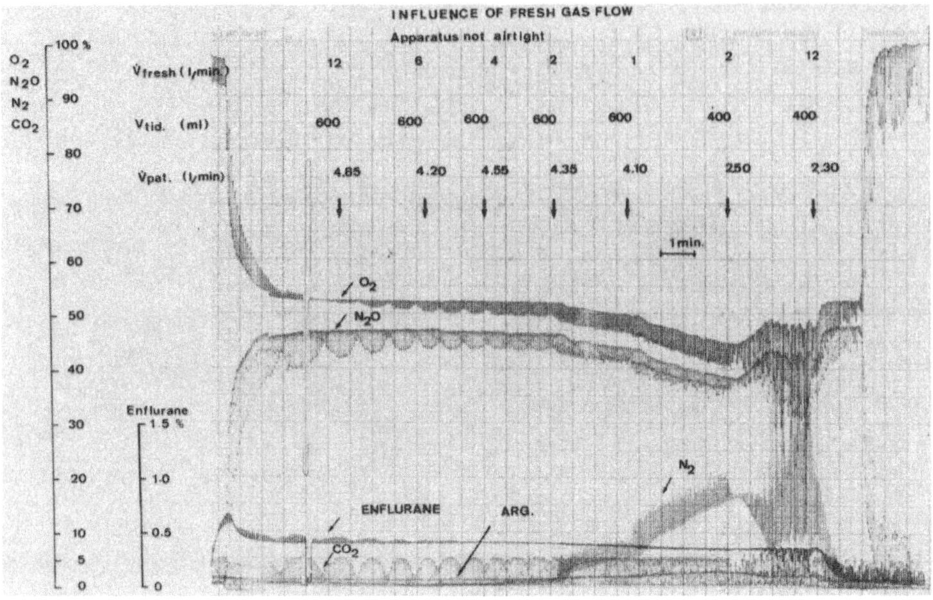

Fig. 12. Low-flow system anaesthesia (apparatus not airtight)

During anaesthesia for breast biopsy, where end-tidal isoflurane concentration is kept at 1% (Fig. 10), the operation is temporarily interrupted for biopsy examination. Meanwhile the end-tidal isoflurane is temporarily lowered by passing the breathing gases twice over active charcoal, resulting in an end-tidal concentration of 0.6% (Fig. 11). As the canister also contains air, N_2 concentration increases by 8% and the N_2O concentration is concomitantly reduced by 8%. For the continuation of surgery, an additional bolus of isoflurane increases the concentration again to the desired 1%.

Apparatuses with a descending bellow, together with controlled ventilation, are frequently used for low-flow, semiclosed anaesthesia. It is known that in this situation the system is not always airtight and unwanted air entrainment can occur. When using a Dräger circuit, together with the Ventilog, this situation can happen, but might go unnoticed at high fresh gas flows. In Fig. 12 it is shown that at a fresh gas flow of 2 litres/min N_2 concentration increases and at 1 litre/min N_2 concentration even rises to 20%. Both O_2 and N_2O concentrations decrease concomitantly. After correcting the air leak, a minimal-flow technique can successfully be applied. When the high-flow technique is then changed to minimal flow, without changing the O_2 concentration of fresh gases, a characteristic proportional increase of N_2O and decrease of O_2 concentrations is noticed (Fig. 13). Nevertheless at a minimal flow of 0.5 litre/min, it becomes impossible to fill correctly the descending bellow, air entrainment occurs with a rise in N_2 and even suction is generated whereby the Vapor delivers a higher enflurane concentration than according to the dial of the vaporizer. These findings suggest that a minimal gas flow technique with descending bellow is not advisable and might even be dangerous. Figure 14 shows that at a 0.5-litre/min fresh gas flow N_2 increase can even be as high as 32%, with decrease of O_2 concentration to 28%, although the O_2 percentage is set at 50% in the O_2/N_2O mixer.

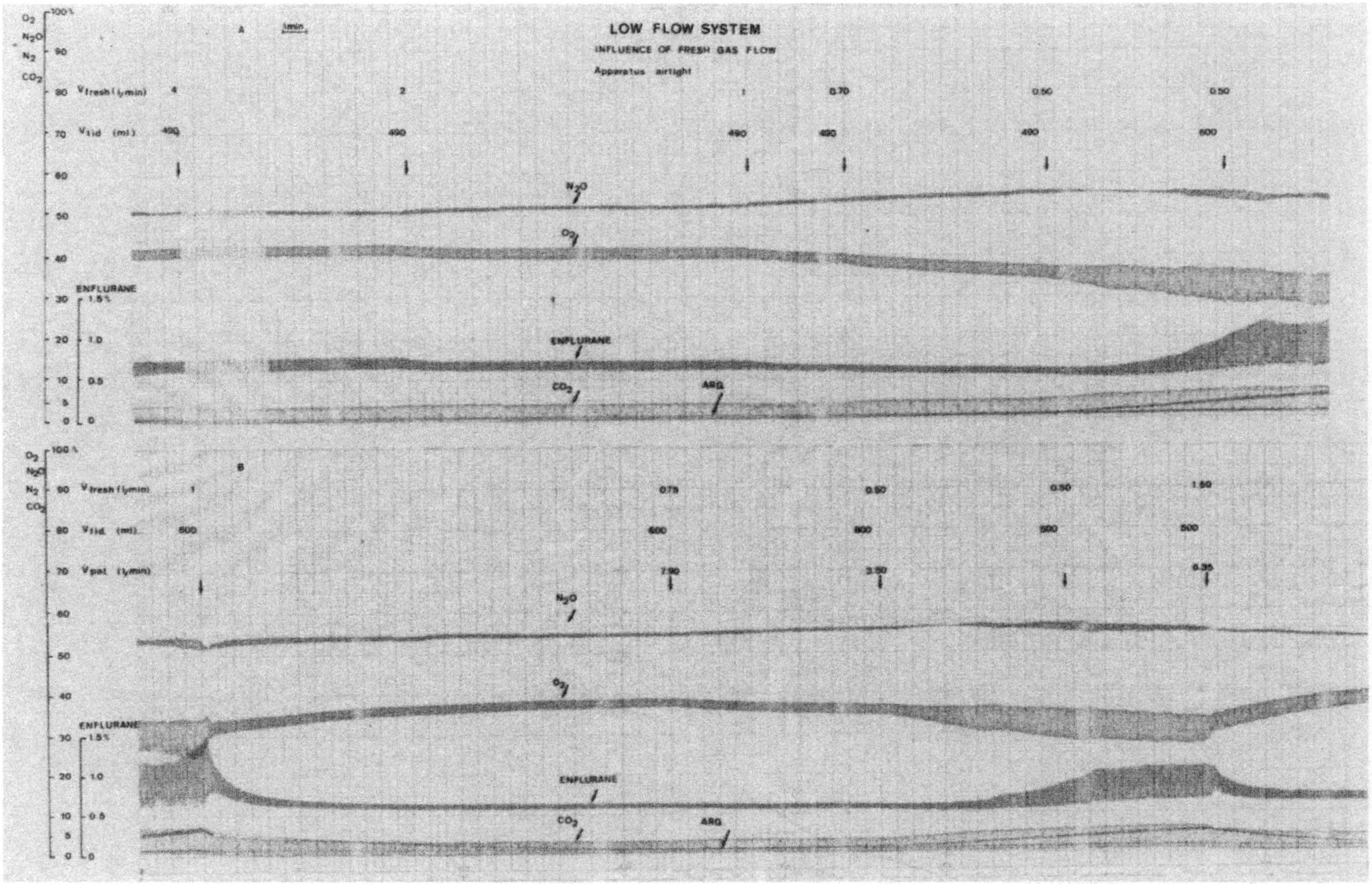

Fig. 13. Low-flow system anaesthesia (apparatus airtight)

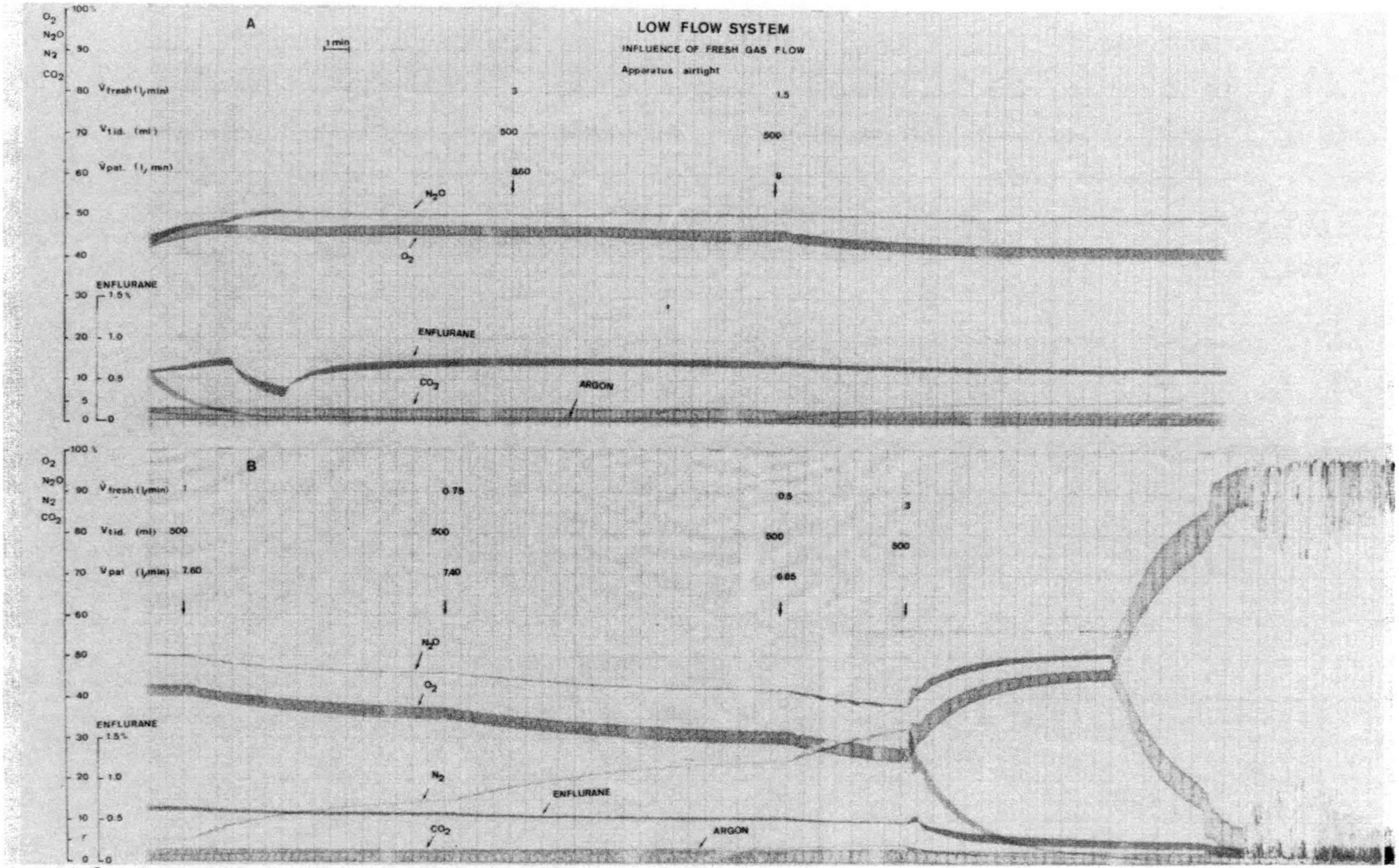

Fig. 14. Low-flow system anaesthesia (apparatus airtight)

These typical examples show clearly that continuous evaluation by mass spectrometer is an important element for a clearer understanding of the behaviour of closed-circuit and low-flow semiclosed anaesthesia. This is even more so if, in addition to potent inhalation anaesthetics, N_2O is used.

References

1. Davis WOM, Spence AA (1979) A modification of the MGA 200 mass spectrometer to enable measurements of anaesthetic gas mixtures. Br J Anaesth 51:987
2. Engström CG, Herzog P, Norlander OP (1961) A method for the continuous measurement of oxygen consumption in the presence of inert gases during controlled ventilation. Acta Anaesthesiol Scand 5:115

Can We Practise Safe, Simple Closed-Circuit Anaesthesia without Extensive Monitoring or Calculus?

C.-Y. Lin

In the past, uncertainty regarding the inspiratory concentration during closed-circuit anaesthesia made the clinical application of closed-circuit unpopular. However, the new concepts in uptake of inhalation anaesthetic [1] including (1) uptake is at its peak at the end of functional residual capacity (FRC) wash-in and remains near constant for a given inspired anaesthetic concentration; (2) uptake depends on inspired concentration– if the inspired concentration increases, uptake increases; and (3) large circuit volume and FRC serve as buffers; allowing closed-circuit anaesthesia to be practiced with simplicity and with minimal requirement of monitoring equipment.

Since Severinghaus's publication on nitrous oxide in 1954 [2], many investigators of inhalation anaesthetics have expressed anaesthetic uptake over time as a power function. For example, the rate of nitrous oxide uptake, according to Severinghaus, is expressed by 1000 (ml) $t^{-1/2}$ and the rate of halothane uptake, according to Lowe and Mapleson [3, 4], is given by 50 (ml) $t^{-1/2}$. However, the approximations made in the derivation of the $t^{-1/2}$ function, in fact, do not separate the functional residual capacity (FRC) wash-in from the true body uptake. When one uses 80% nitrous oxide at the beginning of wash-in a total of 2400 ml nitrous oxide must be administered to fill the average 3000 ml FRC before uptake begins. Severinghaus's measurements do not take this wash-in volume into account. During wash-in of certain anaesthetic gases into the FRC, especially with a large volume or high concentration of an anaesthetic gas such as nitrous oxide, exchange with gases pre-existing in the FRC takes place on a volume-by-volume basis.

If the rate of uptake of inhalation anaesthetics does not follow the square root of time (power function) during the period of wash-in, then what is the time course of uptake of inhalation anaesthetics? Because of the higher solubility partition coefficient of anaesthetic gases, it was believed in the past that no membrane barrier existed for uptake of inhalation anaesthetics. However, we have demonstrated in several experiments that: (1) a membrane barrier does exist; (2) uptake is at its peak at the end of FRC wash-in and remains near-constant for a given inspired anaesthetic concentration; and (3) uptake depends on inspired concentration – if the inspired concentration increases, uptake increases.

To separate the FRC wash-in from the total uptake measured at the mouthpiece, we performed an experiment in which we used a subtraction method. During constant-volume ventilation, inspiratory-expiratory concentration differences represent uptake if one assumes that complete mixing of gases occurred in the lungs. For nitrous oxide uptake, we obtained inspiratory and expiratory ni-

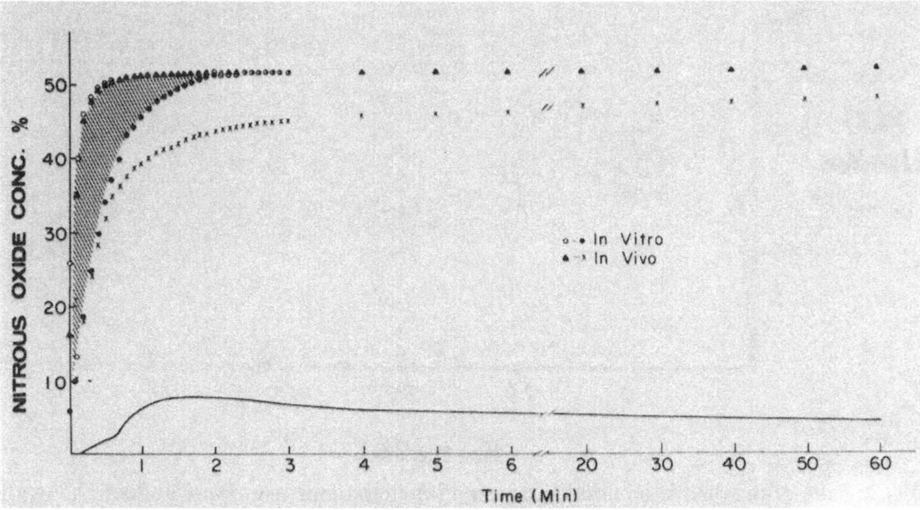

Fig. 1. Results of an experiment conducted in vitro and in vivo, designed to demonstrate the near-constancy of nitrous oxide uptake following FRC wash-in. The *shaded area* indicates in vitro wash-in in an experiment with the FRC of the nitrous oxide wash-in into this simulated lung from the tracing obtained in vivo yields the net body uptake, which is plotted *on the bottom*. This demonstrates the near-constant uptake of nitrous oxide over a 1-h period. In the beginning, the anaesthetic gas mixture is washed into the FRC and must be exchanged with existing gases in the FRC. This produces only limited uptake, because the anaesthetic gas has not reached its peak inspiratory concentration due to dilution by gases pre-existing in the lung

trous oxide concentration curves when nitrous oxide and oxygen were introduced into a circle system with a patient attached. With the same ventilatory rate, ventilatory volume and fresh-gas flow, we then carried out an in vitro wash-in experiment with the FRC of the patient matched by a reservoir bag. Subtraction of the expired nitrous oxide concentration during wash-in into the simulated lung from the expired concentration measured in vivo yielded the net nitrous oxide concentration difference due to actual body uptake of the gas across the alveolar membrane. As shown at the bottom of Fig. 1, nitrous oxide uptake by the blood in the 1st min is less than that in the 2nd or 3rd min. This can be explained by the fact that the inspired concentration of anaesthetic cannot immediately reach a peak at the alveolar level because the anaesthetic gas is diluted by the gases pre-existing in the FRC.

With a similar experimental method, nitrous oxide uptake was measured clinically. As shown in Fig. 2, nitrous oxide uptake was low in the first 2 min; the rate of uptake reached its peak at the 3rd min and declined slowly over the next 60 min. The figure also demonstrates that a 60% inspired nitrous oxide concentration gave a higher average rate of nitrous oxide uptake than did a 50% inspired concentration. In Fig. 3, a comparison is made between Severinghaus's power function approximation of the rate of nitrous oxide uptake and our measured values. A great difference in uptake of nitrous oxide during the 1st 10 min is demonstrated. This discrepancy again reflects that, when an anaesthetic gas mixture is washed into the FRC, it must be exchanged with the gases in the FRC. During the initial time of this exchange, the blood will absorb some of the anaesthetic gas

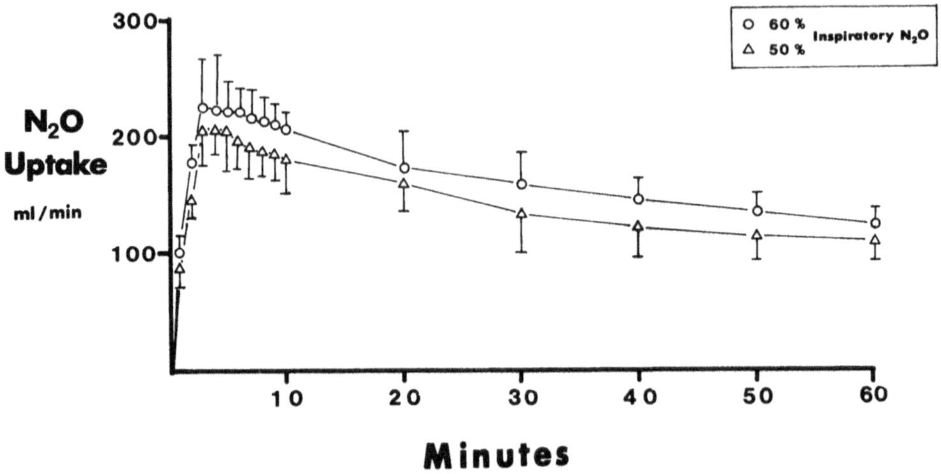

Fig. 2. Rate of nitrous oxide uptake, measured in 50 patients who were undergoing open-heart surgery. Twenty patients received 60% nitrous oxide and 30 patients received 50% nitrous oxide. The rate of uptake reached its peak at the 3rd min and then declined very slowly during the 1st h. The higher inspired concentration (60%) increased the rate of uptake

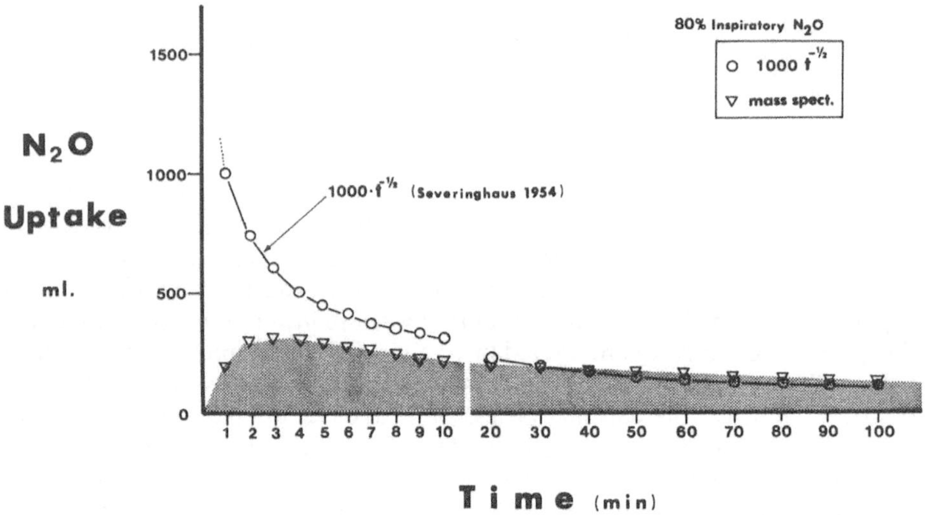

Fig. 3. Schematic comparison of rates of nitrous oxide uptake as measured by mass spectrometry and as approximated with the $t^{-1/2}$ function (Severinghaus) at an inspiratory nitrous oxide concentration of 80%. The disrepancy during the initial phase indicates that the power function approximation overestimates uptake of nitrous oxide because of failure to separate FRC wash-in from true body uptake. (*Shaded area represents uptake*)

mixture from the lungs, but only to a limited degree, because the anaesthetic has not reached its peak inspiratory concentration. In Fig. 4, it is further shown indirectly from measurements on a patient that, initially, nitrous oxide uptake is limited in amount because of the existence of the FRC and the alveolar membrane. After complete preoxygenation, 1500 ml/min nitrous oxide and 250 ml/min oxygen were introduced. After 6 min at this level, the nitrous oxide concen-

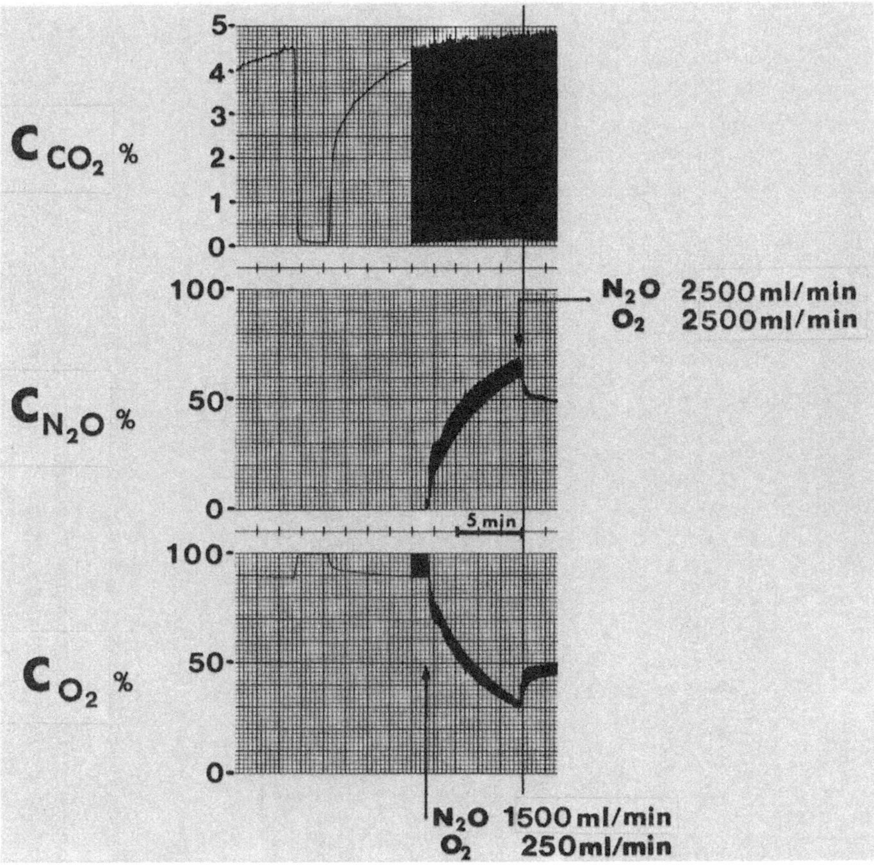

Fig. 4. Mass spectrometric tracings from a patient, showing that the increase in nitrous oxide concentration almost matches the wash-in time constant (6 min) during nitrous oxide administration; this is indicative of limited nitrous oxide uptake in the beginning. (3000 ml FRC plus 6000 ml of circuit equals 9000 ml with 1500 ml/min of nitrous oxide; after one time constant of 6 min, the nitrous oxide concentration will reach 63% if there is no uptake across the alveolar membrane)

tration at the expiratory side of the circuit reached 60%. With 1500 ml/min nitrous oxide introduced into 3000 ml FRC and 6000 ml circuit volume (a total of 9000 ml), after one time constant of 6 min the nitrous oxide concentration will be 63% if none was absorbed. This indicates that very limited nitrous oxide uptake occurred in this 6-min period. If nitrous oxide uptake is a function of the square root of time, there should be a slower rise in the expired concentration of the gas.

In Fig. 5, we illustrate an experiment which we carried out during anaesthesia to demonstrate the existence of a membrane barrier to the uptake of anaesthetic from the lung. The fresh-gas nitrous oxide concentration was increased five times, at 5-min intervals, in steps of 10%; at a total fresh-gas flow of 10000 ml/min, and then was decreased in equal steps every 5 min. With constant-volume ventilation, as was used here, inspiratory-expiratory differences in nitrous oxide concentration again represent uptake of the gas after each brief period of FRC wash-in.

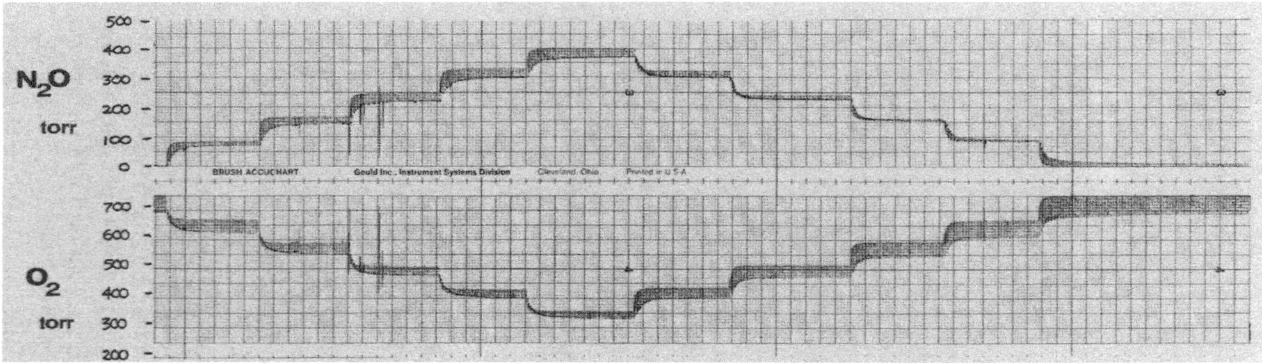

Fig. 5. An experiment was conducted to demonstrate inspiratory-concentration-dependent uptake of nitrous oxide in a patient. The nitrous oxide concentration was increased five times, at 5-min intervals in steps of 10%, at a total fresh-gas flow of 10000 ml/min, and then decreased in equal steps. With constant-volume ventilation, inspiratory-expiratory concentration differences represent the uptake of N_2O after each brief period of FRC wash-in. As the inspired concentration rises, uptake also rises

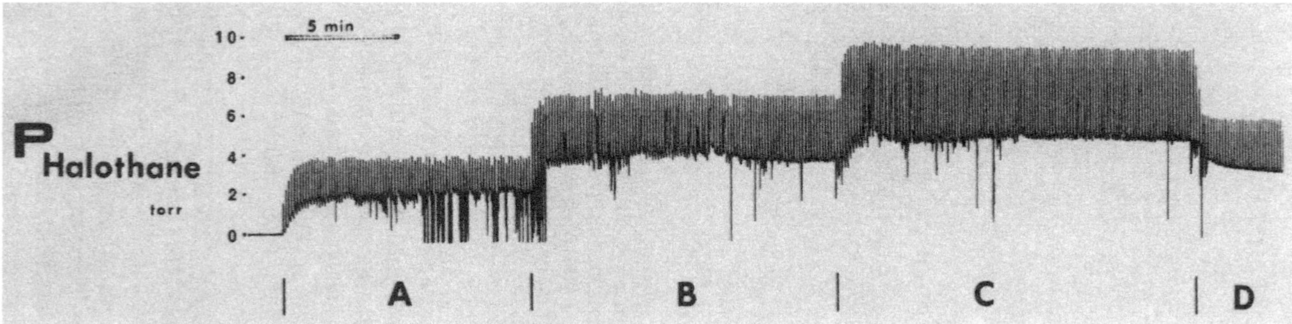

Fig. 6. An experiment was conducted to demonstrate inspiratory-concentration-dependent uptake of halothane in a patient. The halothane concentration was increased three times, at 10- to 15-min intervals, in steps of 0.5% (3.5 torr), at a total fresh-gas flow of 10000 ml/min. With constant volume ventilation, inspiratory-expiratory concentration differences represent the uptake of halothane after each brief period of FRC wash-in. As the inspired concentration rises, uptake also rises

Figure 5 shows that, when the inspired nitrous oxide concentration rises, the uptake rises. This indicates that, provided the cardiac output, ventilatory rate and solubility partition coefficient remain constant, the partial pressure gradient across the alveolar membrane is the sole factor controlling the rate of uptake. This same phenomenon can be demonstrated with other inhalation anaesthetics such as halothane (Fig. 6). When the inspired halothane concentration was raised from 0.5% to 1.5% in 0.5% increments at 15-min intervals, the uptake, again measured as the inspiratory-expiratory concentration difference, doubled at 1% inspired concentration and tripled at 1.5% inspired concentration.

The uptake of an anaesthetic gas through the alveolar membrane commonly follows the Fick principle of diffusion:

$$\text{rate of penetration} = (C_{\text{out}} - C_{\text{in}})\, DAK/x,$$

where C_{out} = concentration outside the membrane, C_{in} = concentration inside the membrane, D = diffusion constant, A = area of membrane, K = partition coefficient and x = thickness of membrane.

The quotient DAK/x is frequently called the permeability constant, P, of the system. Thus, we can rewrite this equation as:

$$\text{rate of uptake} = (C_{\text{out}} - C_{\text{in}})\, P.$$

The permeability constant P is mainly determined by the solubility coefficient of the gas, and in the past it was commonly neglected in consideration of the cardiac output, or, strictly speaking, the pulmonary capillary flow together with diffusion. In Pipper's [5] simple, but useful, model for analysis of blood gas equilibration in the lung, the pulmonary capillary blood is separated from the gas space by a "membrane" representing resistance to diffusion. The degree of equilibration, expressed as the ratio of the alveolar-to-arterial pressure difference to the alveolar-to-mixed venous pressure difference, is a function of the ratio D/BQ (D = diffusion capacity, B = capacitance coefficient, Q = pulmonary capillary blood flow). In the case of anaesthetic gases, no equilibration deficit exists at the membrane ($D/BQ \rightarrow$), and the gas transfer is mainly perfusion limited.

In the past, the rate of uptake was believed to be very high in the beginning, and no barrier to initial uptake was postulated, so that the mixed venous concentration was thought to rise very rapidly because of rapid equilibration of blood-rich organs. In contrast to this viewpoint, one should recognize that the membrane factor exists and that uptake is not diffusion-limited, but perfusion-limited, in the case of inhalation anaesthetics.

In view of these changes in the concept of uptake of inhalation anaesthetics, let us further examine the relationship between end-expiratory or alveolar concentration and inspiratory concentration over time. Eger [6] has employed this relationship to demonstrate the rate of uptake. However, the initial rapid rise of the F_A/F_I curve for nitrous oxide in Fig. 7 is not indicative of a large uptake of nitrous oxide, but represents the FRC wash-in, as described above. In other words, because of the initial limited uptake of nitrous oxide, the alveolar concentration will quickly rise towards the inspired concentration (F_A/F_I). Since uptake of anaesthetics can be measured as the difference between inspired and expired concentration, we conclude that the rate of uptake is best represented not by the F_A/F_I curve, but by the region above the curve, i.e. the difference between inspiratory

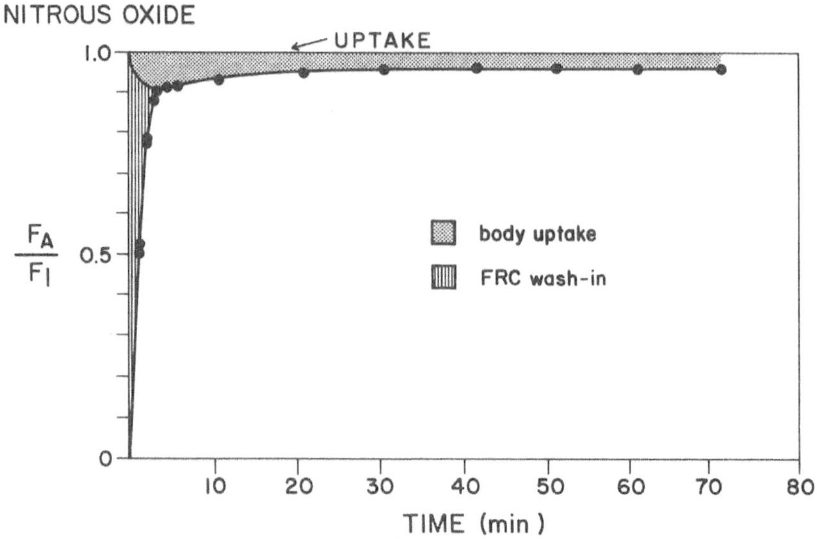

Fig. 7. F_A/F_I curve for nitrous oxide. The initial rapid rise in F_A/F_I indicates FRC wash-in and not a fast build-up of the mixed venous anaesthetic concentration to oppose uptake. Since inspiratory and expiratory anaesthetic concentration differences indicate the anaesthetic uptake during constant-volume ventilation, the rate of true body uptake should be represented by the *shaded area* which shows very limited change over 1 h. The rate of uptake is best expressed by the values above the F_A/F_I curve and not by the F_A/F_I curve itself. The initial lower rate of uptake can be explained by the fact that the inspired concentration of nitrous oxide cannot reach a peak at the alveolar level because nitrous oxide is diluted by the gases pre-existing in the FRC

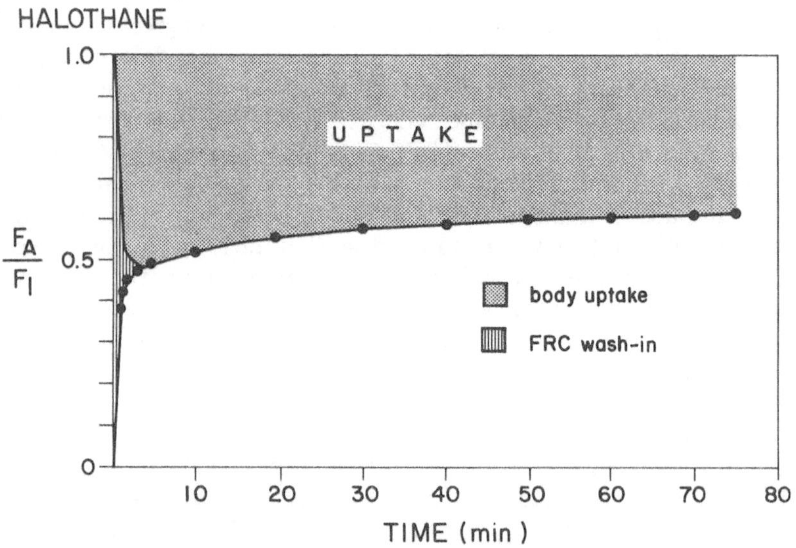

Fig. 8. F_A/F_I curve for halothane. The initial fast rise in F_A/F_I indicates FRC wash-in and not a fast build-up of the mixed venous anaesthetic concentration to oppose uptake (decreased partial pressure differences across the alveolar membrane). The true body uptake is represented by the *shaded area,* which shows a very limited change in the rate of uptake over 1 h. This diagram also demonstrates that, as inspired concentration increases, the rate of uptake increases. Thus, the rate of uptake can be approximated by the expression: inspiratory concentration × fraction of uptake × alveolar ventilation

concentration (F_I) and the F_A/F_I curve. The fractional N_2O uptake at a given time can be expressed as:

$$\text{fraction of uptake} = 1 - F_A/F_I.$$

The same principle can be applied to other inhalation anaesthetics; the curve for halothane is shown in Fig. 8 and that for enflurane (Ethrane) in Fig. 9. The isoflurane (Forane) curve is very similar to that for enflurane because of the similarity in their solubility coefficients. The fraction of uptake for several anaesthetic gases is given in Table 1. As mentioned before, the fact that the fraction of uptake for each of the gases changes very little with time indicates that the uptake of an anaesthetic can be considered to be nearly constant at a given inspired concentration over 1 h (with the assumption of constant cardiac output and constant alveolar ventilation).

As demonstrated by Eger, the F_A/F_I curves vary with ventilation and cardiac output. Much misleading information has been published on this variation in the past because too much emphasis was placed on the value of the alveolar concentration. During shock or when the cardiac output is low, the alveolar concentra-

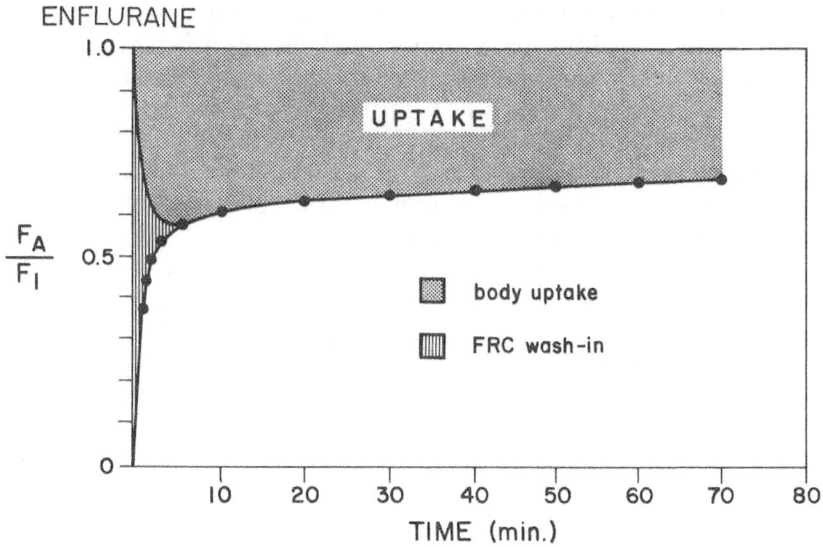

Fig. 9. F_A/F_I curve for enflurane. This again demonstrates the near-constancy of the rate of uptake over 1 h

Table 1. Fraction of uptake[a]

Agent	Initial	60 min	120 min
N_2O	0.13	0.07	0.05
Halothane	0.50	0.40	0.35
Enflurane	0.40	0.35	0.30
Isoflurane	0.40	0.35	0.30
Methoxyflurane	0.80	0.75	0.70

[a] Fraction of uptake $= 1 - \dfrac{F_A}{F_I}$ (after FRC wash-in)

tion rises towards the inspired concentration faster than is the case under normal cardiac output conditions. This may reflect not an increase in the depth of anaesthesia, but a reduction in the fraction of uptake at a given concentration – an indication that anaesthetic uptake is lower. Ventilation also influences the shape of the F_A/F_I curve. A higher ventilation rate results in a higher F_A/F_I curve, and lower ventilation gives a lower curve. Since the rate of uptake of anaesthetic after FRC wash-in can be expressed or estimated as: rate of uptake = inspired concentration × fraction of uptake × alveolar ventilation, altering the rate of ventilation should have a very limited influence on uptake except during the initial wash-in period (if the alveolar ventilation increases, the fraction of uptake decreases).

With these new concepts of uptake of inhalation anaesthetics in mind, do we really require extensive monitoring of the inspired anaesthetic concentration in order to carry out closed-circuit anaesthesia? The answer is certainly "no". Since we always adjust the inspiratory concentration of the potent inhalation anaesthetics based on the responses and haemodynamic condition of individual patients and so the approximate amount of anaesthetic vapour needed to maintain a similar inspiratory anaesthetic concentration can now be calculated with the use of the simple formula given above. Thus, combined with the fact, that the uptake is inspired concentration dependent and that the uptake remains near constant after FRC wash-in with a given concentration, and that the differences between true uptake of anaesthetic and supply of approximated amount of anaesthetic vapour are quite small as compared with the existing volume of circuit and FRC, limited self-feedback control of inspiratory concentration will be activated when the circuit is being closed. In other words, after the initial wash-in period, when the system is closed, one can apply a very simple physics principle – the lower the flow, the longer the time constant. At its extreme, the circuit condition becomes a closed system, and the discrepancy between supply and demand volume becomes extremely small. With the small volume of fresh gas compared with the large circuit volume which we use during closed-circuit anaesthesia, the circuit volume will act as a giant buffer system. Thereafter, original inspiratory anaesthetic concentration will be maintained within a reasonable range. Therefore, with a better understanding of the process of the uptake of inhalation anaesthetic and with a new concept in uptake of inhalation anaesthetic, closed-circuit anaesthesia can be practised with ease and safety, simply, with existing anaesthetic equipment and without extensively monitoring the inspired anaesthetic concentration.

References

1. Lin CY, Mostert JW, Benson DW (1980) Closed circle systems. A new direction in the practice of anesthesia. Acta Anaesthesiol Scand 24:354–361
2. Severinghaus JW (1954) Rate of uptake of nitrous oxide in man. J Clin Invest 33:1183–1189
3. Lowe HJ (1981) The anesthetic continuum in low flow and closed system anesthesia. In: Aldrete JA, Lowe HJ, Virtue RW (eds) Closed Circuit Anaesthesia. Grune and Stratton, New York, pp 11–37
4. Mapleson WW (1973) Circulation-time models of the uptake of inhalation anaesthetics and data for quantifying them. Br J Anaesth 45:319–334
5. Pipper J (1981) Blood-gas equilibration in lungs and pulmonary diffusion capacity. Prog Resp Res 16:115–125
6. Eger EI (1974) Anesthesia uptake and action. Williams and Wilkins, Baltimore

Estimation of Cardiac Output and Lung Tissue Volume in Closed-Circuit (Rebreathing) Systems

P. D. Wagner

Introduction

In 1959, Cander and Forster [1] showed how the rebreathing of a gas of moderate solubility in blood could be used to measure pulmonary tissue volume and pulmonary capillary blood flow. There have been many attempts to improve the technique since then by focussing on one or more details of the method [2–5], but the basic principles are still used today as presented by Cander and Forster. These principles are illustrated in Fig. 1. The left-hand side shows the experimental system consisting of the lung attached to a bag of known volume (V_{bag}). The lung is considered to be homogeneous and is characterized by the variables gas volume, V_{lung}; tissue volume, V_{tissue}, and blood flow, $\dot{Q}$. The bag is filled with a gas mixture such as 1% helium, 1% acetylene, 21% O_2 and 77% N_2 to the volume V_{bag}, and at time zero the lung inhales the gas mixture from functional residual capacity (V_{lung}). For some 10–15 s after the initial inhalation, the lung rapidly exhales and inhales from the bag, the system being closed as in Fig. 1. At the airway opening (between the lung and bag), a rapidly responding gas analyzer such as a mass spectrometer measures the concentrations of the tracer gases (helium and

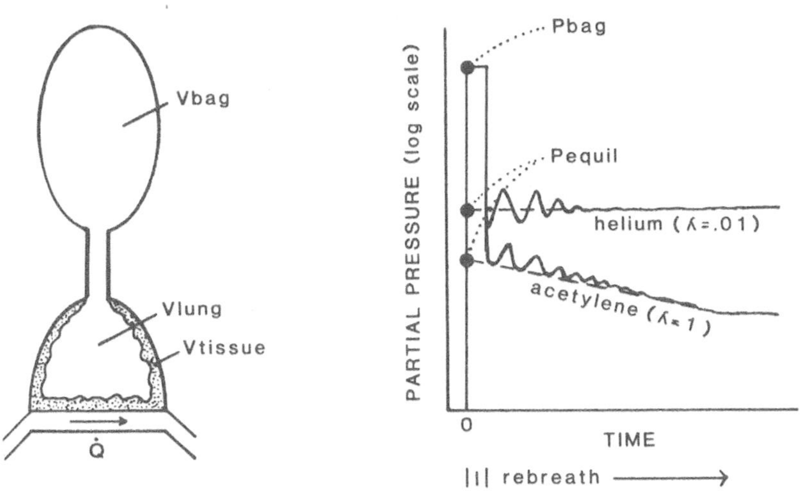

Fig. 1. Scheme for rebreathing estimates of pulmonary gas and tissue volumes and pulmonary blood flow using the insoluble gas helium and the soluble gas acetylene. See text for details

acetylene) continuously in time. The right-hand side of Fig. 1 shows a reproduction of the gas tension recordings against time. Gas tension is on a logarithmic scale, and both helium and acetylene curves are presented. P_{bag} represents original levels of both gases prior to the rebreathing and *P*equil represents the two gas tensions projected back to zero time. Note that the blood:gas partition coefficient of the gases (approximately 0.01 for helium and 1 for acetylene) are different by two orders of magnitude. Helium is essentially insoluble, while acetylene is of intermediate solubility. Mass conservation principles are applied to each gas in turn, and when this is done it is evident that the measurements made in Fig. 1 can be used to estimate lung gas volume (V_{lung}), tissue volume (V_{tissue}) and blood flow ($\dot{Q}$).

The expression for mass conservation for helium is:

$$P_{bag_{He}} \times V_{bag} = Pequil_{He} \times [V_{bag} + V_{lung} + \lambda_{He} \times V_{tissue}]. \quad (1)$$

In this equation the subscript He denotes helium. The LHS expresses the amount of helium present in the bag prior to rebreathing; the RHS represents the same quantity of He, now distributed throughout the bag, lung gas volume and lung tissue volume at a uniform tension ($Pequil_{He}$). The equality depends on having no losses from the system by leaks or by transport out of the lungs in pulmonary venous blood. Because λ_{He} is 0.01, the latter loss of helium is inconsequential over the 10–15 s of the manoeuvre. This is shown by comparing $P_{bag} \times V_{bag}$ (the total amount of helium) with the maximum amount lost to the circulation in one-fourth of a minute if the blood had the same tension P_{bag}. This latter amount is given by $P_{bag} \times \lambda_{He} \times \dot{Q} \times 1/4$. The ratio ($R$) of these two amounts is:

$$R = \frac{\lambda_{He} \times \dot{Q} \times \frac{1}{4}}{V_{bag}}, \quad (2)$$

where λ_{He} is 0.01 as above, and reasonable values for $\dot{Q}$ and V_{bag} are 6 and 3 litres/min respectively. R thus comes to 0.005, indicating a potential error of only 0.5% in making the mass conservation assumption. Also, because $\lambda_{He} \times V_{tissue}$ is approximately 0.01 × 0.6 or 0.006 litres, while $V_{bag} + V_{lung}$ is about 6 litres, the term λ_{He} can also be neglected, incurring only 0.1% error. Since in Eq. (1), $P_{ba\,He}$ and $Pequil_{He}$ are measured (as in Fig. 1) and V_{bag} is also known, V_{lung} is calculated easily as:

$$V_{lung} = V_{bag} \times \left[\frac{P_{bagHe}}{Pequil_{He}} - 1\right]. \quad (3)$$

This gives functional residual capacity. Turning our attention now to acetylene, Eq. (1) is applied to this gas also:

$$P_{bag_{AC}} \times V_{bag} = Pequil_{AC} \times [V_{bag} + V_{lung} + \lambda_{AC} \times V_{tissue}]. \quad (4)$$

In this use of mass conservation, the correct value of $Pequil_{AC}$ to use is that projected back to zero time from the acetylene disappearance curve (Fig. 1): Acetylene is sufficiently soluble that it is removed by blood flow, so that the zero time projection represents the acetylene tension in the lung after mixing but *before* any loss into blood, thus satisfying the mass conservation principle.

Rearranging Eq. (4) gives:

$$V_{\text{tissue}} = \frac{V_{\text{bag}}}{\lambda_{\text{AC}}} \times \left[\frac{P_{\text{bagAC}}}{\text{Pequil}_{\text{AC}}} - 1\right] - \frac{V_{\text{lung}}}{\lambda_{\text{AC}}}. \tag{5}$$

In Eq. (5), P_{bagAC} and $Pequil_{\text{AC}}$ are measured from tracings as in Fig. 1. λ_{AC} and V_{bag} are known, and V_{lung} is known from the helium data and Eq. (3). Thus, all the variables are known and V_{tissue} can be calculated. Note that in Eqs. (4) and (5) the correct value for λ_{AC} is the pulmonary tissue : gas partition coefficient. This is taken to be that of blood since in intact animals or man, λ_{AC} in lung tissue is clearly not measurable. This may introduce errors if blood and tissue solubilities differ, as they do for some gases [6].

Now to analyse the acetylene data in such a manner as to calculate pulmonary blood flow, we proceed as follows:

Another mass conservation equation is written to describe the *dynamic* events during rebreathing:

$$[V_{\text{bag}} + V_{\text{lung}} + \lambda_{\text{AC}} \times V_{\text{tissue}}] \frac{dP}{dt} = -\lambda_{\text{AC}} \dot{Q} P. \tag{6}$$

In Eq. (6), P refers to instantaneous acetylene tension during the rebreathing, and $\frac{dP}{dt}$ to its rate of change with time. The LHS states that the loss from the lungs and bag into the blood is total system volume $(V_{\text{bag}} + V_{\text{lung}} + \lambda_{\text{AC}} V_{\text{tissue}})$ times rate of change of system gas tension $\left(\frac{dP}{dt}\right)$. The RHS equates this loss from the lungs to gain by the blood given by $\lambda_{\text{AC}} \dot{Q} P$ at the same point in time. Equality implies no other way for acetylene to leave the system and also no recirculation of acetylene back to the lungs (which would have the effect of retarding acetylene uptake during rebreathing and cause the disappearance curve to flatten out, as shown at the right-hand side of Fig. 1). This is why the entire manoeuvre must be completed within 10–15 s, since that is the approximate recirculation time in resting man.

Equation (6) is a linear first-order differential equation in P with respect to time, and as such is readily integrated to express P as an explicit function of time:

$$P = P_o \times \text{Exp}(-A x \dot{Q} x t) \tag{7}$$

where P is acetylene tension as a function of time t, P_o is acetylene tension at $t = O$ and A is a constant. A, from Eq. (6), becomes:

$$A = \frac{\lambda_{\text{AC}}}{[V_{\text{bag}} + V_{\text{lung}} + \lambda_{\text{AC}} \times V_{\text{tissue}}]}. \tag{8}$$

If we now take the logarithm of Eq. (7) and rearrange the result we get:

$$\dot{Q} = \left[\frac{V_{\text{bag}} + V_{\text{lung}} + \lambda_{\text{AC}} \times V_{\text{tissue}}}{\lambda_{\text{AC}}}\right] \times \left[\frac{\text{Log}_{(P_0)} - \text{Log}_{(P_1)}}{t_1}\right] \tag{9}$$

In Eq. (9) the term in the first set of brackets is known from Eq. (4). The term in the second set of brackets is a numerical estimate of the slope of the acetylene disappearance curve on a log scale. In Eq. (9) this is taken to be the slope between two points, namely, time zero and any subsequent chosen time t_1. If the volumes are in litres and t_1 is in minutes, $\dot{Q}$ will be in litres per minute.

Assumptions in the Rebreathing Measurements of Tissue Volume and Cardiac Output

Assumptions associated with the use of helium for the rebreathing measurement of lung volume are well known since this is a common laboratory method. In particular, areas of the lung that are very poorly ventilated or unventilated will not be reached by helium, and therefore to the extent that there is any gas volume in such regions, this will be excluded from the number obtained. It is assumed that the gas analyser is linear for helium, and that there are no significant leaks by which helium can escape the bag-lung rebreathing system.

For the estimation of tissue volume and blood flow, additional assumptions to those just listed are required. As mentioned earlier, assuming a value for the tissue: gas partition coefficient of acetylene (or other tracer gas used) is a potential source of error, due both to differences between tissue and blood solubilities in any one case, and to the natural variation of partition coefficients between and within species. It is evident from Eq. (9) that the simple inverse relationship between blood: gas partition coefficient of acetylene and the derived estimate of blood flow leads to a relative error in derived blood flow that will equal the relative error in partition coefficient. In other words, a 20% error in partition coefficient will produce a 20% error in the calculated value of pulmonary blood flow. It is important to complete the rebreathing prior to significant recirculation, since the entire formulation (Eqs. (6)–(9)) is based upon a simple one-compartment lung taking up acetylene without recirculation occurring. Fortunately, recirculation can often be recognized as departure from linearity on the semilogarithmic plot of acetylene disappearance as in Fig. 1. Just as for helium, to the extent that acetylene does not reach poorly ventilated or unventilated areas, the blood flow associated with those areas will not be visualized by the technique, and consequently the value obtained from Eq. (9) will underestimate the real pulmonary blood flow. It is also assumed for acetylene that there is complete diffusion equilibration of the gas between alveolar gas and end-capillary blood. This is certainly a very reasonable assumption under normal, and even pathological, conditions.

In addition to the need to satisfy these assumptions, there are significant experimental pitfalls with the rebreathing method that lead to substantial potential for experimental error in the derived results. This can be seen particularly for the measurement of pulmonary tissue volume by examining Eq. (5). In that equation, the subtraction of 1 from the ratio of initial to equilibrated gas tensions increases the amount of error in the estimate of tissue volume, particularly when that gas tension ratio is reasonably close to unity. In a similar vein, the fact that Eq. (5) represents the difference of two fairly large terms increases the relative error. As a numerical example, suppose that the bag volume is 3 litres, the lung volume is 3 litres, λ_{AC} is 1.0, P_{bag} is 100 units and $P\text{equil}_{AC}$ is 45 units. Substitution of these numbers into Eq. (5) will yield an estimated tissue volume of 667 ml. If now the value $P\text{equil}_{AC}$ of 45 were to be replaced by a value of 46, all other variables unchanged, it can be verified from Eq. (5) that this would reduce the estimated tissue volume from 667 to 520 ml. Thus, a 2% error in the estimated value of $P\text{equil}_{AC}$ produces a 22% error in the derived value of tissue volume. This example examines the effect of a very small error in just one variable in Eq. (5), and when multiple errors occur randomly it is evident that the variability of the measurement of tissue volume by this approach is great, even under the best circumstances.

Perhaps the major limiting factor in the measurement of tissue volume is non-uniformity of function within the lung itself [8]. In the most careful hands, the technique appears to provide useful results in normal subjects and animals [7, 8]. However, the presence of ventilation-blood flow heterogeneity violates the assumptions of the mass balance equations which were derived for a homogeneous lung. As a result, the acetylene disappearance curve will be multiexponential and it will be difficult, if not impossible, correctly to estimate tissue volume. In any event, it would require a quantitative knowledge of the way in which ventilation and blood flow were distributed in relation to lung volume even to attempt a correction for such non-uniformity. This is all the more frustrating when one realizes that the very areas of the lung that one would like to include in the tissue volume measurement are those with the most extravascular lung water and, in turn, it is just these areas that are likely to be most poorly ventilated and thus least accessible to the technique.

It is worth pointing out that a specific problem is the determination of zero time, which is seen to be critical to the measurement of the extrapolated acetylene value to be used in Eq. (5). Various approaches have been proposed [5, 6], but the important point to remember is that small errors in estimating this value produce large errors in tissue volume, and so extreme care must be used when dealing with this particular issue.

As is evident from Eq. (9), errors in the estimation of pulmonary blood flow are potentially less. No extrapolation procedure is needed beyond that of estimating tissue volume which appears in the numerator of Eq. (9), but as can be seen from Eq. (9), this is only one portion of the numerator of that equation, and so errors in tissue volume will not have as great an effect as otherwise. The slope of the disappearance curve, as long as it is monoexponential, can be estimated with considerable accuracy from direct recordings, and so the main sources of error for the determination of pulmonary blood flow reside in the assumption of the blood: gas partition coefficient for acetylene appearing in the denominator of Eq. (9), and the problems mentioned above with respect to violations of the assumptions of functional homogeneity within the lung.

Summary

Closed-circuit (rebreathing) systems such as those used in closed-circuit anaesthesia are well suited to physiological measurements of pulmonary gas volume, pulmonary tissue volume and pulmonary blood flow, all by the use of insoluble and soluble inert gases. The techniques are well established and have been in use for some 25 years. The measurements are entirely non-invasive and are relatively straightforward in terms of data acquisition. The theory behind the techniques is well established,but depends critically upon functional homogeneity. This problem, together with the intrinsic susceptibility to experimental error which can be understood by examining the basic equations presented in this review, leads to the need for extreme caution when making such measurements and using them as part of clinical decision-making processes.

References

1. Cander L, Forster RE (1959) Determination of pulmonary parenchymal tissue volume and pulmonary capillary blood flow in man. J Appl Physiol 14:541–551
2. Burma GM, Saidel GM (1983) Pulmonary blood flow and tissue volume: model analysis of rebreathing estimation method. J Appl Physiol 55:205–211
3. Hook C, Meyer M (1982) Pulmonary blood flow, diffusing capacity and tissue volume by rebreathing: theory. Respir Physiol 48:255–279
4. Petrini MR, Peterson BT, Hyde RW (1978) Lung tissue volume and blood flow by rebreathing: theory. J Appl Physiol 44:495–802
5. Sackner MA, Markwell G, Atkins N, Birch SJ, Fernandez RJ (1980) Rebreathing techniques for pulmonary capillary blood flow and tissue volume. J Appl Physiol 49:910–915
6. Young IH, Wagner PD (1979) Solubility of inert gases in homogenates of canine lung tissue. J Appl Physiol 46(6):1207–1210
7. Overland ES, Gupta RN, Huchon GJ, Murray JR (1981) Measurement of pulmonary tissue volume and blood flow in person with normal and edematous lungs. J Appl Physiol 51:1375–1383
8. Peterson BT, Petrini MF, Hyde RW, Schreiner BF (1978) Pulmonary tissue volume in dogs during pulmonary edema. J Appl Physiol 44:782–795

Controlled Respiration with He-O_2 Mixtures Using a Semi-open and a Closed System

K.-W. Fritz, K. Lundin, K. Zettergren, M. Tabbert, J. Mottner, and D. Patschke

Introduction

It has been demonstrated in animal experiments that rising inspiration pressure during artificial ventilation can cause a pulmonary barotrauma [4]. These results show the need for methods to be developed which may positively influence this parameter [4, 5]. High-frequency positive-pressure jet ventilation (HFPPV) is one possibility [5]. With this method humidification and elimination of CO_2 is the main problem and one which still has not been solved.

In our investigations we used He-O_2 and N_2-O_2 mixtures (F_iO_2 = 0.3 in both cases) for controlled respiration of polytraumatic patients, all suffering from an injury of the lung or the chest (e.g. rib fractures, aspiration, contusion, haemato- or pneumothorax). In 1936 Barach used He-O_2 mixtures (F_iO_2=0.2) in the treatment of patients suffering from severe asthma [2]. Some years later Segal reported the survival of four asthma patients, who were treated as an *ultima ratio* with the help of He-O_2 mixtures [29]. The main difference between using He-O_2 mixtures and N_2-O_2 mixtures for controlled respiration is the laminar flow pattern in the upper airways [2, 3, 10, 12, 14, 22, 23]. It is dependent on the low density of this inert gas [22, 23, 32]. It can also be demonstrated by the Reynold (Re) number and other physical laws [9, 12, 22]. As haemodynamics and respiration are also connected we also recorded cardiac and circulation parameters [30]. We wanted to demonstrate in this investigation with the use of similar mixtures of He-O_2 and N_2-O_2 (F_iO_2 = 0.3) that it is possible to influence ventilatory mechanics positively by using an inert gas (He). It was also important to have no negative side effects in haemodynamics or in pulmonary gas exchange.

Methods

Investigations were performed in 19 patients with multiple injuries (♂ = 16, ♀ = 3; average age, 29.6 years) requiring ventilatory support. All the patients were suffering from a trauma of the chest or the lung which caused reduced ventilatory mechanics and troubled pulmonary gas exchange. Gas checks before controlled respiration could not be demonstrated because a tube was applied immediately after the accident in the ambulance. After collecting the patients in the ICU, a Swan-Ganz catheter (Edwards) was applied via the jugular vein with the help of pressure monitoring (transducer, Bentley; pressure monitor, Hellige Servomed).

We recorded the cardiac output directly (*CO*; litres/min) (Fischer computer), central vein pressure (*CVP;* mm Hg), mean pressure in the pulmonary artery ($\bar{p}_{AP}$; mm Hg) and pulmonary capillary pressure (p_{CP}; mm Hg; "wedge pressure"). Mixed venous blood was taken from the pulmonary artery for calculating the oxygen consumption (O_2; ml/min) and the intrapulmonary right-left shunt (*Qs*/*Qt*; %). With the help of the directly registered parameters we were able to calculate: total systemic resistance (*TSR; PVR;* dyn · s · cm^{-5}) and the stroke volume (*SV;* ml). Blood pressure was measured in a radial artery (*MAP* = mean arterial pressure; mm Hg). Blood from this vessel was also used for blood gas analysis (Corning-Analyzer).

All the patients were respirated with a Servo-Ventilator 900 B (SV 900B; Siemens-Elema), which was calibrated for both gases. In addition to this ventilator a calculation unit (compliance-resistance Calculator; CO_2 analyzer, Siemens-Elema) was used for the minute volume (*MV;* litres/min), inspiration pressure (p_{max}; cm H_2O), pressure during inflation hold (p_{plat}; cm H_2O), inspiratory resistance (R_{insp}; cm H_2O/litre per second), expiratory resistance (R_{exsp}; cm H_2O/litre per second) and the compliance of the total ventilatory system (*Compl;* ml/cm H_2O) [21, 26, 28].

We began our investigations in positive end expiratory pressure (*PEEP*) O using a minute volume which demonstrated an alveolar normoventilation ($pCO_2 \sim$ 40 mm Hg; end-expiratory $CO_2 \sim$ 4.2–4.6 vol.%) [8]. For all the other PEEP manoeuvres (5, 10, 15 cm H_2O) the minute volume was not corrected. There was an interval between the different PEEP conditions in order to achieve a "steady state". A similar interval was maintained when we changed the gases. We used a constant flow continuously. From all the results mean values $\bar{x}$ and the mean error ($s_{\bar{x}}$) of the standard deviation were calculated and demonstrated graphically. Statistics were drawn up using Student's *t*-test for paired values. Results were significant at $P<0.05$. Circulation parameters are demonstrated.

Results

Minute Volume (*MV*; litres/min)

The initial value of the *mv* (*PEEP* O) using N_2-O_2 was 10.25 litres/min compared with 8.5 litres/min with He-O_2. The difference is about 1.75 ≙ 17.5%. When the *PEEP* increases the *mv* reduces by the same extent in both gases (Fig. 1).

Inspiration Pressure (p_{max}; cm H_2O)

At the beginning a difference in p_{max} was observed in favour of He-O_2 of about 20.1% ($p<0.0005$). In *PEEP* 10 and 15 cm H_2O this value reduces (13.6% and 16.6%) (Fig. 2).

Inflation Hold Pressure (p_{plat}; cm H_2O)

As expected less difference was observed in p_{plat}, especially in *PEEP* O, in favour of He-O_2 (N_2-O_2, 15.3 cm H_2O; He-O_2, 13.7 cm H_2O). When the *PEEP* increases the difference becomes greater (Fig. 3).

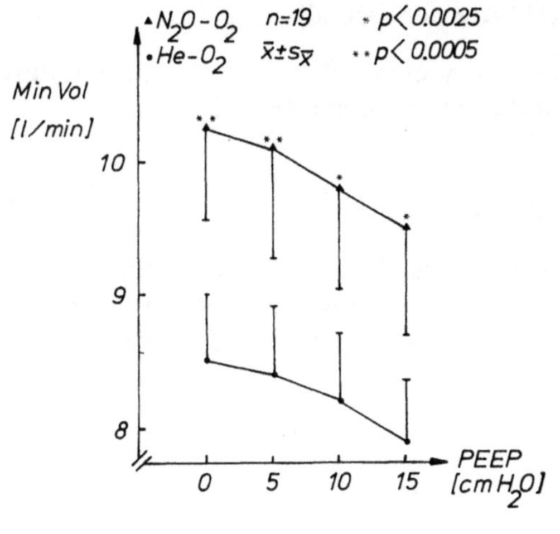

Fig. 1. Minute volume (*Min Vol*) (litres/min)

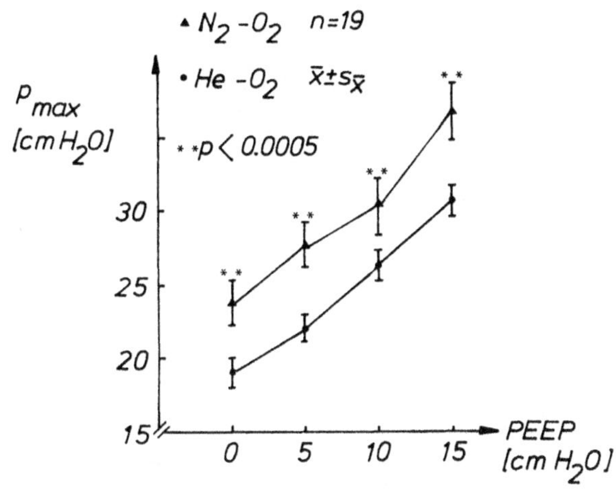

Fig. 2. Inspiration pressure (p_{max}) (cm H_2O)

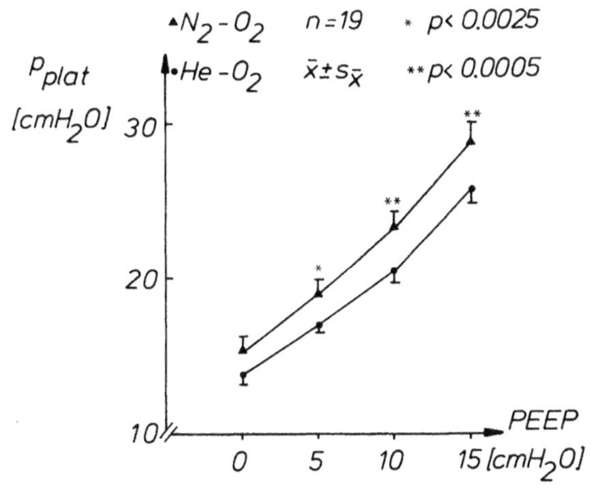

Fig. 3. Inflation hold-pressure (p_{plat}) (cm H_2O)

Inspiratory Resistance (R_{insp}; cm H_2O/litre per second)

The results range with N_2-O_2 in all PEEP manoeuvres from 13 to 15 cm H_2O/litre per second (He-O_2, 10.4–10.89 cm H_2O/litre per second) (Fig. 4).

Expiratory Resistance (R_{exsp}; cm H_2/litre per second)

The initial value when ventilating with He-O_2 is about 6.2 cm H_2O/litre per second and reduces to *PEEP* 15 cm H_2O (5.56 cm H_2O/litre per second). With N_2-O_2 a range of between 6.85 and 7.0 cm H_2O/litre per second is continuously observed (Fig. 5).

Compliance (*Compl*; ml/cm H_2O)

As expected all the results are similar in both gases (Fig. 6).

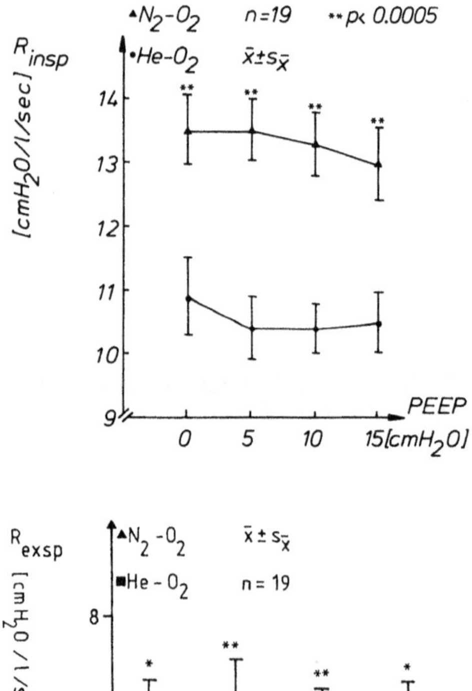

Fig. 4. Inspiratory resistance (R_{insp}) (cm H_2O/litre/s)

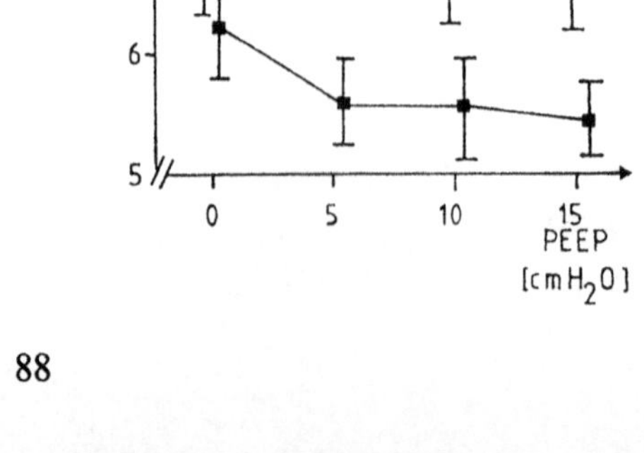

Fig. 5. Expiratory resistance (R_{exsp}) (cm H_2O/litre/s);*$P<0.05$;**$P<0.01$

Blood-Gas Analysis

The arterial gas check continuously demonstrates an alveolar normoventilation (pCO_2 ~ 40 mm Hg), which is accompanied by normoxia (Fig. 7).

Haemodynamics

All the parameters demonstrate similar results except for cardiac output and stroke volume (Table 1). Therefore only these differences are explained in detail.

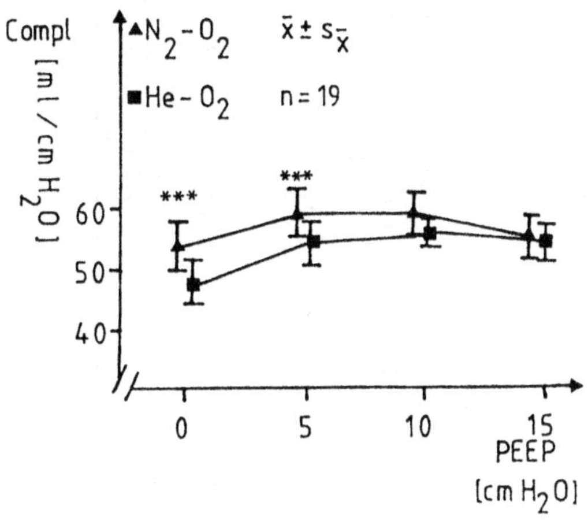

Fig. 6. Compliance (*Compl*) (ml/cm H_2O)***$P<0.005$

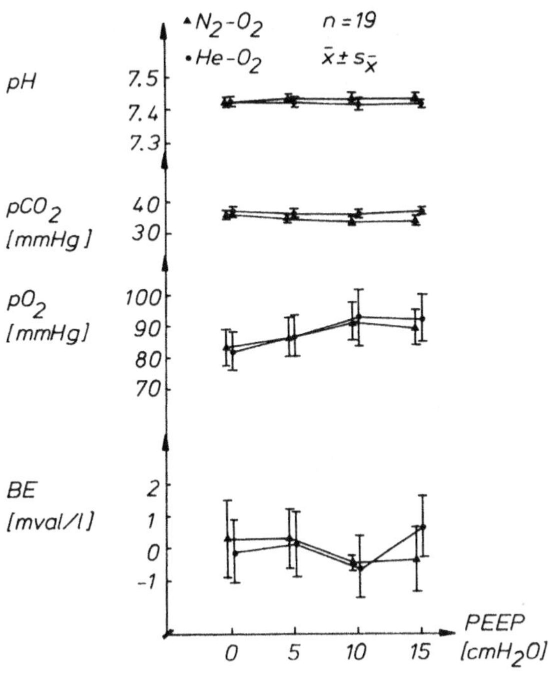

Fig. 7. Gas check

Table 1. Haemodynamics in controlled respiration with $He\text{-}O_2$ and $N_2\text{-}O_2$ mixtures ($n=18$)

PEEP (cm H_2O)	0		5		10		15	
Gas mixtures	$N_2\text{-}O_2$	$He\text{-}O_2$	$N_2\text{-}O_2$	$He\text{-}O_2$	$N_2\text{-}O_2$	$He\text{-}O_2$	$N_2\text{-}O_2$	$He\text{-}O_2$
HR (min^{-1})	106 ± 4.74	108 ± 5.30	106 ± 4.90	109 ± 5.40	106 ± 5.04	109 ± 5.90	110 ± 5.61	112 ± 6.69
$MAP=\bar{p}_{art}$ (mmHg)	82.0 ± 3.02	78.0 ± 4.98[a]	82.8 ± 2.33	82.3 ± 2.60	81.0 ± 2.61	81.5 ± 2.81[a]	77.0 ± 3.01	81.3 ± 3.09
CO (litres/min)	8.47 ± 0.56	8.42 ± 0.55	7.71 ± 0.50	7.85 ± 0.54	6.72 ± 0.47	7.33 ± 0.51	6.09 ± 0.43	6.61 ± 0.43[a]
CVP (mmHg)	6.40 ± 0.93	6.47 ± 1.07	8.20 ± 0.90	7.45 ± 0.98	10.10 ± 0.97	9.62 ± 0.91	11.80 ± 0.95	12.30 ± 0.89
$\bar{p}_{ap}$ (mmHg)	19.3 ± 1.56	19.4 ± 1.61	20.2 ± 1.36	21.0 ± 1.50	21.6 ± 1.29	21.8 ± 1.31[a]	23.5 ± 1.21	23.9 ± 1.20
p_{CP} (mmHg)	9.10 ± 0.95	8.86 ± 0.86	10.30 ± 0.79	10.30 ± 0.68	11.50 ± 0.75	10.80 ± 0.63[a]	13.10 ± 0.76	12.00 ± 0.76[a]
TPR (dyn · s · cm^{-5})	769 ± 58.3	775 ± 63.2	831 ± 55.0	822 ± 60.0	916 ± 63.9	852 ± 64.0	901 ± 56.7	895 ± 61.5
PVR (dyn · s · cm^{-5})	99.37 ± 8.61	101.80 ± 9.87	106.00 ± 9.62	99.40 ± 8.60	130.00 ± 12.80	125.20 ± 12.30	153.00 ± 16.40	153.40 ± 12.30
SV (ml)	82.7 ± 6.43	81.6 ± 6.70	76.0 ± 6.24	75.7 ± 6.32	66.7 ± 6.30	70.2 ± 6.60	59.1 ± 6.03	64.8 ± 6.72
O_2 consumption (ml/min)	343 ± 23.0	326 ± 25.4	331 ± 23.1	321 ± 22.8	315 ± 22.6	329 ± 25.3	318 ± 22.2	323 ± 20.1
Q_s/Q_t (%)	16.3 ± 3.00	20.3 ± 4.36[a]	14.7 ± 2.37	17.1 ± 3.09	11.8 ± 1.92	14.0 ± 2.47	10.6 ± 1.49	11.5 ± 1.62

[a] $p<0.05$

The initial value of CO ($PEEP$ O cm H_2O) was similar in both gases (8.5 litres/min). When the $PEEP$ increases a reduction was observed in both cases. The drop was significantly lower in He-O_2 than in N_2-O_2. The same tendency was seen with stroke volume.

Discussion

Results of animal experiments on spontaneous respiration using He-O_2 mixtures (80%–20%) were published in 1936 by Barach [2]. He demonstrated that respiratory work and peak expiratory flow are significantly improved by He-O_2 mixtures compared with N_2-O_2 [2]. These differences in favour of He-O_2 increased when a stenosis was fixed in the trachea of the dogs via a tracheostomia [2].

Similar effects were recorded in patients suffering from an obstructive disease of the upper airways [2]. For therapy the mixture was used as suggested by Segal [31]. He reported four cases of patients suffering from severe asthma. The reason for survival was the application of He-O_2 mixtures. Similar results were demonstrated by Ishikawa [19]. Harder used He-O_2 mixtures for bronchoscopy especially when he performed a bronchial lavage in patients receiving long-term artificial respiration who were also suffering from narrow airways caused by viscid mucus [17]. Grimrath and Smidt noticed improved pulmonary diffusion of N_2-O_2 (80%–20%) compared with He-O_2 (80%–20%) mixtures [16]. The differences demonstrated are minimal. In other comparative investigations the contrary is reported [18]. Better distribution of He-O_2 in particular is observed [18]. "He" became very important during the "sea-lab" programme of the American Navy. Only by using He-O_2 mixtures is it possible to dive into the deep sea [3, 24, 27, 29]. Initial animal experiments in controlled respiration with He-O_2 mixtures were performed in 1978 by Ehehalt et al. [10] using anesthetized dogs, lying in a glass box which was used as a body plethysmograph. The main problem in these experiments was to seal the glass box. Therefore the results were not as favourable as demonstrated in physical calculations. Investigations by our group began in 1979 using the SV 900B and the calculation unit. The ventilator was checked for use of both gases. It was demonstrated that there was no difference in the range we needed [14].

Minute volume in the SV 900B is measured with a modified pneumotachograph. He-O_2 and N_2-O_2 mixtures as used in our experiments have a different density [32]. Therefore calibration must be performed [32].

Our investigations must be performed in patients with multiple injuries although it is well known that asthma patients are more suitable. These patients were treated in another ICU. Although we used the same flow in both mixtures ($F_iO_2 = 0.3$), we demonstrated better results for He-O_2 of about 15%–20% in the parameters minute volume (MV), inspiration pressure (p_{max}) and inspiratory and expiratory resistance (R_{insp}, R_{exsp}) in all $PEEP$ manoeuvres. A lower difference was seen during inflation hold (p_{plat}) ($\sim$10%).

These favourable results are caused by the laminar flow pattern of the He-O_2. It guarantees reduced resistance in the upper airways. No differences were seen in the compliance ($Compl$) and the gas check. These results were similar in both mixtures.

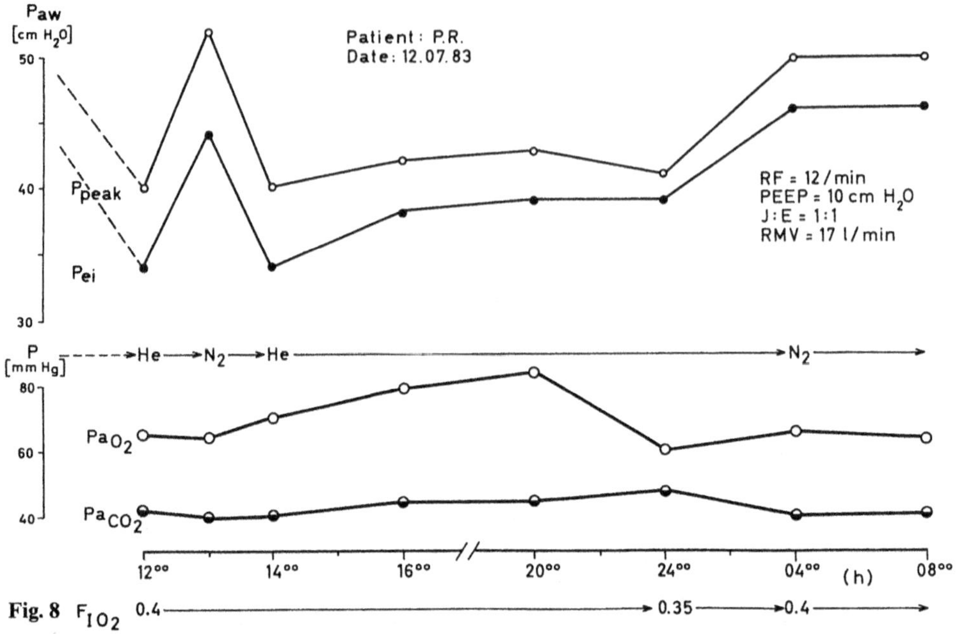

Fig. 8

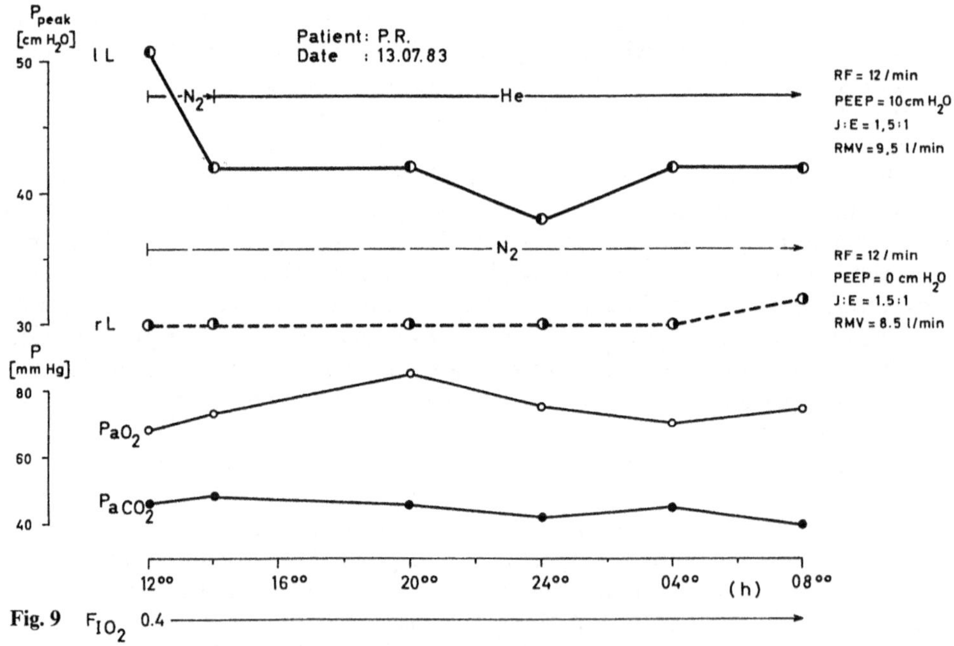

Fig. 9

Figs. 8, 9, 10. Results of controlled respiration with He-O_2 mixtures using a closed system

Another problem in controlled respiration is the side effect in haemodynamics especially when using high *PEEP*. In this case cardiac output drops because increasing intrathoracic pressure reduces the venous flow back to the heart. In addition pulmonary vascular resistance rises [1, 7, 25]. In some cases of adult respiratory distress syndrome a respiration method is required which is called "in-

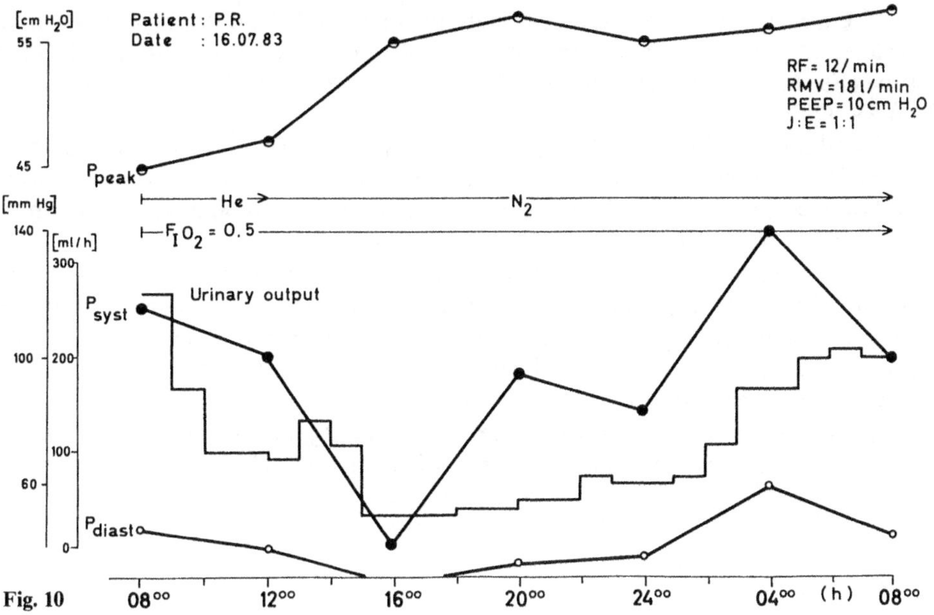

Fig. 10

versed ratio ventilation" (IRV) [6, 13]. Gaseous exchange is favoured in such a manoeuvre, but cardiac output and blood pressure drop. In some cases catecholamines must be applied (e.g. dopamine or dobutamine for maintaining sufficient diuresis) [6, 7].

In our investigations we demonstrated that cardiac output was better with He-O_2 mixtures especially with increasing *PEEP* manoeuvres. He-O_2 mixtures are more dependent on lower intrathoracic pressure than N_2-O_2 mixtures. All the other haemodynamic parameters behave similarly in both gases as demonstrated in Table 1.

Finally the results of these investigations can be explained as follows:

1. Compared with N_2-O_2 mixtures, He-O_2 mixtures ($F_i\,O_2 = 0.3$) guarantee a laminar flow pattern is produced in the bronchial system [9, 12, 22, 23].
2. The distribution of the inert gas in the alveolar space may be much improved, as demonstrated by other authors; airway-closed areas may be ventilated again [18].
3. The diffusion of CO_2 in an He atmosphere is six times better than in an N_2 atmosphere [22].
4. In the lower part of the bronchial system there is gas flow; cardiac action alone is not responsible for the gaseous exchange in the pre-alveolar space ("cardiogenic mixing") [11, 22, 23, 33].

Helium is very expensive. Therefore a closed system was constructed which can be connected to the SV 900B for recycling He. In one case of differential-lung ventilation (DLV) this new system was used (Patschke D., personal communication). A female, suffering from acute respiratory distress syndrome (ARDS), was initially ventilated by use of an SV 900C.

The end-expiratory pressure was about 15 cm H_2O; the minute volume was in a range between 15 and 20 litres/min. Subsequently a peak inspiration pressure of 50 cm H_2O was seen. Blood pressure dropped and the diuresis stopped completely. We changed the normal tube and ventilated the patient via a Rob-Shaw tube (Fa. Mallinckrodt). The sick lung was respirated by He-O_2 mixtures using an SV 900B.

Ventilation of the normal lung was performed conventionally by N_2-O_2 mixtures. Peak pressure and minute volume were reduced. The blood pressure arose and diuresis began again. This manoeuvre was used for some days. The main results are shown in Figs. 8–10.

We were able to demonstrate that it was possible to recycle helium into the respirator. The most important problem when using this closed system is humidification. The expiratory volume is recycled and the inspiration gas becomes saturated. The result is that there is always a lot of water on the inspiration side. This problem must be solved in the near future.

Recommendations in the literature to use He-O_2 mixture in certain cases of lung disease are reason to perform further investigations [34].

References

1. Ashbaugh DG, Petty TL, Bigelow DB, Harris TM (1979) Continuous positive pressure breathing (CPPB) in adult respiratory distress syndrome. J Thorac Cardiovasc Surg 57:31
2. Barach AL (1936) The effect of inhalation of helium-mixtures with oxygen on the mechanics of respiration. J Clin Invest 15:47
3. Bartels H (1975) Gaswechsel (Atmung). In: Keidel WD (ed) Kurzgefaßtes Lehrbuch der Physiologie, 4th edn. Thieme, Stuttgart
4. Benzer H (1969) Respiratorbeatmung und Oberflächenspannung. In: Bergmann H et al. (Hrsg) Anaesthesiologie und Wiederbelebung, vol 38. Springer, Berlin Heidelberg New York
5. Baum M, Benzer H, Geyer A, Haider W, Mutz N (1980) Forcierte Diffusionsventilation (FDV). Grundlagen und Anwendung. Anaesthesist 29:586
6. Baum M, Benzer H, Mutz N, Pauser G, Tonczar L (1980) Inversed ratio ventilation (IRV). Die Rolle des Atem-Zeit-Verhältnisses in der Beatmung beim ARDS. Anaesthesist 29:592
7. Benzer H, Haider W, Pauser G (1976) Zur Technik der Respiratorbeatmung. Intensivbehandlung 4:157
8. Breuching E, Altemeyer KH, Dietz W (1981) Droperidol-Ketamin Untersuchungen zur intravenösen Narkose für periphere Eingriffe im Kindesalter. Anaesthesist 30:107
9. D'Ans J, Lax A (1949) Taschenbuch für Physik und Chemie. Springer, Berlin
10. Ehehalt V, Tabbert M, Mottner J (1980) Die Verminderung von Strömungswiderständen bei Beatmung mit He-O_2-Gemischen. Vortrag anläßlich der Jahrestagung des DGAI 1978 in Würzburg. In: Weis KH, Cunitz G (eds) 25 Jahre DGAI. Springer, Berlin Heidelberg New York (Anaesthesiology and intensive care medicine, vol 130)
11. Engel LA, Wood LDH, Utz G, Macklem PT (1973) Gas mixing during inspiration. J Appl Physiol 35:18
12. Fritz KW, Kramer K, Tabbert M, Mottner J (1982) Ehehalt V, Hendrickx HH, Patschke D (1982) Physikalische und experimentelle Grundlagen einer He-O_2-Beatmung. MTA-Praxis 28:305
13. Fritz KW, Zinck B, Lüllwitz E (1981) Die Behandlung des adult respiratory distress syndrom (ARDS) bei der akuten nekrotischen Pankreatitis. Intensivmed Prax 4:23–26
14. Fritz KW, Tabbert M, Mottner J, Patschke D (1982) Die Beatmung polytraumatisierter Patienten mit He-O_2 und N_2-O_2-Gemischen. I. Atemmechanik und pulmonaler Gasaustausch. Anaesthesist 31:323–329

15. Giordano J, Harden A (1975) Effect of continuous positive pressure ventilation on cardiac output. Am Surg 41:221
16. Grimrath V, Smidt U, von Nieding G, Krekeler H (1978) Respiratorischer Gasaustausch bei Atmung von 20,9% Sauerstoff in verschiedenen Inertgasen. Respiration 35:15
17. Harder HJ (1972) Tracheo-bronchiale Lavage. Anaesthesist 21:413
18. Herzog P, Norlander OP (1968) Distribution of alveolar volumes with different types of positive pressure gas-flow patterns. Opusc Med 13:37
19. Ishikawa S, Segal M (1974) Re-appraisal of helium-oxygen therapy on patients with chronic lung disease. Ann Allergy 31:536
20. Ito A (1975) Simulated multiday underwater habitation in hyperbaric helium-oxygen environment. Bull Tokyo Med Dent Univ 21:281
21. Jonson B, Nordström L, Olsson SG, Akerback D (1971) Monitoring of ventilation and lung mechanics during automatic ventilation. A new device. Bull Eur Physiopathol Respir 11:729
22. Kalide W (1980) Einführung in die technische Strömungslehre. Hanser, München
23. Kramer K, Ehehalt V, Tabbert M, Mottner J, Fritz KW (1979) Die Herabsetzung von Strömungswiderständen bei der künstlichen Beatmung mit He-O_2-Gemischen. Biotechn Umsch 3:366
24. Linaweaver PG (1969) Saturation diving. J Occup Med 11:223
25. Morgan BC, Crawford EW, Gutheroth WG (1969) The hemodynamic effects of changes in blood volume during IPPV. Anesthesiology 30:297
26. Osswald RM, Hartung HJ, Klose R, Spier R (1981) Die Wirkung von verlängerter Inspirationszeit und PEEP auf die Compliance und den Gasaustausch bei der mechanischen Ventilation. Anaesthesist 30:71
27. Overrath G, Matthys H, Bühlmann AA (1969/70) Saturation experiment at 31 ata in an oxygen-helium atmosphere. Helv Med Acta 35:180
28. Prakash O, Jonson B, Mey S, v.d. Vorden S, v.d. Kolk J, Hugenholtz PG, Bos E, Nauta J, Olsson SG (1977) Measurement of cardiopulmonary function during anaesthesia and intensive care. Curr Top Crit Care Med 3:60
29. Robertson WG (1967) Study of man during a 56-day exposure to an oxygen-helium atmosphere at 258 mm Hg total pressure: VII. Respiratory function. Aerospace Med 37:578
30. Schorer R (1965) Auswirkungen der Atmung auf den Kreislauf. In: Bergmann H (ed) Anaesthesiologie und Wiederbelebung, vol 10. Springer, Berlin Heidelberg New York
31. Segal MS (1943) Inhalational therapy in the treatment of serious respiratory disease. N Engl J Med 278:1355
32. Ulmer WT, Reichel G, Nolte D (1976) Die Lungenfunktion. Thieme, Stuttgart
33. Worth H, Takahashi H, Willmer H, Püper J (1976) Pulmonary gas exchange in dogs ventilated with mixtures of oxygen with various inert gases. Respir Physiol 28:1
34. Mathewson HS (1982) Helium – Who needs it? Resp Care 11:1400

Technical Conception of an Anaesthesia System with Measurement and Semiautomated Dosage of Gases and Vapours

C. F. Wallroth

Introduction

The inhalational anaesthesia machines in today's hospitals are with few exceptions used with a semiclosed or semi-open breathing system. The delivery of respiratory gas and anaesthetic vapours exceeds the amount consumed by the patient. The consumption could be estimated by exact measurement of the concentration differences between inspiratory and expiratory gases and vapours. However, this would be difficult to measure.

When using a closed-circuit anaesthesia machine the breathing system with complete CO_2 absorption receives only as much oxygen, anaesthetic gas and anaesthetic vapour as the patient is supposed to consume or to absorb.

The closed-circuit anaesthesia systems in use today are based on components which are also used in semiclosed systems. They can be complemented by monitoring devices, e.g. for oxygen. The simplest type of a closed system is described by Droh [1] and consists of the following components which have to be monitored and controlled manually:

1. Precise delivery of oxygen by low-flow-metering tubes
2. Precise delivery of nitrous oxide by low-flow-metering tubes
3. Delivery of anaesthetics by calibrated precision vaporizers
4. Manual ventilation

Presently available flow metering devices are, e.g. based on needle valves and flowmeter tubes, which are optimized for semiclosed anaesthesia applications.

Today's precision vaporizers are only of limited use in closed circuits, e.g. the amount of the anaesthetic delivered can only be approximated from gas flow, concentration and time of application. The accuracy of the delivered concentration at low gas flows is also unsatisfactory.

There are systems described in the literature, e.g. by Spiess [2], which use anaesthetic ventilators where probable leakages will have to be compensated. Monitoring and manual readjustments are also necessary.

Lowe [3] developed a system with the liquid anaesthetic being added to the breathing system by an externally controllable syringe. This system differs from the two described above in that the anaesthetic is given in absolute quantity per unit, i.e. millilitres of anaesthetic, and not as a percentage of the volume.

The concentration indicates the instantaneous amount of anaesthetic being delivered, whereas the system of Lowe keeps track of the amount of anaesthetic delivered from the start of the anaesthesia.

Delivery of anaesthetic gas and anaesthetic vapours is subject to non-linear laws and thus does not remain constant with time, which in turn necessitates the systems to be monitored and controlled by the anaesthesiologist. In our opinion this special effort is one of the reasons why closed-circuit anaesthesia is being applied only by a small number of experts.

With today's technological capabilities the majority of the monitoring and controlling efforts can be automated. First steps in this direction have been taken by Westenskow [4, 5]. Necessary prerequisites are appropriate sensors, signal processing and controller elements.

Technical Conception

The ideas presented have been incorporated in the conception of an anaesthesia system for measurement and semiautomated dosage of anaesthetic gases. The operational modes for the proposed anaesthesia system are shown in Fig. 1. Via simple switchover, the operational mode of a semiclosed and a closed system can be chosen. For each mode spontaneous breathing, manual ventilation or automatic ventilation can be selected with a single breathing system suitable for adults as well as for children.

This system contains, besides others, the following functional components (Fig. 2):

1. Sensors
2. Anaesthetic gas supply
3. Anaesthetics supply
4. Respiratory gas reconditioning

The sensors can be divided into inspiratory and expiratory sensors (Fig. 3):

1. Inspiratory
   a) Anaesthetic concentration
   b) O_2 concentration
   c) Respiratory gas temperature

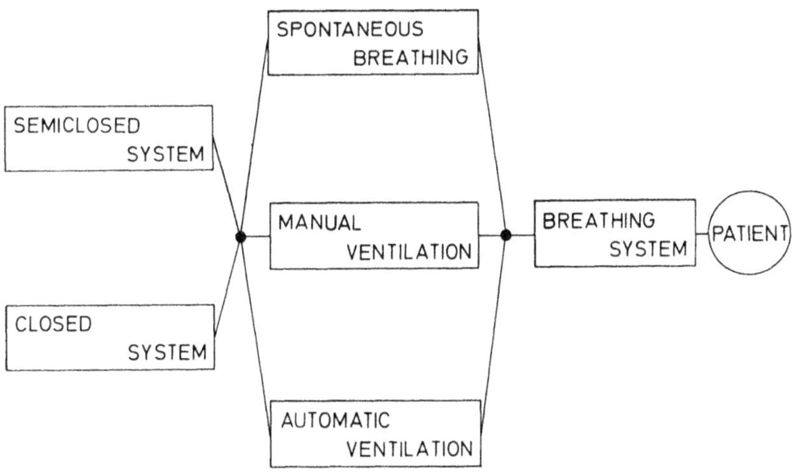

Fig. 1. Operational modes for a proposed anaesthesia system

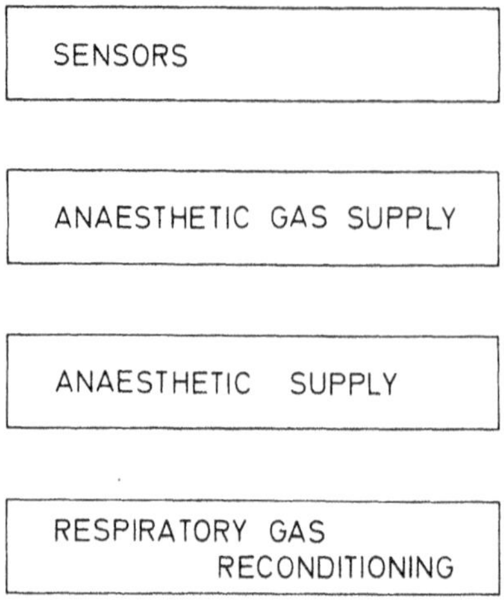

Fig. 2. Functional components for a proposed anaesthesia system

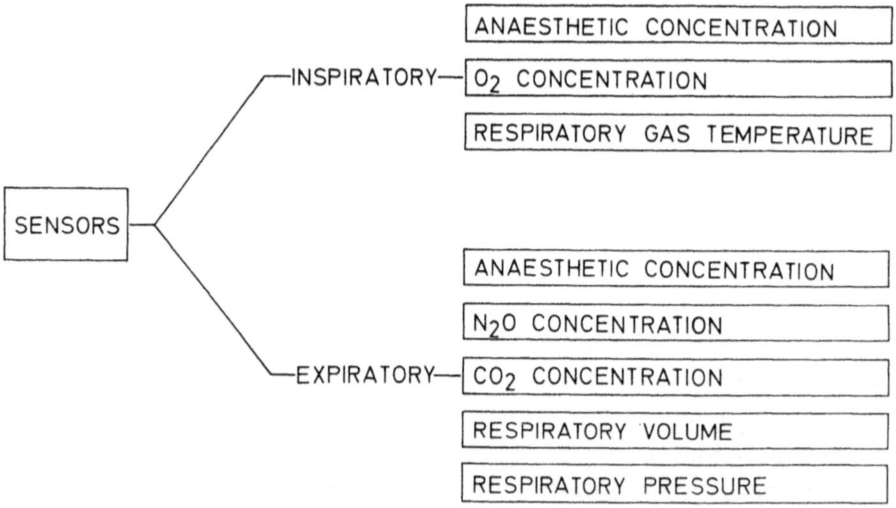

Fig. 3. Sensors in the proposed breathing system

2. Expiratory
   a) Anaesthetic concentration
   b) N_2O concentration
   c) CO_2 concentration
   d) Respiratory volume (tidal volume, minute volume)
   e) Respiratory pressure

The inspiratory concentration measurements are intended for monitoring the anaesthetic delivery and the inspiratory oxygen concentration; they thus represent in part a redundant safety aspect.

The expiratory concentration measurements are used to monitor or to control the anaesthetic gas and anaesthetics supply. Open loop control can be achieved either by a time law given by the user, e.g. a square root of time function, or by a user-selected step function. Closed-loop control can be directed, for instance, towards maintenance of a constant alveolaric concentration.

End-expiratory CO_2 measurements can be used for controlling respiration. The measurement of the tidal volume, e.g. at the ventilator bellows can be used for control of the gas delivery and for compensation of possible leakages. Temperature measurement and pressure and volume measurements in the breathing system are used for patient monitoring and protection.

The application range for the anaesthetic gas delivery has to cover gas flows of only few millilitres per minute up to about 10 litres/min. For the automatic control and regulation of the gas dosage system digitally controllable elements are required. A possible principle of the gas dosage system was reported by von dem Hagen [6], which is presented in Fig. 4.

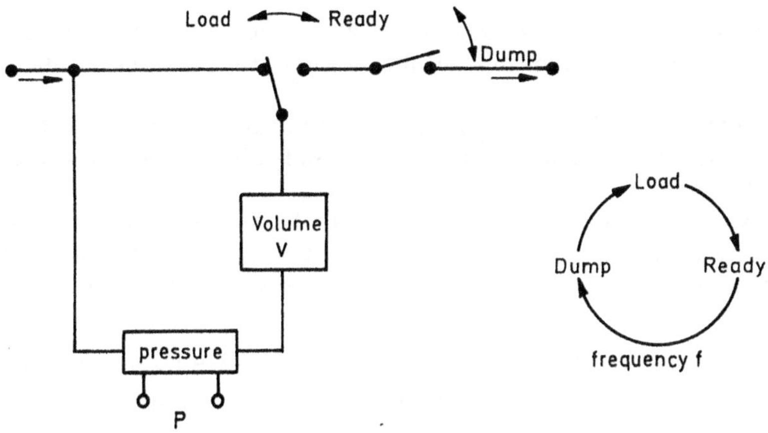

Fig. 4. Anaesthetic gas dosage scheme

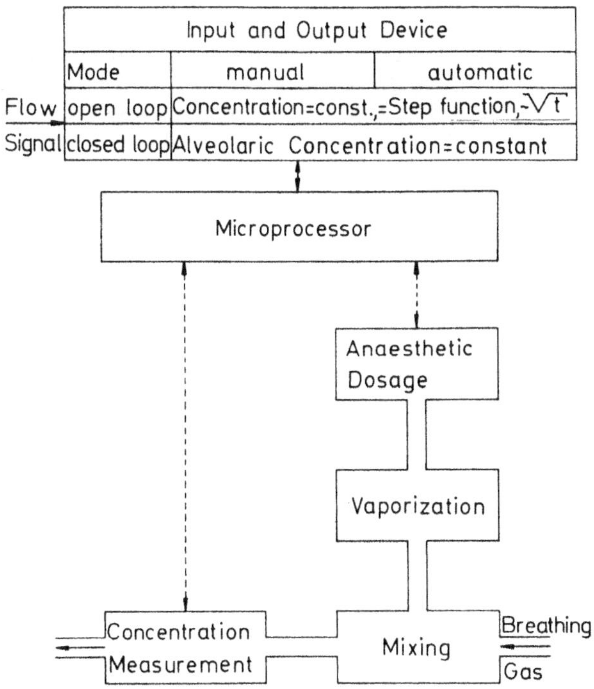

Fig. 5. Anaesthetics system scheme

For the delivery of the anaesthetics a digitally controllable system is required for minimal delivery of a few microlitres. The principle is shown in Fig. 5. The anaesthetic concentration can be measured with an infrared analyser, which was described earlier by Hattendorff [7].

For longer-lasting anaesthesias the breathing system can be flushed from possible metabolites, according to a suggestion of Lowe, by a short opening of the circuit. Alternatively, Ernst [8] suggests the use of a charcoal filter. By means of digital control elements the short flush can be done under computer control and the previous concentration can be reinstalled automatically.

Because of safety and technological considerations the system is designed for redundancy:

1. Redundancy in monitoring of the anaesthetic application by means of inspiratory and expiratory measurements and registration of the amount of anaesthetic injected
2. Redundancy in monitoring of the oxygen and nitrous oxide concentrations and metering by measurement of concentration and volume as well as optical control of the flow
3. Redundancy in patient monitoring by measuring the oxygen uptake from the amount of oxygen delivered, by CO_2 measurement, temperature measurement of the respiratory gas, measurement of pressure and volume in the breathing system

There are provisions manually to override the open or closed loop operations, e.g. the gas delivery can be done by conventional flow control valves.

Prototypes

The presented technical concept of a closed-circuit anaesthesia system is shown in Fig. 6, which is being implemented under the sponsorship of the Bundesministerium für Forschung und Technologie. The first step is the development of an

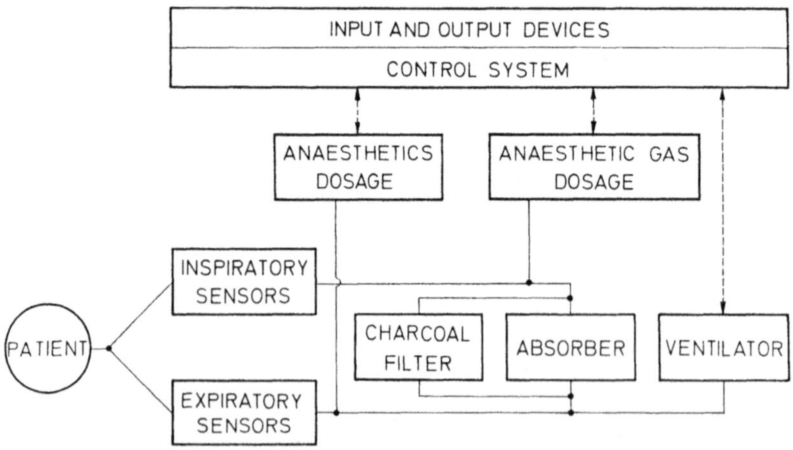

Fig. 6. Anaesthesia system scheme

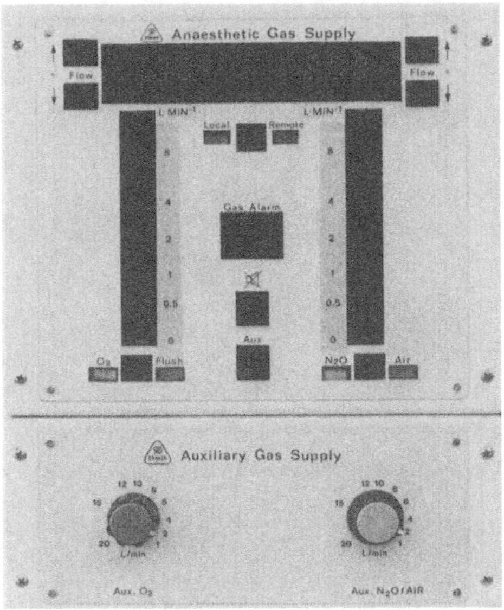

Fig. 7. Anaesthetic gas supply prototype

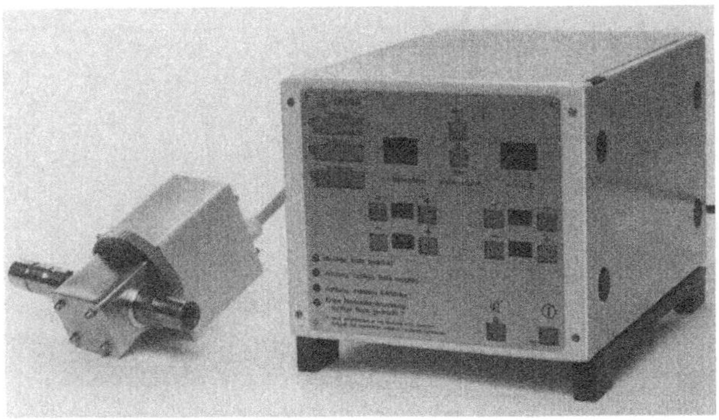

Fig. 8. Irina readout unit and sensor

automatic gas supply system. A prototype is presented in Fig. 7. The next step is the development of reliable sensors for anaesthetics (a prototype is shown in Fig. 8); innovative anaesthetic delivery systems (see Fig. 9) and respiratory systems will be necessary as well. However, before any of the different control mechanism can be implemented, they will have to be tested and confirmed or modified by clinical investigations.

All those components will have to be integrated into an ergonomical system simply to operate in order to elevate the acceptance of this technical conception in clinical use. A prototype is shown in Fig. 10.

The variable application range of the described system will enable the anaesthesiologist to approach closed-circuit anaesthesia stepwise and thus lead almost automatically to an introduction and further advancement of this form of anaesthesia.

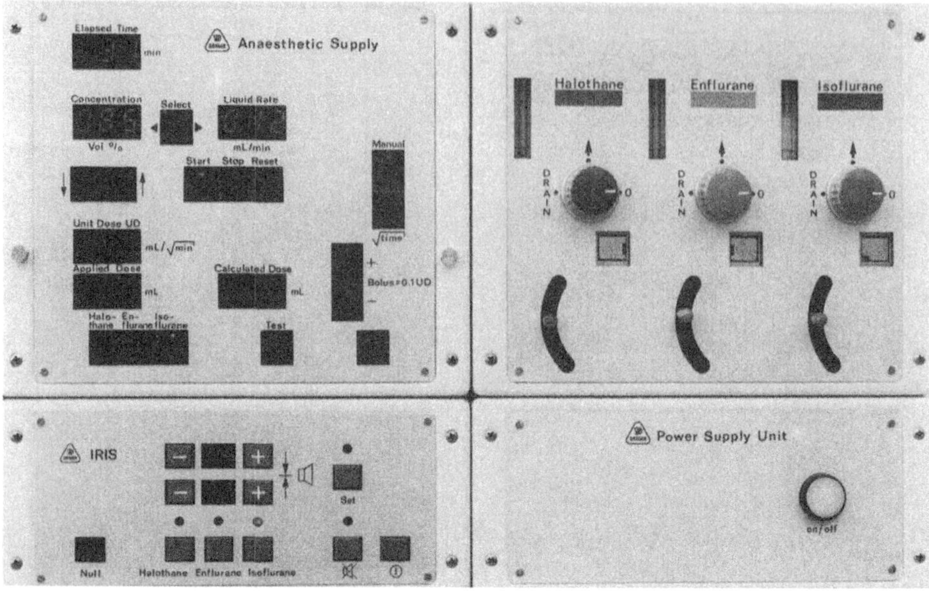

Fig. 9. Anaesthetic supply prototype

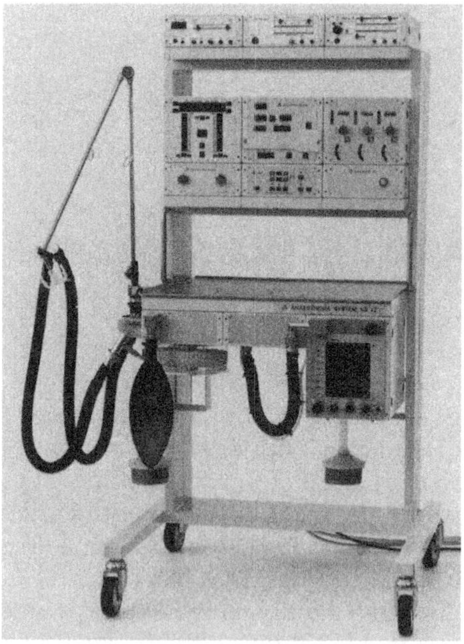

Fig. 10. Anaesthesia system AS 1.2 prototype

References

1. Droh R, Rothmann G (1977) Das geschlossene Kreissystem. Anaesthesist 26:461–466
2. Spiess W (1977) Narkose im geschlossenen System mit kontinuierlicher inspiratorischer Sauerstoff-Messung. Anaesthesist 26:503–513
3. Lowe HJ, Ernst EA (1981) The quantitative practice of anaesthesia. Williams and Wilkins, Baltimore
4. Westenskow DR, Jordan WS, Genulin DS (1979) Electronic feedback control and measurement of oxygen consumption during closed circuit anaesthesia. In: Aldrete JA, Lowe HJ, Virtue RW (eds) Low-flow and closed system anaesthesia. Grune and Straton, New York, pp 135–150
5. Westenskow DR, Jordan WS, Hayes JK, East TA (1983) Computer control of anaesthesia delivery. In: Prakash O, Meg SH, Patterson RW (eds) Computing in anaesthesia and intensive care. Martinus Nijhoff, pp 269–278
6. von dem Hagen T, Kleinschmidt L (1983) Principles of low flow measurements for closed circuit systems. Symposium: Innovations in management and technic and pharmacology. 13–15 May, Lüdenscheid, West Germany
7. Hattendorff HD, Wallroth CF (1983) Principles for measurement of anaesthetic concentrations in closed circuit systems. Symposium: Innovations in management and technic and pharmacology. 13–15 May, Lüdenscheid, West Germany
8. Ernst EA (1982) Use of charcoal to rapidly decrease depth of anaesthesia while maintaining a closed circuit. Anaesthesiology 57:343

Discussion I

J. W. R. McIntyre: This is just a question to Dr. Rolly. He adsorbs isoflurane or any other halogenated agent onto activated charcoal to get it out of the circuit. Have you had any experience of reintroducing it into the circuit from the charcoal?

R. Rolly: No. Maybe Dr. Schepp has more information on that point with reference to the Narcocon.

R. Schepp: We never have recovered the anaesthetic agent. The amount of charcoal we use is 100–200 ml in the absorber canister. It is many hours before you see any level of isoflurane coming out, and some 20 or 30 ml fluid of isoflurane would need to be added before any real backpressure could build up. It takes many hours of anaesthesia and many patients before you see any isoflurane coming from the charcoal.

J. R. W. McIntyre: I understand what you are saying.

We were interesting in this for military purposes about 15 years ago, when halothane was to be used within small tents and we wished to remove the halothane from the environmental atmosphere. So we used charcoal to remove it. We were interested to see whether or not we could regain the halothane for additional anaesthesia purposes. We found that using any kind of a simple pump we could revaporize halothane.

R. Schepp: But that is in an open system. And here you cannot get a higher partial pressure.

E. A. Ernst: To follow up with a question to Dr. Rolly. From your data I noted that when you turned on the charcoal filter your circuit concentration did not go to zero. This is what I remember. It was around 0.5% or 1%, and I do not know where you sample in and why the concentration did not fall to zero.

R. Schepp: These pictures were taken when I was Dr. Rolly's guest with my equipment for 2 or 3 weeks. I have since had more experience with the system. In fact, it was charcoal that had already been used several times, and in these circumstances you cannot go lower than 0.2%. If you want to go further you must flush your system. But without opening the system we could reduce it from 1% as far as 0.2% in a few breaths. If you use fresh charcoal then you can reduce the concentration to an almost undetectable level.

E. A. Ernst: A part of the answer to your question, Dr. McIntyre, is that charcoal has a temendous adsorption capacity. We put our charcoal on the inspiratory side so we can lower the concentration, as Dr. Rolly showed very nicely, or wake the patient up with a completely closed circuit. But there is no indicator in the Narcocon to show when you start desorbing and putting charcoal back into the line. We use a mass spectrometer as indicator on the inspiratory line after the charcoal and when we start seeing that break through then we know the time has come to change our charcoal.

R. Schepp: We use the Normac analyser and as soon as we cannot go back to our zero line we can very simply change the canister.

E. A. Ernst: Right.

R. Rolly: The initial clinical data you asked for: We wanted to lower it a little, so we just introduced the charcoal for one breath.

E. A. Ernst: If you have a really good valve and really good charcoal, then, with one or two breaths the inspiratory concentration would go to zero?

R. Rolly: Yes. Of course, that switch valve is very important.

E. A. Ernst: It is interesting we have all this discussion on charcoal when it was hardly mentioned in the lectures!

M. Paloheimo: Let me point out that the enormous capacity of this system to absorb the anaesthetic agent during a very short time depends on the blower, which flushes 120 l/min through the charcoal all the time. This is the secret of the large capacity.

R. Droh: Dr. Ernst, if we review all we said this morning, would you agree with me that measuring is better than estimating the halothane concentration and the CO_2 concentration? We ourselves measure as much as possible. We know that our equipment is not as fast as it should be. So for instance we lose about 18–20 s by measuring the oxygen concentration. But I still think it is much better to measure the oxygen, CO_2, N_2, etc. What do you think?

E. A. Ernst: More is always better. Of course we need better information faster, but we have to be practical. We must get accurate information quickly now. We need to know quantities; we need to measure whatever we can. If you use a closed circuit and you put N_2O into the circuit you absolutely have to measure the oxygen concentration. But on the other hand, many other people know that the priorities do not change so fast in anaesthesia. I think we will have to be able to demonstrate whether we need to go to all the expense entailed in reducing the time lag in measurement to a millisecond.

P. Wagner: I have a question to Dr. Schepp. According to some of the work that John West did some time ago in our laboratory, I was impressed by the effect of a leak on these equilibration curves; it strikes me that it would be pretty important to try to fit the data to some log-normal distribution.

R. Schepp: At the moment we can deal with it. However, in an open system it is much more difficult to get an idea of how big your leak actually is. If you are working in the intensive care unit with a low-pressure cuff – and such cuffs are notoriously leaky how can you get an idea of how big the leak actually is?

P. Wagner: That is a different question. I was just asking how you cancel the leak in your system; because you did show how sensitive these equilibration curves appear to be.

R. Schepp: Well, normally in my system there is a leak of 10–20 ml/min at a pressure of 20 cmH_2O. And we can actually calculate the leak. So it is assumed that after 100 breaths there must be an equilibrium from then on. Any fall in concentration would indicate a leak. You can calculate the leak, extrapolate back, and correct for it.

E. A. Ernst: Do you use CO_2 as your leak indicator?

R. Schepp: No, I do not use CO_2 as a leak indicator. We use N_2O, N_2 or helium, because CO_2 is very difficult to use as a leak indicator.

E. A. Ernst: Loss or gain?

R. Schepp: Any leak would be a loss, not a gain.

E. A. Ernst: Well, not necessarily. That opens up another question about leaks. Leaks can be inward and outward. You are proceeding on the assumption that they are always outward.

R. Schepp: Yes.

P. Wagner: I would like to make another comment. You have done what lots of people do with physiological data, which is to fit a model to the data; and that can be useful. But it is my experience, and that of a lot of people that I work with, that it is important to look at what other models might also fit to the data. There are several ways of doing this. I am wondering to what extent you have looked at what other kinds of models might be compatible with the data.

R. Schepp: We are not yet as far as that. This is our first attempt because it is the easiest model.

P. Wagner: I was not being critical.But there may be different models, different interpretations, that you can place on the same data. I think it is important to evaluate all of those. I hope you will not stop at one log-normal distribution.

R. Schepp: No.

P. Wagner: Good.

T. Mostert: Dr. Spintge, in some microcomputersystems the memory is held in the Read Only Memory, or ROM, while in others it is not. I am wondering what happens in the case of power failure? Do you have to restore the operating system to the computer, or is it permanent in the ROM of the Narcocon?

R. Spintge: It is permanently stored in the ROM module.

P. A. Foster: What is the advantage of a Rolling Seal? Why not use a bellows?

R. Spintge: The advantage of the Rolling Seal is that you have complete separation between any ventilator you might use and a closed and airtight patient circuit. This is one technique; there may be others. But we have tested nearly every pressure-controlled ventilator available in Germany. Not a single one could be used in closed-circuit ventilation, because they leaked at least 1 litre/min.

E. A. Ernst: But if your ventilators do function there should be no communication between the ventilator-driving gas and the circuit gas. Perhaps the Rolling Seal might cause less resistance to movement, or you might have a mechanism for more accurate measurement of displacement of the bellows or of the volume. But if you have a properly constructed ventilator we should be able to separate these two gases.

R. Spintge: So far in Germany we have no ventilators in which the part of the patient circuit placed inside the ventilator is airtight. They have a leak of at least 1 litre/min on the patient side!

R. Schepp: Our purpose was to measure uptake of gases not averaged over several minutes but actually from breath to breath. We had to define a system which could very stable and could very reproducibly measure end-tidal differences of as little as 1 ml. We tried, and we compared this Rolling Seal spirometer and a spirometer from a lung function laboratory for volume accuracy and reproducibility of volume indication. And the instability of the spirometer balloons, in particular, yields lower resolution of breath-by-breath volume measurement than the Rolling Seal does. Furthermore, the resistance of the Rolling Seal is much smaller than in any other bellows. The prices are not all that different. So, these mechanical properties also influenced us in our selection of the Rolling Seal.

P. A. Foster: In other words, the wall of your spirometer and the wall of your bellows are rigid, and therefore you can predict the compliance much more accurately than you can with a rubber bellows.

C. Y. Lin: Do you think that with such high volumes in the circuit system breath-by-breath measurement of oxygen consumption is necessary?

R. Spintge: You need this breath-by-breath measurement, for example, for non-invasive determination of O_2 pulse, O_2 availability and cardiac output.

E. A. Ernst: Indeed, we have to measure concentration and volume breath by breath over quite a long time. There is no way round this. I think this is what this seminar is all about: where our limits are and how we can attempt to reach them.

D. W. Lübbers: How big is the leak in your machine? Does it come about because you have a rubber membrane and some degree of leak, or is this a specially prepared membrane?

R. Spintge: It is a specially prepared membrane, covered with aluminium.

E. A. Ernst: The leak is zero?

R. Spintge: As far as we can measure the leak is zero.

E. A. Ernst: So it is really a tight system.

R. Spintge: Yes, it is, because the patient circuit is tight, the Rolling Seal is tight; and this makes us independent of any leak in any driving ventilator.

T. J. A. Tamsma: I have a question about the requirements and the possibilities of measuring end-tidal or inspiratory flushin of inhalational agents. There are people who say there is no need to measure those values. Today we have heard a lot about the possibilities of measurement, as presented by Dr. Wallroth, for example. What is Dr. Ernst's opinion about that?

E. A. Ernst: I don't know whether I can answer that question, but I am somewhat confused by the simplifications in references to the use of injection techniques. Dr. Lin, you were talking about introducing the anaesthetic agent in a constant manner without monitoring it, because your hypothesis is that after you get this initial washin the uptake is minimal and the system is so large that it will realy take care of any variability, and that there is really no need to worry about any decrease in the rate of uptake in a closed system. What bothers me is that some of the arguments you use rest upon models from open systems, that is to say, nonrebreathing systems. And all the data we saw are based on such models. For instance, you mentioned the partial pressure in the alveoli over the inspiratory concentration. Your formulation was: Given an infinite supply of gas (F_I), how long would it take for the F_A to reach 1? In the closed circuit we are asking just the opposite question. We are saying let the alveolar concentration be constant, so that we have a constant arterial concentration. And let us introduce the agent in such a way that alveolar concentration and arterial concentration remain constant. So, I do not know how you can use this type of information in the closed-circuit system, because we do not have an infinite supply of agent and we are completely turning the question around. So it bothers me to think that you envisage being able to introduce the same amount of agent per unit of time and maintain a constant level of anaesthesia. I do not know whether that was related to the question that was asked or not. But these are some of my problems with it.

C. Y. Lin: I think the biggest controversy in this matter between Dr. Eger's or Dr. Servinghaus's uptake series and mine or Dr. Lowe's is that question about the $\sqrt{t}$. The main problem is that the assumption about the approximation of $\sqrt{t}$ neglects the fact of functional residual capacity (FRC) wash-in. The term of this $\sqrt{t}$ function is actually distribution-side uptake and not supply-side uptake. You cannot instantaneously equilibrate to the point you want in a closed system. And so the distribution side, or maybe the tissue-uptake side in this approximation can be wrong. If you maintain inspired concentration in a circuit using high flow then you can see there is a change in uptake over 1 h. Even Dr. Eger agreed that there is not much fluctuation over time in terms of the rate of uptake in a closed system.

E. A. Ernst: That is simply because you have got most of the muscle compartment saturated and all you have now is uptake into fat, which is perfusion limited, and so it does become linear.

T. E. J. Healy: I just like to ask Dr. Lin whether he has taken any notice at all during surgery of the fact that either N_2 is lost at a large tissue-wound interface or that in fact N_2 may be absorbed. This means there may be changes in the closed-circuit levels of these gases; in other words, once the surgeon has made a large incision the closed-circuit system is no longer closed.

C. Y. Lin: There is a loss of N_2O through the skin, through the intestinal wall and through any abdominal wound.

J. R. W. McIntyre: The topic of your presentation was: "Can we practice safe simple closed-circuit anaesthesia without extensive monitoring or calculus?" The answer still evades me.

C. Y. Lin: In the over 7000 cases we have anaesthetized in this way, mass spectrometry has shown that after FRC wash-in the rate of uptake does not change. So we now measure only oxygen concentration. Mostly it is even not really necessary to monitor oxygen concentration, but from a medicolegal standpoint I think this oxygen monitoring is still necessary.

H. Schwilden: Dr. Lin, I do feel that there is actually no real difference between Severinghaus's and Lowe's opinion and yours. I feel there is some misunderstanding. The point Lowe and Severinghaus are making is not that the rate of uptake is $\sqrt{t}$; rather they are saying that if you keep the alveolar concentration constant the uptake is one over the square root of time. And looking at your figures, at most times I have not seen constant alveolar concentration. In general your curves started at an FA/FI ratio of zero. So there seems to be some misunderstanding. The transfer to the tissues is described by perfusion divided by a virtual volume of distribution. The delivery from the tissue to the blood again is given by perfusion × blood gas partition coefficient and something else, I do not remember what at the moment. That is the relationship. So, one would not expect that with a constant inspiratory concentration you could measure an uptake which is proportional to one over the square root of time ($\sqrt{t}$). There is no evidence of that, and that is not what Lowe and Severinghaus state.

C. Y. Lin: I completely disagree, simply because I have already shown you the discrepancy between my results and Dr. Severinghaus's. To reach equilibration takes 12 breaths, even with good alveolar ventilation. That means, assuming ten breaths per minute you need more than one minute, during which uptake is much lower than at the end of FRC wash-in. I am thinking in terms of constancy of the alveolar concentration; given a constant volume you do not need sophisticated monitoring equipment.

E. A. Ernst: At one stage I saw an arteriovenous difference. How far are you into anaesthesia at that time? 3 hours? And you still have a flow of 150 ml for nitrous oxide?

C. Y. Lin: Yes.

E. A. Ernst: That is a very high uptake. Are you sure your system is closed?

C. Y. Lin: Yes, for sure.

E. A. Ernst: It is interesting that you report still having this much uptake after 3 hours.

C. Y. Lin: But this is something which Dr. Healy already mentioned: The nitrous oxide loss from the skin and also from the intestinal cavity. There we have a tremendous nitrous oxide loss.

T. E. J. Healy: I think it is equally important to remember that there is quite a considerable nitrogen uptake from that area as well. And this could therefore – since you are not actually aware what oxygen you are giving your patient in your mixture in the closed circuit – make it important for you to measure oxygen concentrations, not only for medicolegal reasons, but also to know that you are giving the patient a reasonable oxygen concentration for your own satisfaction. You need to know what you are giving the patient. You are losing nitrous oxide from one end of the patient and you are absorbing nitrogen from the same end of the patient, so you have lost all contact with reality unless you are actually monitoring something. And the one thing you have to monitor is oxygen.

C. Y. Lin: I do not think nitrogen is really accumulating to such an extent in the circuit. We have measured more than 500 cases in the past. I do not think nitrogen accumulation ever exceeded the 5% level after the initial FRC washin with high flows.

Non-invasive Monitoring

Non-invasive Monitoring of $tcpO_2$ and $tcpCO_2$ in Patients with Normal and Compromised Circulation

R. Lemke, D. Klaus, and D. W. Lübbers

Transcutaneous oxygen and carbon dioxide measurements are successfully applied in non-invasive monitoring of newborn children. Recent reports on its applicability in adults are quite encouraging, not only as a continuous monitoring of arterial blood gas analysis in patients with stable circulation, but also for patients in shock [1–11].

The transcutaneous pO_2 ($tcpO_2$) represents the balance of oxygen delivery to the skin, which is determined by the ratio of oxygen consumption to oxygen offer. Since oxygen offer is determined by blood flow and blood O_2 content, both factors determine the $tcpO_2$.

Under normal conditions the $tcpO_2$ on the skin is close to zero, due to vascular regulation of blood supply, which keeps the blood flow small compared with oxygen consumption. With the application of local heat (43°–45 °C) local vascular reactions can be abolished and with normal circulation the oxygen offer becomes large compared with the O_2 comsumption. pO_2 measured with abolished vascular reactions and with local maximal vasodilation is called "transcutaneous pO_2". Figure 1 shows the factors which influence $tcpO_2$ measurements:

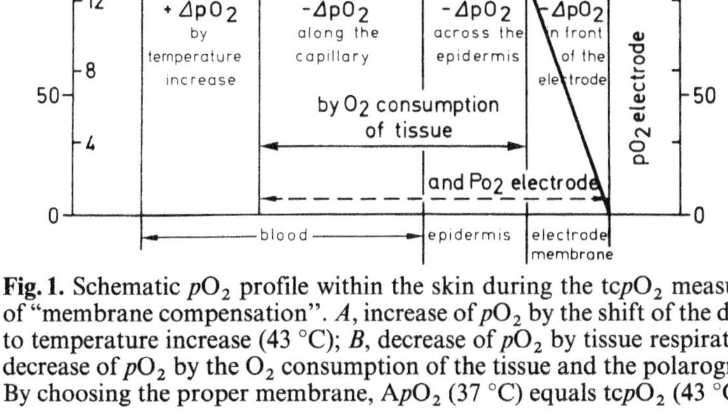

Fig. 1. Schematic pO_2 profile within the skin during the $tcpO_2$ measurement. Mechanism of "membrane compensation". *A*, increase of pO_2 by the shift of the dissociation curve due to temperature increase (43 °C); *B*, decrease of pO_2 by tissue respiration (*hatched line*). *C*, decrease of pO_2 by the O_2 consumption of the tissue and the polarographic pO_2 electrode. By choosing the proper membrane, ApO_2 (37 °C) equals $tcpO_2$ (43 °C)

A The shift of the O_2 dissociation curve with increase of temperature increases blood pO_2.
B The tissue respiration of the epidermis decreases tcpO_2 (Fig. 1, hatched line).
C Oxygen consumption of the platinum electrode and O_2 consumption along the capillary as well as across the epidermis decrease tcpO_2.

In *A* the tcpO_2 is increased, but by choosing a suitable membrane for the electrode, the effect of *A* can be compensated by *B* and *C* ("membrane compensation"). Satisfactory "membrane compensation" can, however, only be achieved at maximal vasodilation and with a heat-induced increase in arterial pO_2 (ApO_2). Under these special conditions tcpO_2 (43 °C) equals ApO_2 (37 °C) [2–4].

In shock peripheral blood flow is small, due to diminished perfusion pressure. Flow may become even smaller, because of vasoconstriction of the major vessels of the skin, which cannot be abolished by application of local heat at the measuring site. Due to lower flow values there is increased oxygen shunt diffusion from the arterial to the venous limb of the capillary loop. As a consequence tcpO_2 may be extremely low [4].

Transcutaneous carbon dioxide (tcpCO_2) measurements can be carried out with a small heated pCO_2 electrode. Since CO_2 is produced in the tissue and washed out by the blood flow, the tcpCO_2 is larger than the arterial pCO_2. tcpCO_2 increases with decreasing blood flow, so an increase of tcpCO_2 compared with $ApCO_2$ indicates a decrease of blood flow [4].

Methods

The following measurements were performed:

1. Arterial pO_2 (ApO_2) and pCO_2 ($ApCO_2$), either from the radial artery or from the hyperemic ear lobe
2. Transcutaneous pO_2 and pCO_2 at the volar side of the forearm

The following values were calculated:

1. The factor tcpO_2/ApO_2 was calculated for the different patient groups to characterize the behaviour of tcpO_2.
2. The tcpCO_2 which was measured at 44 °C was first corrected to 37 °C with the following formula: tcpCO_2 (44 °C)/1.37 = tcpCO_2 (37 °C).
3. A factor tcpCO_2 (37 °C)/$ApCO_2$ was then calculated for the different patient groups to characterize the behaviour of tcpCO_2.
4. Additionally, a differences D = tcpCO_2 (37 °C) − $ApCO_2$ was calculated for the different patient groups.

Results

We present two different patient groups to discuss the possibilities and limitations of the transcutaneous measurements of pO_2 and pCO_2.

1. Stable patients on artificial respiration
2. Patients in cardiogenic shock

1. Fourteen patients on artificial respiration

pO_2 values: (Fig. 2)
1. Mean tcpO_2 $= 87.4 \pm 43.7$ mmHg
   Mean ApO_2 $= 93.3 \pm 41.9$ mmHg
2. tcpO_2/ApO_2 $= 0.95 \pm 0.19$ mmHg
3. Correlation coefficient $R = 0.9413$

pCO_2 values:
$ApCO_2$ $= 39.8 \pm 4.47$ mmHg
tcpCO_2 (37° C) $= 43.3 \pm 4.66$ mmHg
D $= 4.1 \pm 3.16$ mmHg
tcpCO_2/$ApCO_2$ $= 1.108 \pm 0.079$ mmHg

The results of the pO_2 and pCO_2 values are similar to those of outpatients and volunteers. There is a good correlation between the tcpO_2 and ApO_2. The factors tcpO_2/ApO_2 and tcpCO_2 (37 °C)/$ApCO_2$ are close to unity. The difference, D, between tcpCO_2 and $ApCO_2$ is small (compared with group 2b). These results are in agreement with those in the literature [2, 4].

2. a) Nine patients in moderate cardiogenic shock

pO_2 values: (Fig. 3)
1. Mean tcpO_2 $= 38.1 \pm 7.55$ mmHg
   Mean ApO_2 $= 52.8 \pm 11.2$ mmHg
2. tcpO_2/ApO_2 $= 0.74 \pm 0.15$ mmHg
3. Correlation coefficient $R = 0.61$

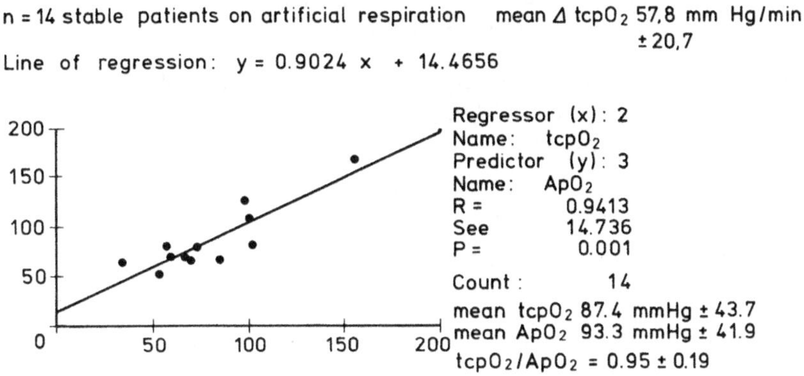

Fig. 2. Correlation between tcpO_2 and ApO_2 in 14 patients on artificial respiration

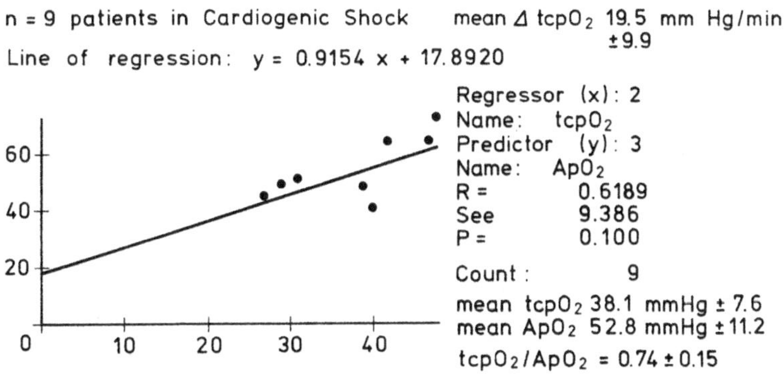

Fig. 3. Correlation between tcpO_2 and ApO_2 in nine patients with moderate cardiogenic shock

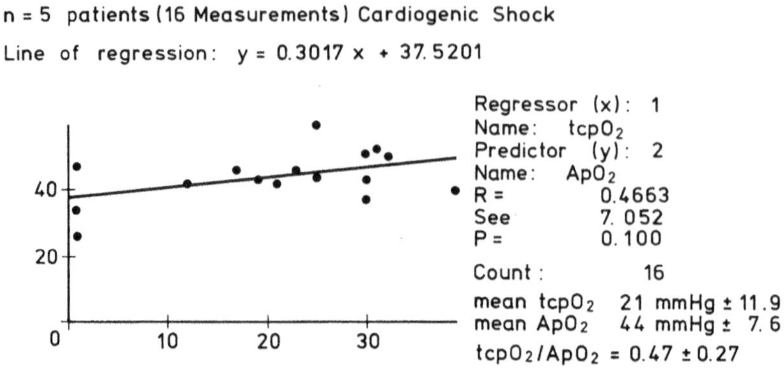

Fig. 4. Correlation between tc$p$O$_2$ and ApO$_2$ in five patients in serious cardiogenic shock

The results demonstrate a loss of correlation between tc$p$O$_2$ and ApO$_2$ and a reduction of the tc$p$O$_2$/ApO$_2$ factor.

2. b) Five patients in serious cardiogenic shock (four of the five died).

pO$_2$ values: (Fig. 4)
1. Mean tc$p$O$_2$ = 21.06 ± 11.9 mmHg
   Mean ApO$_2$ = 44.1 ± 7.6 mmHg
2. tc$p$O$_2$/ApO$_2$ = 0.47 ± 0.27 mmHg
3. Correlation coefficient $R = 0.46$

The results demonstrate an extremely low tc$p$O$_2$ compared with the ApO$_2$, shown by the decrease of the tc$p$O$_2$/ApO$_2$ factor. There was an extremely poor correlation between tc$p$O$_2$ and ApO$_2$.

pCO$_2$ values:
ApCO$_2$ = 43.9 ± 10.6 mmHg
tc$p$CO$_2$ (37° C) = 66.9 ± 12.9 mmHg
D = 23 ± 12.46 mmHg
tc$p$CO$_2$/ApCO$_2$ = 1.74 ± 0.455 mmHg

The results show a very high tc$p$CO$_2$ compared with ApCO$_2$, demonstrated by the increase of the factor tc$p$CO$_2$/ApCO$_2$ as well as the increase of the difference, D, due to low tissue perfusion.

Discussion and Conclusion

Stable patients on artificial respiration are good candidates for continuous transcutaneous blood gas monitoring. The factors tc$p$O$_2$/ApO$_2$ and tc$p$CO$_2$/ApCO$_2$ are close to unity. The difference, D, between tc$p$CO$_2$ and ApCO$_2$ is small; these patients need only infrequent invasive controls.

Patients in cardiogenic shock demonstrate, in coincidence with the severity of their symptoms, a disproportionatey decreasing tc$p$O$_2$ and, thus, a decrease of the factor tc$p$O$_2$/ApO$_2$, while tc$p$CO$_2$ reaches insufficiently high values, demonstrated by the increase of the factor tc$p$CO$_2$/ApCO$_2$ and the difference, D. These patients need frequent invasive blood gas controls.

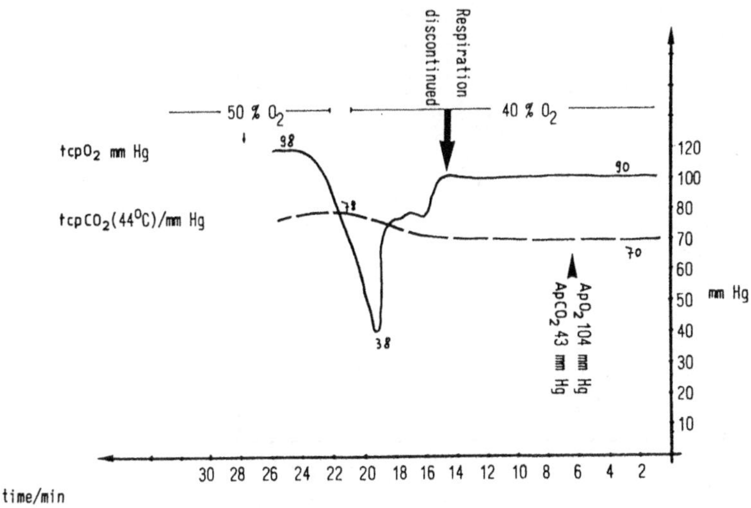

Fig. 5. Patient on artificial respiration. The ventilation is discontinued for suction. There is a steep drop of tcpO_2 and a small delayed increase in tcpCO_2

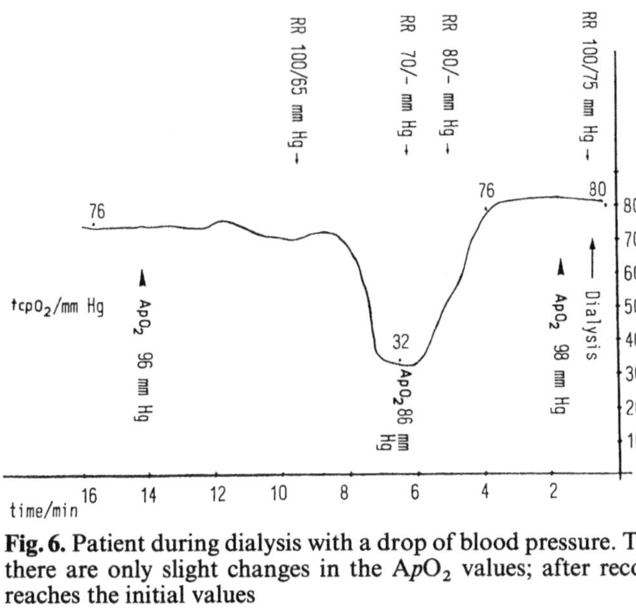

Fig. 6. Patient during dialysis with a drop of blood pressure. There is a steep drop of tcpO_2; there are only slight changes in the ApO_2 values; after recovery, tcpO_2 rises again and reaches the initial values

The last figures demonstrate that continuous measurements are distinctly superior to discontinuous measurements, because of monitoring transient events.

1. Figure 5 shows a patient on tracheal suction, where the drop of tcpO_2 and increase of tcpCO_2 provide information which is usually missed by the discontinuous arterial measurements.
2. Figure 6 shows a patient at the beginning of dialysis, who has a sudden drop of blood pressure. There is a steep drop of tcpO_2 due to diminished local blood flow at the measuring site with only slight changes in ApO_2.

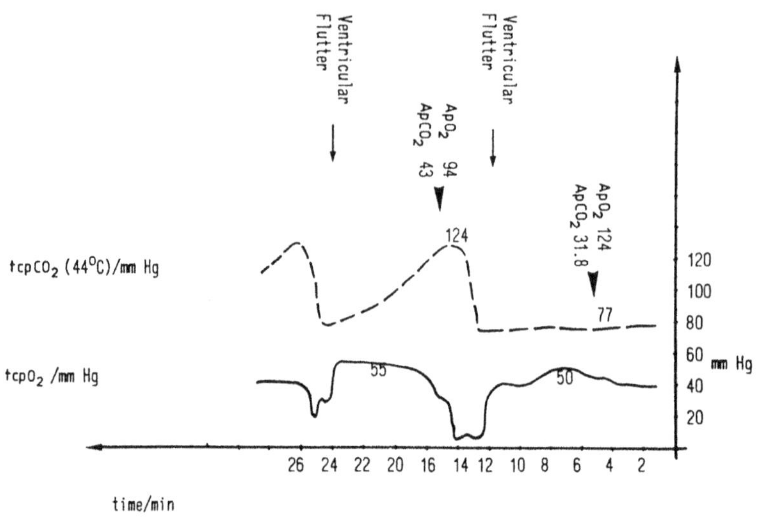

Fig. 7. Patient in cardiogenic shock with high tcpCO_2 and low tcpO_2, compared with arterial measurements. Transcutaneous values deteriorate greatly during ventricular flutter. Arterial pO_2 and pCO_2 values change only slightly

3. Figure 7 shows a patient with ventricular flutter or fibrillation, where tcpO_2 reaches extremely low values and tcpCO_2 reaches extremely high values, due to decreasing local flow with small changes in ApO_2 and $ApCO_2$ values.

Reports on patients in haemorrhagic shock prove the tcpO_2 to be a very sensitive indicator for the prognosis of a patient as well as for the success of resuscitation [5, 8]. Low tcpO_2 values and especially a decreasing factor tcpO_2/ApO_2 may indicate deterioration of circulation, even in patients with adequate blood pressure and arterial pO_2.

Disproportional increase in tcpCO_2 is less sensitive and appears later in the clinical course of shock, when tcpO_2 is already extremely low. This could be demonstrated in our patients in serious cardiogenic shock.

The measurements demonstrate clearly, that tcpO_2 and tcpCO_2 are measuring values in their own right. They can provide additional information about the quality of tissue perfusion in patients with haemodynamic instability.

References

1. Brünstler I, Enders A, Versmold HT (1982) Skin surface PCO_2 monitoring in newborn infants in shock: effect of hypotension and electrode temperature. Pediatrics 100:454–457
2. Huch R, Huch A, Lübbers DW (1981) Transcutaneous PO_2. Thieme-Stratton, New York Thieme, Stuttgart
3. Lübbers DW, Grossmann U (1983) Gas exchange through the human epidermis as a basis of tcPO_2 and tcPCO_2 measurements. In: Huch R, Huch A (eds) Continuous blood gas monitoring. Dekker, New York
4. Lübbers DW (in press) Transcutaneous PO_2 in shock
5. Nolan LS, Shoemaker WC (1982) Transcutaneous O_2 and CO_2 monitoring of high risk surgical patients during the perioperative period. Crit Care Med 10:762–764

6. Rithalia SVS, George RJD, Tinker J (1981) Continuous tissue pH and transcutaneous PO_2 measurement as an index of tissue perfusion in critically ill patients. Resuscitation 1:67–74
7. Schober JG, Stübing K (1983) Arterial and transcutaneous PCO_2 monitoring in cardiogenic shock. In: Huch R, Huch A (eds) Continuous blood gas monitoring. Dekker, New York
8. Tremper KK, Shoemaker WC (1981) Transcutaneous oxygen monitoring of critically ill adults, with and without low flow shock. Crit Care Med 9:706–709
9. Versmold HT, Linderkamp O, Holzman M, Strohhacker I, Riegel KP (1978) Limits of $tcPO_2$ monitoring in sick neonates: relation to blood pressure, blood volume, peripheral blood flow and acid base status. Acta Anaesthesiol Scand 68:88–90
10. Waxman K, Sadler R, Eisner ME, Applebaum R, Tremper KK, Mason ER (1983) Transcutaneous oxygen monitoring of emergency department patients. Am J Surg 146:35–38
11. Yip WCL, Tay ISH, Wong HB, Ho TF (1983) Reliability of transcutaneous oxygen monitoring of critically ill children in a general pediatric unit. Clin Pediatr 22:431–435

A Microsystem to Measure Respiratory and Anaesthetic Gases During Surgery

G. Jibelian, G. Yates, and B. Taylor

Estimation of the concentration of light and volatile anaesthetic gases in the operating arena is usually achieved either with a series of discrete analysers or with a specially designed time-shared mass spectrometer. The cost and maintenance of either system, as well as the bulk of instrumentation and the time-consuming calibration of each device, have been deterrents to their widespread use. A low-cost system, simpler to calibrate, to operate and to maintain has been designed. It operates on the principle of chromatography but without the usual slow response-time, and the dependency on technical skill. The overall system incorporates two separate microanalysers: one dedicated to the analysis of volatile anaesthetics, the other to permanent gases. Unlike commercially available chromatographs, this system allows analysis of physiological levels of carbon dioxide in the presence of large concentrations of nitrous oxide. Total analysis time for all gases is within 60 s, and the sample volume is less than 0.25 ml. The analysers are designed to be microcomputer compatible, and a built-in autozeroing circuit ensures a virtually drift-free baseline. Once calibrated prior to use, no periodic calibration is required throughout the duration of a case. Because of their microdimensions, the gas analyzers with their inherent power supplies can be housed in a utility drawer found in any conventional anaesthesia cart, making the overall system unobtrusive during routine use.

Several gas mixtures of varying concentrations were analyzed to study the detector response as a function of gas concentration. In the case of volatile anaesthetics 2% isoflurane (Forane) was used as the test gas. In the concentration range of 0%–2% the detector displayed a linear behaviour. Analysis of the data using the linear regression method yielded a straight line connecting all the points with the origin. The coefficient of determination r^2 was better than 0.99.

In the case of light gases, detector response was linear for CO_2 in the 0%–10% concentration range, with the regression line passing through zero, and r^2 equal to 1.

For O_2 and N_2O, detector response was curvelinear. In the commonly used levels of oxygen (20%–60%) the regression equation yields a straight line with r^2 better than 0.99. In the case of N_2O, the detector response is linear from 0% to 40%. Beyond 40%, the regression line changes slope, but remains linear in the 40%–65% range, with $r^2 = 0.99$.

Since most commonly delivered oxygen and nitrous oxide levels are within 40%–60%, and the volatile organic gas levels between 0%–2%, a single calibration tank with 45% N_2O, 5% CO_2, 2% volatile anaesthetic and 3% nitrogen can be used to calibrate the system without the need for tedious calibration charts.

The performance of the microprocessors in estimating the magnitude of each gas component was evaluated by simultaneously recording on an analogue strip chart recorder the response of the detector to different concentrations of isoflurane. Analysis of the paired results showed excellent correlation (1.00). Comparison of computer and manual estimation of concentration by the paired *t*-test showed no significant difference (*P*, 0.01).

We conclude that analysis of light and anaesthetic gases using micro gas chromatographs and a microcomputer placed on each anaesthesia delivery cart is technically feasible and offers significant advantages over commercially available systems. Such a system can be efficient, accurate, portable, compact, easy to operate and very cost-effective. It can eliminate the expense of laying cables between different operating rooms and a central analyser system, providing total independence to individual clinicians.

References

1. Harry LV, Beckham LM (1964) Determination of volatile organic anesthetics in blood. In: Szymanski HA (ed) Biomedical applications of gas chromatography, 2nd edn. Plenum, New York, p 307
2. Adlard ER, Hill DW (1960) Analysis of anesthetic mixtures by gas chromatography. Nature 186:1045
3. Dressler DP, Mastio GJ, Allbritten FF (1960) Clinical application of gas chromatography to analysis of respiratory gases. J Lab Clin Med 55:144
4. Dýfrerman A, Sjovall J (1962) Estimation of fluothane by gas chromatography. Acta Anesthesiol Scand 6:171

On-Line Estimation of Cerebral Oxygenation

N. S. Faithfull, H. T. van der Zee, M. H. Kuypers, K. Dhasmana, and W. Erdmann

Kwan and Fatt [6] have pointed out that the palpebral conjunctiva is a particularly suitable position in which oxygen tension (PO_2) may be sensed. This structure, which assists in the oxygenation of the cornea when the latter is not exposed to the surrounding air, possesses a dense vascular bed with the conjunctival capillaries located very close to the surface layers, hence minimizing the distance over which oxygen must diffuse.

The above authors developed and tested an early conjunctival electrode. This had a response time of as much as 2 min and was therefore unsuitable for detection of rapid acute changes in PO_2. The clinical use of a conjunctival PO_2 electrode has recently been described by Yelderman [11], but no mention of response speed was made. The conjunctival PO_2 ($PconO_2$) was always lower than arterial PO_2 (PaO_2) and the sensor was able to follow the trend of the changes in arterial oxygen tension.

By application of solid-state technology, it has been possible to produce a miniature membrane-covered polarographic Clark cell. A low-cost, mass-produced, O_2 sensor chip has recently been produced by Honeywell Medical Electronics [3] and this paper describes our initial experiences with this device.

Materials and Methods

Studies were performed on anaesthetized Wistar rats, in which unconsciousness had been produced using a gas mixture of 33% oxygen in nitrous oxide to which halothane vapour had been added from a Cyprane Fluotec Mark III vaporizer. A tracheostomy was performed and the animals were ventilated with 0.5% halothane vaporized in a nitrous oxide/oxygen mixture using a Loosco Amsterdam infant ventilator. Respiratory rates and tidal volumes were adjusted to achieve normal end-tidal CO_2 values, as measured on a Godart type 1467 capnograph. A Braun Melsungen Perfusor apparatus was adjusted to deliver the non-depolarizing relaxant, pancuronium bromide, at a rate of 0.4 mg/h.

Blood was intermittently withdrawn from a 1-mm-diameter catheter that was inserted into the femoral artery and estimation of blood gases and acid/base status were performed using a Radiometer ABL 1 acid base laboratory. This cannula was connected to a Gould P23 pressure transducer and, after amplification by a Grass 7B polygraph, systemic arterial pressures were recorded on a Grass ink-writing oscillograph. The electrocardiogram was continuously monitored.

The O_2 sensor was applied between the upper eyelid and cornea, the chip facing the palpebral conjunctiva. The eyelid were sewn closed to ensure a tight apposition of the sensor to the conjunctival tissues. The inspiratory oxygen concentration (FiO_2), measured using an Instrumentation Laboratory Oxygen Monitor 404, was varied between 0.2 and 0.5. Arterial blood samples were taken for blood gas analysis at the end of a 15-min period of ventilation at each FiO_2.

In some animals, hypotension was induced to investigate further the responses of the sensor. In addition the animals were, in some cases, hyperventilated or hypoventilated to ascertain whether changes in cerebral circulation (which would be produced by changes in the partial pressure of carbon dioxide) would be reflected in the oxygenation of the palpebral conjunctival capillary bed.

The Conjunctival Oxygen Sensor

The sensor is constructed using the principle of the ring-shaped cathode system as described by Kimmich and Kreuzer [4] and was incorporated by constructing two rectangular spirals [5]. In this manner it was possible to combine the small width of the cathode, which determines the sensitivity of the polarographic cell to oxygen flux, with a relatively large total cathode area, and thus stronger electrode current. This has several advantages, such as small zero current and improved stability – two factors which are difficult to achieve in miniaturized microelectrodes.

The gold cathode and the silver anode are vapour-deposited on a silicon substrate, while a silicon-oxide layer is used for insulation between the electrodes. A porous cross-linked polymer matrix between the cathode/anode system and the rubber membrane serves as carrier for the electrolyte. The polymer matrix, the electrolyte and the membrane were all applied by spin coating. The electrode is activated just prior to use by equilibrating in saline. This procedure has several advantages, but it obviously restricts applicability of the cell for the measurement of oxygen in a completely fluid medium.

The cable is only 140 µm in diameter, protected by a Teflon tube and fastened to the chip by ultrasonic bonding techniques. The dimensions of the chip are

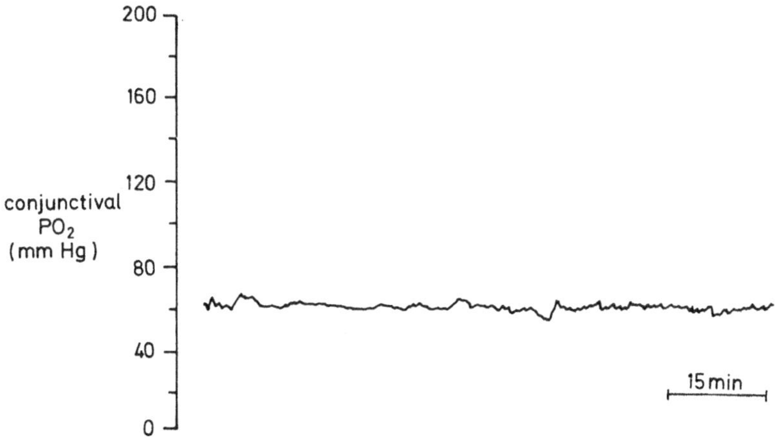

Fig. 1. Conjunctival partial pressure of oxygen in the rat in the presence of 20% inspired oxygen concentration

0.7 × 3.7 mm and it has a thickness of 0.4 mm. The whole is embedded in a flap of silicon rubber in such a way that the membrane of the chip is in direct contact with the inner surface of the eyelid. This flap is 45 mm long, 4 mm wide and 0.5 mm thick, thus enabling it to be fixed directly onto the skin adjacent to the eye. The soft surface of the pliable rubber is in contact with the eyeball so there is no danger of damaging the surface of the eyeball.

Prior to application, the O_2 sensor was calibrated in 0.9 NaCl equilibrated with air. The electrode current was fed into a Philips XV 1506 amplifier system, and conjunctival oxygen tension was continuously recorded using a Philips PM 822 pen recorder.

Results

The sensor was stable for extended periods, both in vitro and in vivo. An in vivo recording of $PconO_2$ in an animal ventilated with a gas mixture containing 20% oxygen is shown in Fig. 1 and it can be seen that the output from the sensor remained constant for more than 1½ h. An example of the results obtained (from two sensors, one in each eye), when stepwise alterations in the inspired oxygen concentration (FiO_2) are made, can be seen in Fig. 2. The response time of the sensor was rapid and after about 10–20 s a new steady-state $PconO_2$ could be obtained.

The arterial PO_2 is plotted against $PconO_2$ in Fig. 4 and the regression line has been drawn. There is a very significant overall correlation, with a correlation coefficient of 0.93 ($n=33$). The conjunctival PO_2 would appear to give a better indication of PaO_2 in the normal and hypoxic range than in the hyperoxic range of arterial oxygen tensions. In Fig. 3 two regression lines have been drawn and, although in both instances the correlation coefficient is 0.81 (this is statistically significant), the slope is 0.93 in the lower range but only 0.55 in the hyperoxic range.

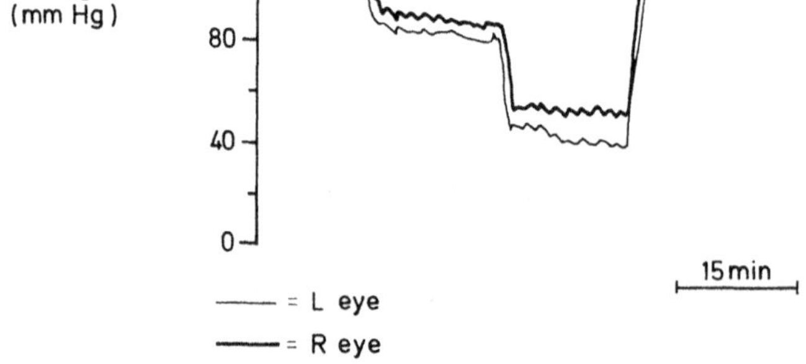

Fig. 2. Responses of the subconjunctival oxygen sensor to stepwise alterations in fractional inspired oxygen concentrations (FiO_2)

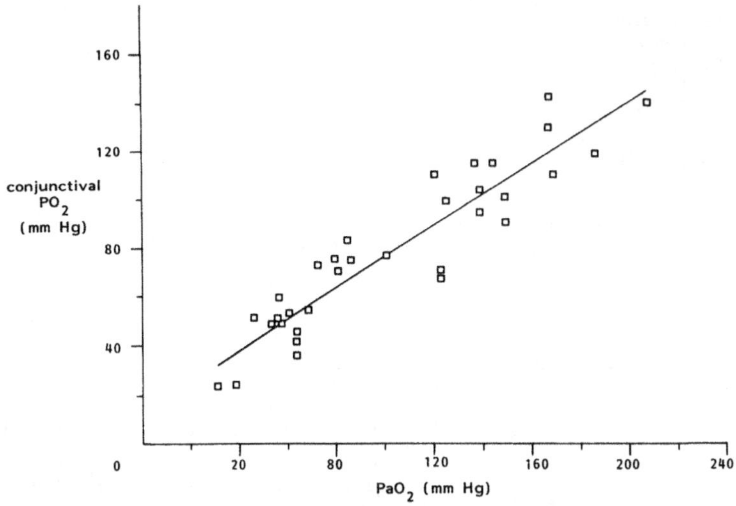

Fig. 3. The relationship between arterial oxygen tension (PaO_2) and conjunctival oxygen tension. The regression line is drawn in. The correlation coefficient is 0.93

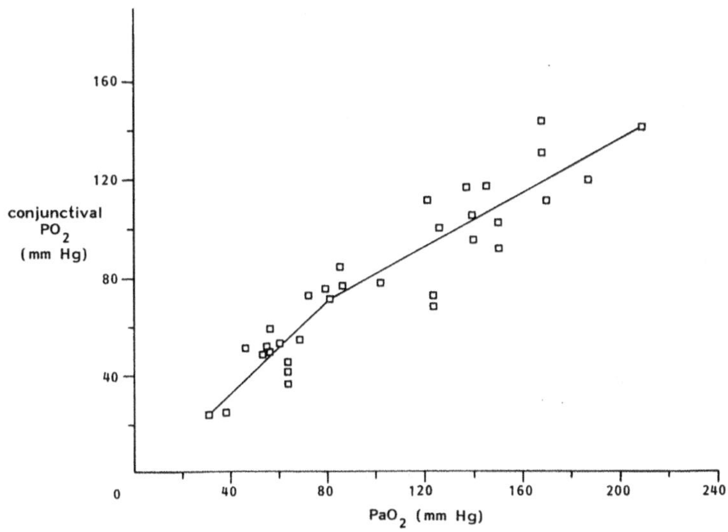

Fig. 4. The relationship between arterial oxygen tension (PaO_2) and conjunctival oxygen tension. The regression lines are drawn for PaO_2s of 100 mmHg and below and for 100 mmHg and above. Correlation coefficients and slopes of the regression lines are discussed in the text

Figure 5 demonstrates the responses of the O_2 sensor to injection of ketamine into the cisterna magna, infusion of 0.9% saline solution and withdrawal and subsequent reinfusion of blood. It can be seen that $PconO_2$ closely parallels the ensuing changes in mean arterial pressure that were to be observed.

The effects of hyperventilation, hypoventilation and temporary apnoea are demonstrated in Fig. 6. Hyperventilation, induced by an increase in the tidal volume, results in a rise of $PconO_2$, reflecting an improvement of tissue oxygenation. However, continued hyperventilation does not maintain this improvement in ox-

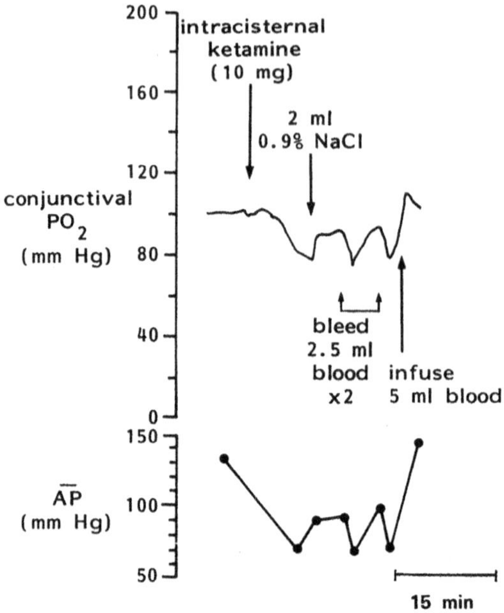

Fig. 5. The influence of intracisternal ketamine, intravenous administration of 0.9% NaCl, bleeding and reinfusion of blood on the mean systolic pressure ($\overline{AP}$) and on conjunctival PO_2

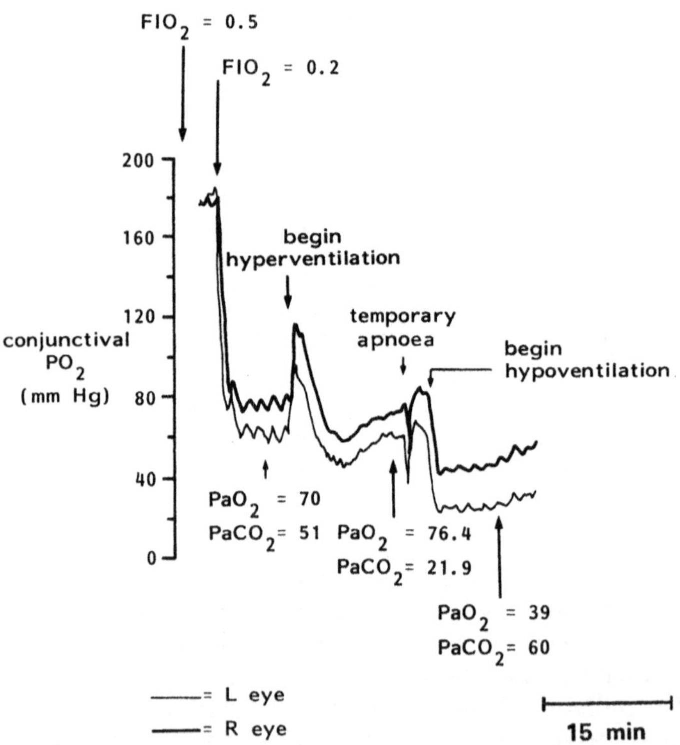

Fig. 6. The effects on subconjunctival oxygen tension of hyperventilation, apnoea and hypoventilation

ygenation of the conjunctival tissue and one can observe a slow decline to below the original baseline level. This may be the result of a vasoconstrictor effect of low carbon dioxide tensions on the cerebral circulation ($PaCO_2$ decreasd from 50 to 20 mm Hg). It is interesting to note that this effect reached a maximum value and was followed by a slight increase in conjunctival PO_2 reading. Possibly this may indicate an altered vascular response to very low $PaCO_2$ (hypoxic vasodilation). Also demonstrated in this figure is a temporary apnoea producing an immediate drop in $PconO_2$ response. Following hyperventilation, the animal was hypoventilated, resulting in a PaO_2 of 39 mm Hg and a $PaCO_2$ of 60 mm Hg. An immediate decrease of the conjunctival PO_2 value was seen, followed by a slow increase which was probably due to the vasodilatory effect of the rising $PaCO_2$.

Discussion

Since the introduction of the first membrane-covered polarographic cell by Clark in 1956 [1], oxygen polarography has undergone such refinement that PO_2 measurements can now be carried out with greater accuracy in almost any situation. Measurement of respiratory gas tensions in blood are routine, but the intermittent and invasive nature of the estimations has highlighted the need for on-line measurement of arterial oxygen partial pressure (PaO_2) in the critically ill patient. The method should preferably be non-invasive and the apparatus needed should be compact and simple to operate.

Continuous transcutaneous monitoring of oxygen tensions has gained considerable popularity and is widely practised in the neonatal period [8]. This method has also been employed in adults [9] but it has been shown that, though transcutaneous oxygen tension reflects the PaO_2 in patients with a normal cardiovascular status, this is not necessarily so in shock and low-flow conditions [10].

The solid-state O_2 sensor used in our experiments proved to be a reasonably accurate sensor of the state of conjunctival tissue oxygenation and there was a fairly high correlation between $PconO_2$ and PaO_2. It could be postulated that the lower correlation between the $PconO_2$ and PaO_2 in the hyperoxic range could be explained on the basis of the presence of autoregulatory vasoconstrictive mechanisms similar to those occurring in the cerebral circulation. This would appear reasonable considering the anatomical origin of the ophthalmic circulation.

In practice, a very useful feature of the O_2 sensor is its rapid response time of 10–20 s. This is much shorter than the early conjunctival electrodes of Kwan and Fatt [6]. The electrode that we used is therefore much more suitable and changes in tissue oxygenation, secondary to changes in oxygen flux, can be rapidly and accurately assessed allowing rapid therapeutic intervention in the clinical situation.

From the manner and the degree to which the sensor responds to alterations in PaO_2 and haemodynamic conditions, it is suggested that the electrode is reflecting changes in cerebral oxygen flux. Kwan and Hunt [7] have maintained that a change in the oxygen-carrying capacity of the blood has no effect on the $PconO_2$. However, it is quite possible that, in their studies employing haemodilution with low molecular weight dextran, the cardiac output of the experimental animals (rabbits) was, due to the decrease in blood viscosity, increased to the extent that total cerebral oxygen flux was unchanged.

The ciliary artery, which supplies the conjunctiva, carries blood coming from the internal carotid artery. It should therefore be possible to gain some idea of the adequacy of the cerebral circulation by the use of bilateral conjunctival oxygen electrodes. This should increase the margin of safety during, for instance, surgery for the relief of partial obstruction of the carotid artery. The instrument may also find useful application in neurosurgical practice, where it might give early warning of vascular compression or of vascular insufficiency during clamping of cerebral aneurisms. In addition, the sensor may be used as a research tool for investigating pharmacological action of drugs on the cerebral vascular smooth muscle.

References

1. Clarke LC Jr (1956) Monitor and control of blood and tissue oxygen tension. Trans Am Soc Artif Intern Organs 2:41–48
2. Dhasmana KM, Erdmann W, Salt PJ, Saxena PR (1982) Analysis of ketamine induced central and peripheral cardiovascular effects in the anaesthetized rats. Proceedings of 23rd Dutch Federation Meeting. Dutch Foundation, Amsterdam, p 94
3. Engels JML, Kuypers HM (1983) Medical applications of silicon sensors. J Phys [E] 16:987–994
4. Kimmich HP, Kreuzer F (1969) Oxygen pressure recordings in gases, fluids and tissues. Karger, Basel 10–100
5. Kimmich HP (1978) In: International workshop on biomedical transducers. Ko, Madrid, p 17
6. Kwan M, Fatt I (1971) A non-invasive method of continuous arterial oxygen tension estimation from measured palpebral conjunctival oxygen tension. Anesthesiology 35:309–314
7. Kwan MR, Hunt TK (1973) Continuous tissue oxygen tension measurements during acute blood loss. J Surg Res 14:420–425
8. Peabody JL, Willis MM, Gregory GA, Tooley WH, Lucey JF (1978) Clinical limitation and advantages of transcutaneous oxygen electrodes. Acta Anaesthesiol Scand [Suppl] 68:76–82
9. Sacci R, McMahan JL, Miller WF (1978) Oxygen tension monitoring with transcutaneous electrodes in adults. Med Instrum 10:192–194
10. Tremper KK, Waxman K, Bowman R, Shoemaker WC (1980) Continuous transcutaneous oxygen monitoring during respiratory failure, cardiac decompensation, cardiac arrest and CPR. Crit Care Med 8:377–381
11. Yelderman M (1983) Transconjunctival oxygen measurements in critical care medicine. Anesthesiology 59:266–267

A Continuous Non-invasive Blood Pressure Measurement Which is Controlled by Finger Plethysmography

J.C. Dorlas, J.A. Nijboer, W.T. Butijn, A.W. Cuiper, K.H. Wesseling, G.M.A. van der Hoeven, and J.J. Settels

A non-invasive method of measuring blood pressure in the finger continuously was developed by Penaz in 1976 [2]. Since then the method has been further developed by Wesseling et al. [3] to produce an instrument which is easy to use in the clinical setting. [1]

The resulting device produces a calibrated arterial pressure wave and has been given the name "Finapres" (*fin*ger *a*rterial *pres*sure). The instrument measures pressure variations in an inflatable cuff which is wrapped around the middle phalanx of a finger (Fig. 1). The cuff is connected to a source of compressed air. It also contains the transducer of a photoelectric plethysmograph of which the light source and the detector cell are applied at opposite sites of the finger. The resulting plethysmogram records the blood volume pulsations of the arteries under the cuff and is used to control the degree of inflation of the cuff. For this control the source of compressed air and the plethysmograph are linked together by a fast-reacting servo system and an electropneumatic transducer which enable the pressure in the cuff to be varied rapidly in such a way that the plethysmographic excursions are kept to a minimum. This indicates that the pressure difference across the arterial wall (the transmural pressure) is kept constant throughout the measurement. Thus cuff pressure follows the arterial pressure pulsations instanta-

[1] Recently we came across an article by Yamakashi [4] presenting a similar instrument to be applied at the rat's tail.

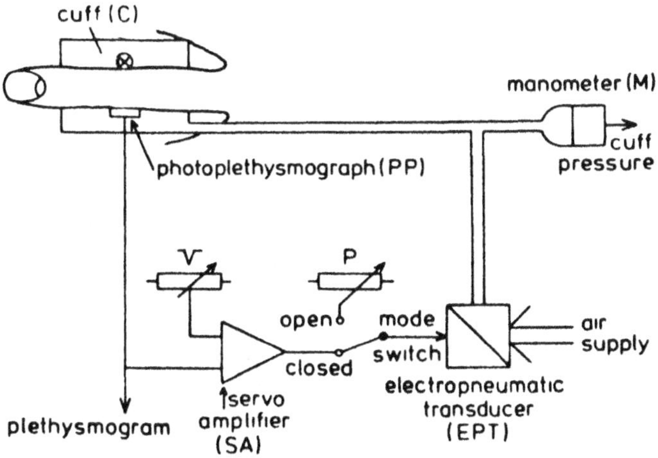

Fig. 1. Block diagram of the Finapres

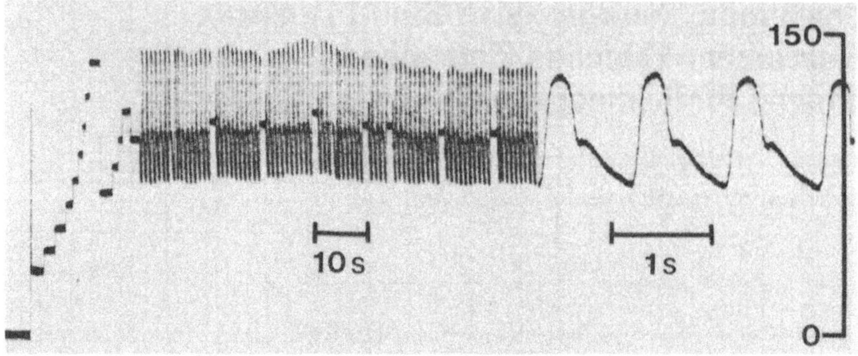

Fig. 2. Finger blood pressure curve recorded by the Finapres. It also shows a calibration staircase and the skipped beats occurring during the automatic calibration procedures. The vertical scale is in millimetres of mercury

neously. For calibration purposes a special automatic procedure is incorporated which momentarily brings cuff pressure stepwise to the level at which the plethysmographic amplitude is maximal. Since this means that cuff pressure is equal to mean arterial pressure, the system is calibrated. This procedure is repeated frequently during the measurement and the end result is that the variations in cuff pressure are at all times identical with the arterial pressure pulsations (Fig. 2).

Comparison of the Finapres with other methods of measuring blood pressure has been performed in other clinical centres. Wesseling at al. [3] compared the Finapres with Riva-Rocci-Korotkov measurements in the upper arm in healthy volunteers and Molhoek et al. [1] made a comparison with invasive brachial artery measurements in awake patients suspected of having hypertension. In both studies a good correlation was found when the normal gradient in pulse pressure along the arterial vascular bed of the arm was taken into account.

However, in contrast to the studies in awake resting subjects reactive vasoconstriction of the peripheral vascular bed often occurs during administration of anaesthetics for surgical procedures. Such a vasoconstriction, meaning an increase in vascular smooth muscle tone, is already contra-acting the intravascular pressure. It might be expected therefore that during vasoconstriction less pressure would be needed in the finger cuff to keep the plethysmographic excursions to a minimum. Since the Finapres only measures the pressure in the cuff, it is to be expected that during peripheral vasoconstriction its readings will be erroneously low. Therefore we have compared the Finapres with upper arm blood pressure in six female patients undergoing gynaecological surgery under general anaesthesia. Volatile anaesthetics were avoided and anaesthesia was deliberately maintained at a light level, so that reactive vasoconstrictions would occur frequently. To assess the occurrence of vasoconstriction the reflection plethysmogram was recorded from the end phalanx of a finger adjacent to the finger in which the blood pressure was measured with the Finapres. A decrease in amplitude of this end phalanx plethysmogram was interpreted as peripheral vasoconstriction. Upper arm pressure was measured at the contralateral side with the Dinamap oscillometric technique. The Dinamap cuff was inflated every 2 min and the precise timing of the Dinamap measurements was established from another plethysmogram recorded distal to the Dinamap cuff.

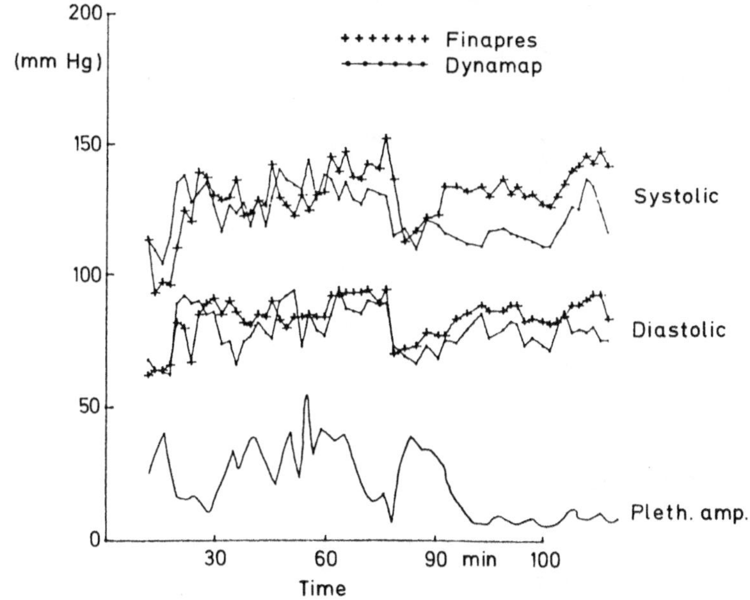

Fig. 3. Computer plot of blood pressures and amplitude of the end phalanx plethysmogram in one patient

Figure 3 shows a typical example of the results obtained in one patient. From this example it may be noted in the first place that the amplitude of the plethysmogram decreased repeatedly and irregularly, indicating the occurrence of peripheral vasoconstriction. Furthermore it may be seen already that during the periods of vasoconstriction the finger pressures deviated from the upper arm values and that the difference in systolic pressure became particularly prominent.

This figure also indicates that approximately 60 sets of pressure values were collected. For each patient these sets of paired pressure differences between finger and upper arm were averaged and tabulated. Table 1 shows the average Dinamap readings for each patient together with the deviations of the Finapres. The results of 378 readings show that the diastolic and mean pressures in the finger are on average 9–10 mm Hg below those in the upper arm and that the systolic pressure in the finger is found to be ± 7 mm Hg above that in the upper arm. Since these results are not grossly at variance with textbook teaching, it may be concluded that, contrary to our theoretical expectations, the Finapres does not give erroneously low readings when peripheral vasoconstriction occurs.

For the explanation of this unexpected result, it must be remembered that the plethysmographic transducer of the Finapres is surrounded by an inflated cuff. We believe that the externally applied pressure around the finger produces a change in the underlying vascular bed which prevents the occurrence of vasoconstriction reactions under the cuff, so that the plethysmogram controlling the Finapres is not affected and the measuring is not disturbed.

Having concluded and explained in this way that the Finapres readings are not disturbed by vasoconstriction, it must be remembered that in all patients the systolic pressure in the finger was not only not lowered but even exceeded the pressure in the upper arm. To study whether this discrepancy was connected with the

Table 1. Deviations of the averaged Finapres readings with respect to the upper arm values

Patient	Systolic			Diastolic			Mean			n
	$\bar{p}$	m	s	$\bar{p}$	m	s	$\bar{p}$	m	s	
443	127	−3.3	9.5	91	−14.2	5.6	103	−15.3	4.5	63
444	125	4.3	11.8	76	−10.5	7.0	96	−14.3	7.2	55
445	122	6.5	12.2	78	4.2	7.5	97	−3.8	6.5	58
446	118	9.9	12.4	79	−10.3	7.3	92	−8.6	8.5	61
447	134	18.0	14.5	94	−18.2	8.8	107	−10.8	10.1	64
448	133	4.1	7.4	85	−5.5	3.6	98	−5.7	4.9	77
Mean	127	7.0	11.0	84	−9.1	7.0	99	−10.0	7.0	Total 378

$\bar{p}$, average Dinamap pressure during the operation; m, mean difference in mmHg; s, standard deviation of the difference; n, number of readings

Table 2. Correlation coefficient (r) of the linear regression between the paired pressure differences and the corresponding amplitudes of the end phalanx plethysmogram

Patient	n	ΔSystolic r	ΔDiastolic r	ΔMean r
443	63	−0.58[a]	−0.33[a]	−0.03
444	55	−0.42[a]	+0.06	−0.03
445	58	−0.54[a]	−0.15	−0.35[a]
446	61	−0.52[a]	−0.41[a]	−0.41[a]
447	64	−0.38[a]	−0.12	−0.18
448	77	−0.59[a]	−0.20	−0.45[a]

[a] significant at $P=0.01$

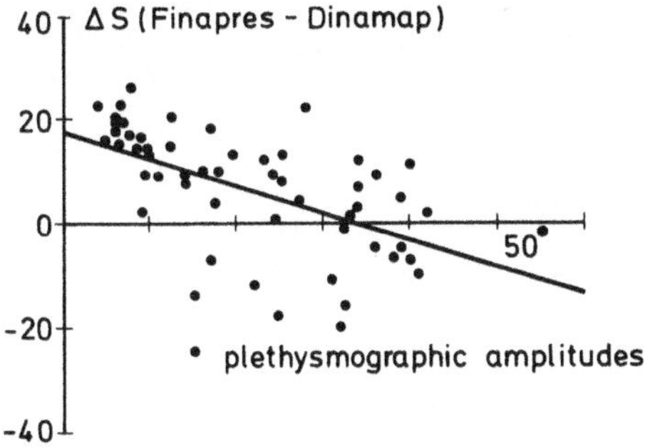

Fig. 4. Scattergram of the paired systolic pressure differences between Finapres and Dinamap versus the simultaneously obtained plethysmographic amplitudes

occurrence of vasoconstriction the paired pressure differences between finger and upper arm were compared with the simultaneously recorded amplitude of the end phalanx plethysmogram. Figure 4 gives the scattergram of this comparison. The slope of the linear regression line shows that with an increasing degree of peripheral vasoconstriction the arterial pressures in the finger had the tendency to rise more than those in the upper arm and even exceeded them by 20 mm Hg (and sometimes even by 30 or 40 mm Hg).

When for each patient the linear regression coefficients for systolic, diastolic and mean pressures were computed (Table 2), it was found that only for the systolic pressure differences were all coefficients significant at the 1% level. This means that the rise in systolic pressure in the finger was significantly more than that in the upper arm.

An increase in systolic pressure from proximal to distal along an arm has been described by other investigators and is attributed to reflection of the pressure waves against the peripheral vascular bed. The reflected pressure wave produces an amplification effect which affects systolic pressure most. Since during peripheral vasoconstriction the reflected wave will become enhanced, systolic pressure in the finger will rise more than that in the upper arm. Therefore it may be expected that the high systolic values indicated by the Finapres during vasoconstriction indeed represent the real pressure in the finger.

On the other hand when peripheral vasoconstriction has such an influence on the systolic pressure difference along an arm, vasodilatation must have an opposite effect. Figure 5 shows an example of our present studies, in which volunteers are riding a bicycle-ergometer. Blood pressure was again measured with the Finapres in the finger and with the Dinamap in the upper arm. From another finger an end phalanx plethysmogram was recorded. It may be noted from this figure that both systolic pressures at first rose in parallel but that at a given moment a marked deviation occurred. This moment always coincided with the moment the patient began the feel hot and to perspire. The discrepancy remained until the maximum exertion was reached and it then rapidly disappeared. We think that the systolic pressure in the finger lagged behind because of the occurrence of a pronounced vasodilatation in the fingers which is needed to conduct the produced heat away. The rise in plethysmographic amplitude indeed suggests a dilatation in the precapillary arteries, but in view of the enormous deviation in systolic pressure we think that the arteriovenous anastomoses participate to a large extent (see Dorlas, this volume, "New approaches of photoelectric plethysmography").

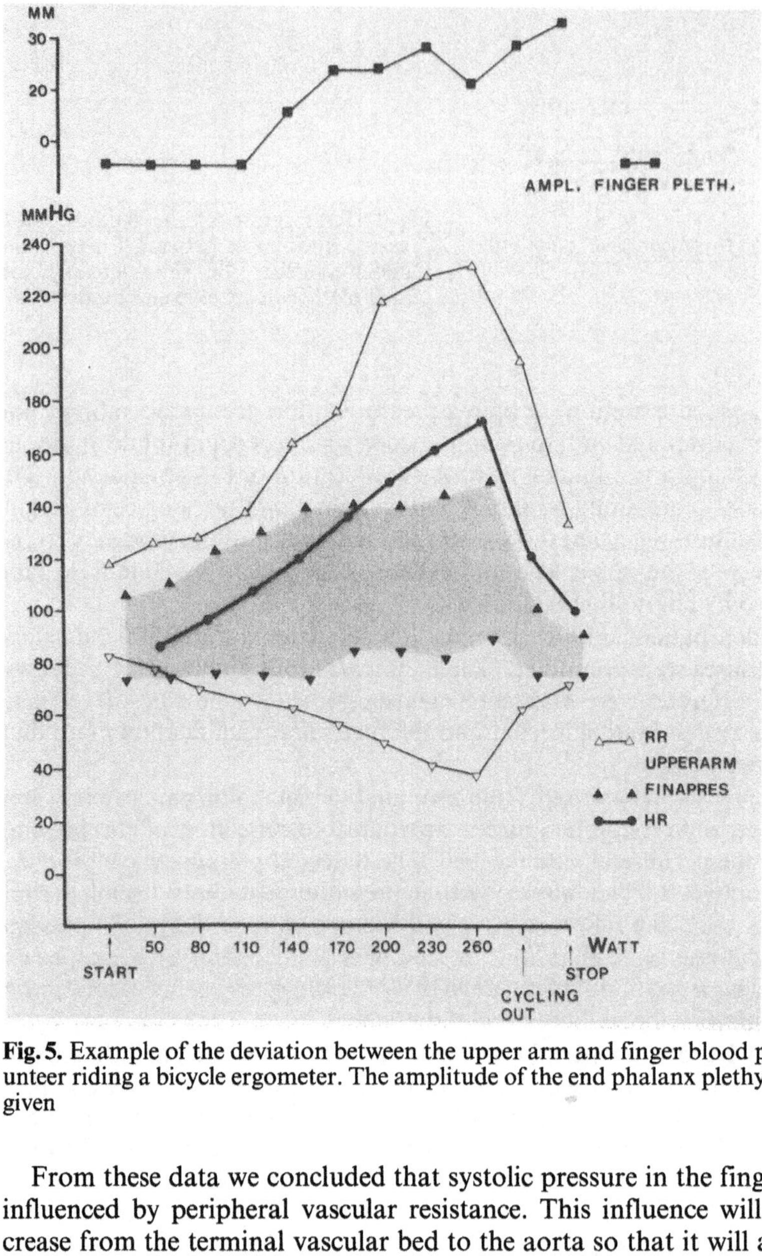

Fig. 5. Example of the deviation between the upper arm and finger blood pressure in a volunteer riding a bicycle ergometer. The amplitude of the end phalanx plethysmogram is also given

From these data we concluded that systolic pressure in the finger is markedly influenced by peripheral vascular resistance. This influence will gradually decrease from the terminal vascular bed to the aorta so that it will also be present in the radial artery, which is the most distal site accessible for invasive blood pressure measurement. Since in anaesthesia the radial artery is also most often used for this purpose, the pressure at this site should be used to give reference values in a further study to determine the accuracy and precision of the Finapres.

In conclusion this study shows that the Finapres continues to function well during peripheral vasoconstriction. However, for the interpretation of blood pressures measured distally it must be realized that a change in peripheral vascular resistance may produce a real shift in the ratio between central and peripheral blood pressure.

References

1. Molhoek PG, Wesseling KH, Arntzenius AC, Settels JJ, van Vollenhoven J, Weeda HWH (1983) Initial results of noninvasive measurement of finger blood pressure according to Penaz. Automedica 4:241–246
2. Penaz J, Voigt A, Teichmann W (1976) Beitrag zur fortlaufenden indirekten Blutdruckmessung. Z Gesamte Inn Med 31:1030–1033
3. Wesseling KH, Wit de B, Settels JJ, Klawer WH (1982) On the indirect registration of ginger blood pressure after Penaz. Funkt Biol Med 1:245–250
4. Yamakashi Ken-Ichi, Hideaki Shimazu, Tatsuo Togawa (1979) Indirect measurement of instantaneous arterial blood pressure in the rat. Am J Physiol 237(5):H632–H637

A New Approach to Photoelectric Plethysmography

J.C. Dorlas, J.A. Nijboer, S.J. Edema, and J.O.J. Prins

Photoelectric plethysmography has already been used for a very long time to monitor the circulation during anaesthesia, because it is a non-invasive method which can be applied easily and rapidly. Because of the accessibility during anaesthesia it is almost exclusively applied to the skin of the fingers, toes or ears. During the past few years much more knowledge has been acquired about the background of the method and in this paper we intend to present a review of our research with this method in approximately 500 patients. In particular the difference between the plethysmograms recorded from finger and earshell will be discussed. The review is preceded by an explanation of the basic principles.

The principle of the method is quite simple (Fig. 1). A small light source is attached to an appropriate part of the skin. The emitted light is multiply scattered and partly absorbed in the tissues. Another part of the light emerges again through the skin and is detected by a photosensitive detector (photoelectric cell) which is applied either besides or opposite to the light source. This results in the reflection or transmission method respectively. The intensity of the light detected by the photo cell is determined by the optical density of the solid tissues such as skin, connective tissue and bone and that of the varying amount of blood in the vascular bed. Since blood has a higher light absorption coefficient than the surrounding tissues, variations in the amount of blood give rise to alterations in the

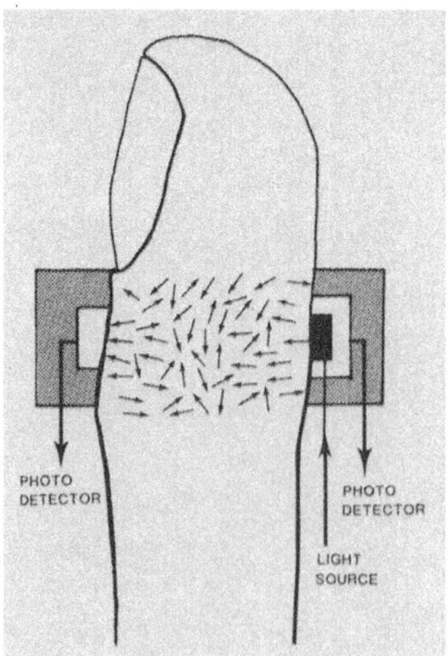

Fig. 1. Sketch of a photoelectric transducer in the reflection and transmission mode

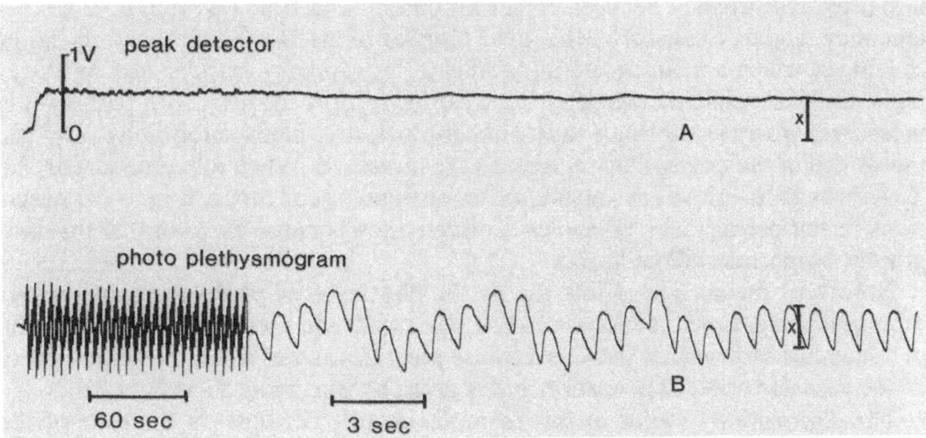

Fig. 2. Photoelectric finger plethysmogram recorded with two paper speeds. B, rapid arterial pulse waves and slower ventilatory waves. *On the right side* the ventilation is stopped temporarily. A, arterial pulse amplitude calculated by a new peakdetector which is not influenced by ventilatory waves. I, height of the arterial pulsations

total amount of light detected. These variations are only small and are proportional (1%–2%) to the total amount of light detected. Only these variations in light are amplified and converted to a voltage signal which can be continuously displayed and recorded as a plethysmogram. In most plethysmographs a decrease in light is recorded as an upward reflection in the plethysmogram.

Figure 2 B shows the plethysmogram of an anaesthetized patient recorded with two different paper speeds. Two wave forms can be distinguished. The rapid excursions run synchronously with the heart action and are called arterial pulsations. The slower waves run synchronously with the ventilation and are caused by volume changes in the venous vascular bed brought about by changes in intrathoracic pressure. The arterial pulse wave is generally used for monitoring purposes, because its amplitude indicates to what extent the arterial blood pulsations reach the periphery. However, during anaesthesia the amplitude of the arterial pulsations is often very difficult to distinguish from the ventilatory waves, which become especially prominent during artificial ventilation, airway obstruction and hypovolaemic states. Therefore a new kind of peak detector is developed which eliminates the ventilatory waves and which indicates the amplitude of the arterial pulsations only (Fig. 2 A). For the interpretation of changes in the arterial amplitude it must be realized in the first place that in fact changes in light are measured which are proportional to the total amount of light detected and which cannot be calibrated. Therefore the amplitude of the photoelectric plethysmogram does not give the height of the arterial pulse wave in a quantitative way. On the other hand it has been proved that changes in the amplitude occurring during one uninterrupted registration correlate very well with changes in blood volume.

Several investigators have reported that the changes in amplitude also correlate well with changes in total blood flow. We have checked this correlation during anaesthesia by a comparison between the changes in finger amplitude and in total blood flow in the finger, measured by venous occlusion plethysmography. Although this study also showed a good correlation in most of the cases, sometimes a marked discrepancy between finger amplitude and flow was found. This discrepancy might be caused by the great number of arteriovenous anastomoses in the finger, which are connected in parallel to the capillary vascular bed. With venous occlusion plethysmography the total blood flow through both pathways is measured, whereas we think that with photoelectric plethysmography only the pulsations in the precapillary arterioles are measured. When for some reason the flow through arteriovenous anastomoses changes out of proportion to the pulsations in the precapillary arterioles a discrepancy between flow and plethysmographic amplitude will be found.

However, irrespective of this theory the photoelectric plethysmogram always represents pulsations of blood volume. Its amplitude therefore depends on the pressure variation within the vessel (pulse pressure) as well as on the distensibility of the vascular wall. This relationship is given by Burton as $\Delta V = D \cdot \Delta P$.

The distensibility factor in this formular mainly depends on the tone of the vascular smooth muscles which is controlled by impulses of the autonomic nervous system. The influence of the vascular smooth muscles is so strong that the effect of vasoconstriction or vasodilatation can completely predominate the effect of pulse pressure in several regions of the body.

Although these principles hold for both the finger and the ear plethysmogram, a striking difference in their response to various stimuli is found during anaesthesia. Figure 3 shows the plethysmograms from finger and earshell recorded simultaneously during the beginning of an anaesthetic. *Upon induction* the most striking phenomenon is the marked rise in amplitude which occurs in the finger plethysmogram and which does not occur in the ear plethysmogram. The increase in finger amplitude we have recorded in 95% of inductions independent of the induction agent used. Furthermore it is independent of pulse pressure which in particular does not rise. Therefore the increase in finger amplitude has to be attributed to a decrease in vascular smooth muscle tone, i.e. a vasodilatation. Since this vasodilatation is found particularly in the fingers, where the vascular walls are

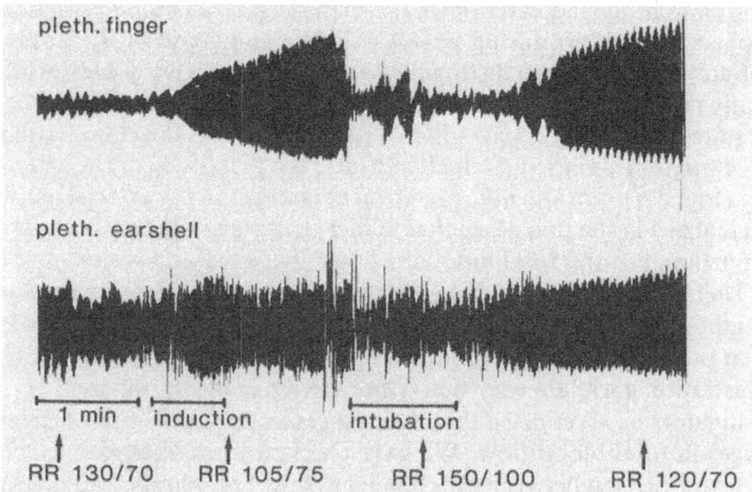

Fig. 3. Photoelectric plethysmograms recorded simultaneously from finger and earshell during the beginning of the administration of an anaesthetic

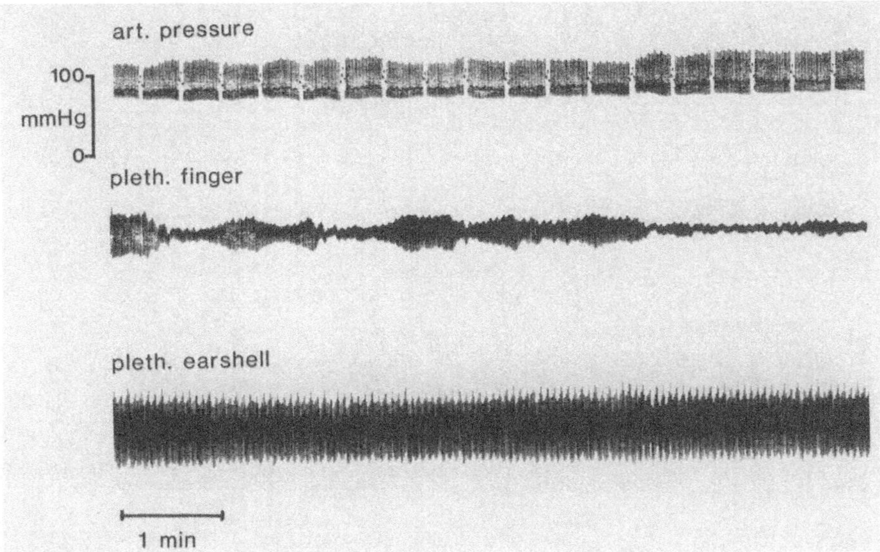

Fig. 4. Responses to stressful surgical stimuli occurring simultaneously in finger and ear plethysmogram and in arterial blood pressure

only α-sympathetically innervated, it is explained by a loss of sympathetic tone – induced at cerebral level – by the suppression of psychic stimuli. Therefore we call it an induction sympatolysis. *The intubation period* on the other hand produces a profound fall in amplitude which is also typical for the finger plethysmogram and which does not occur in the ear plethysmogram. Since this fall in amplitude is not accompanied by a fall in pulse pressure it has to be caused by constriction of the vascular smooth muscles under the influence of sympathetic impulses. In fact pulse pressure even rises during intubation, which shows that the constriction of the vascular smooth muscles even predominates the effect of pulse pressure (after intubation the dilatation in the finger plethysmogram resumes its cause and ventilatory waves become prominent).

During surgery shorter or longer periods of finger vasoconstriction arose in ±75% of our recordings (Fig. 4). They were always accompanied by a small rise in systolic blood pressure but the ear plethysmogram remained all but stable. In analogy to the intubation effect these reactions have to be due to α-adrenergic responses to stressful stimuli during surgery. *Towards the end of surgery* a gradual fall in amplitude has been found in ±80% of our recordings (Fig. 5). It is not accompanied by a decrease in ear amplitude and it can be explained neither by a rise in expiratory CO_2 nor by a fall in pulse pressure. It therefore has to be caused by a vasoconstriction, i.e. a rise in sympathetic tone during a lighter plane of anaesthesia.

From these observations it is evident that amplitude changes in the responsive finger plethysmogram are determined by variations in distensibility of the cutaneous finger vessels under the influence of sympathetic stimuli.

However, Fig. 6 shows that the reactivity of the finger plethysmogram can be inhibited by several anaesthetic agents, as is shown here for dehydrobenzperidol (DHB), which prevents the vasoconstriction reactions from occurring. Similar ef-

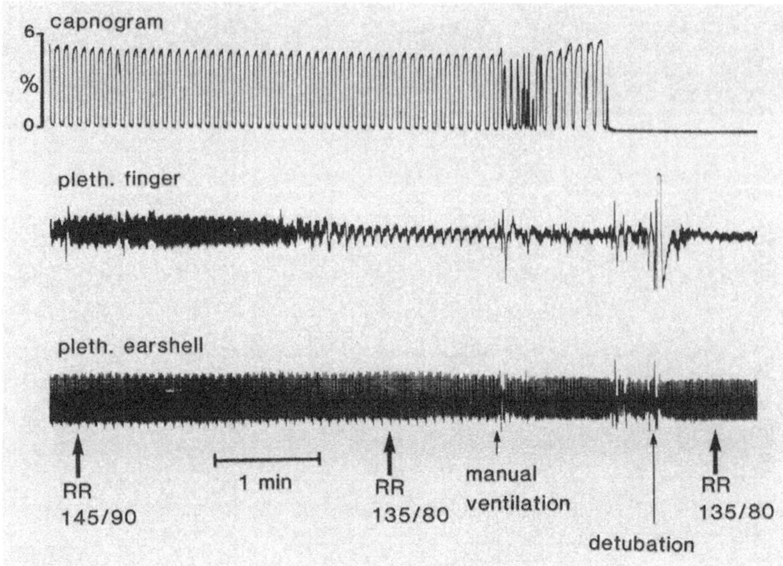

Fig. 5. "Normal" pattern in the period of regaining consciousness

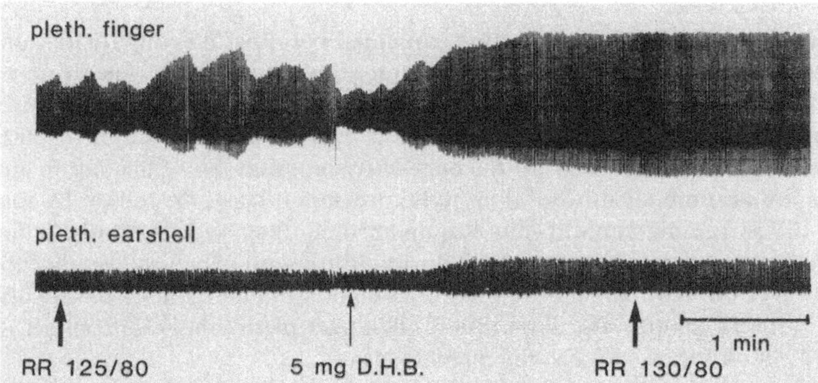

Fig. 6. Effect of dehydrobenzperidol on the reactivity of the finger plethysmogram

fects can be seen with, e.g. halothane, fentanyl and pethidine. The blocking effect of these agents is dose dependent and varies from patient to patient. Therefore it is our opinion that the amplitude pattern of the finger plethysmogram may also be used to monitor the effect of "stress-free" anaesthesia. However, it must be realized then that, depending upon the degree of blockade, the finger amplitude will respond more and more to changes in pulse pressure only. As to the ear plethysmogram we have already seen that vasoconstriction reactions to α-adrenergic stimuli hardly ever occur. Therefore it might be expected that the ear amplitude would always respond to pulse pressure only. Figure 7 indeed shows a gradual fall in ear amplitude which is accompanied by a decrease in systolic blood pressure whereas the finger amplitude and the expiratory CO_2 remain all but stable. This sometimes happens directly after the beginning of a laparotomy and placing of

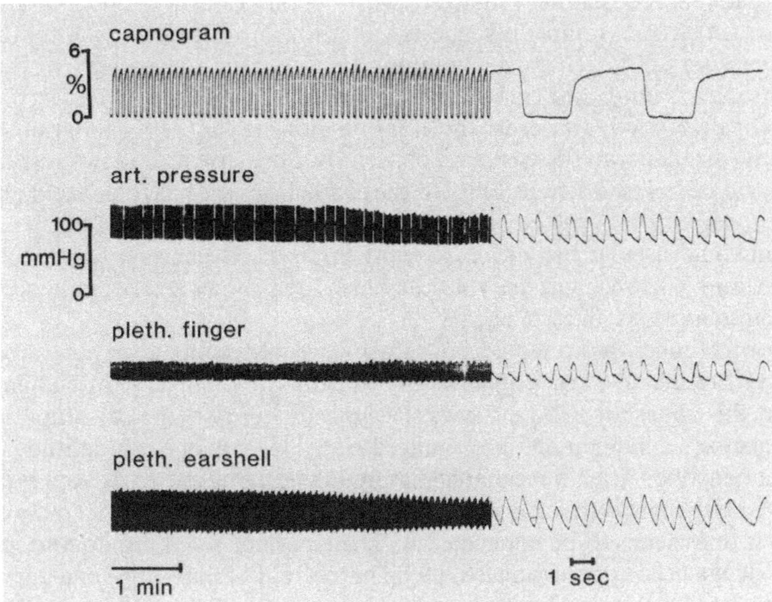

Fig. 7. Decrease in amplitude of the ear plethysmogram in comparison with some other variables at the onset of intra-abdominal manipulations

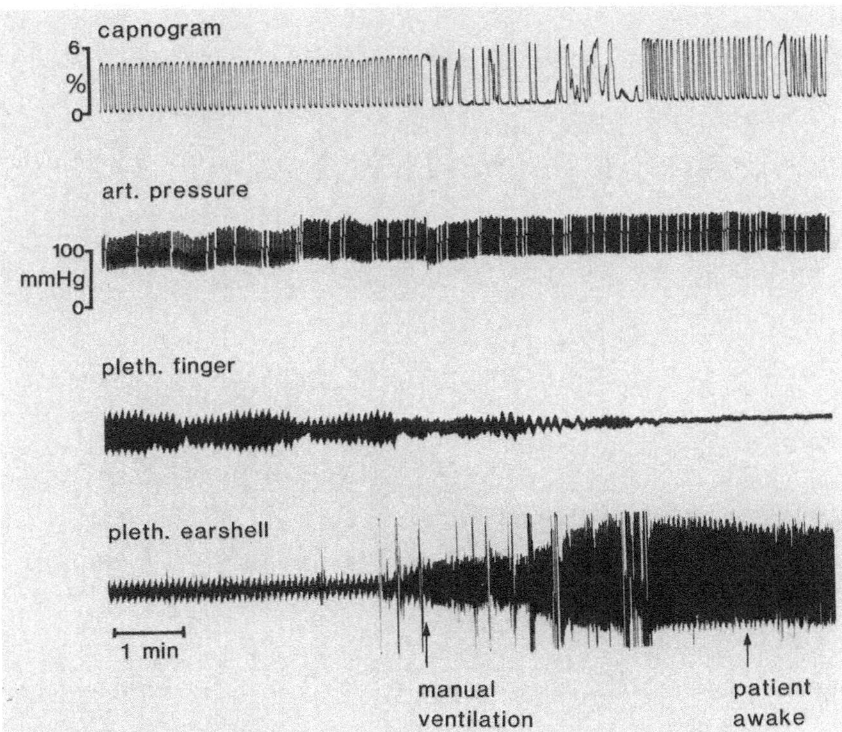

Fig. 8. Example of a sudden and marked rise in ear amplitude which sometimes occurs when the patient is regaining consciousness

abdominal pads. Since this may interfere with venous return, producing a decrease in cardiac stroke volume, it suggests a relationship between ear amplitude and pulse pressure (and even stroke volume). However, in a retrospective study of 100 recordings a significant correlation between ear amplitude and pulse pressure could not be proved. Therefore the amplitude of the ear plethysmogram has to depend on vascular wall distensibility as well. But because it does not respond to α-adrenergic stimuli the distensibility of the earshell vessels has to be controlled by a different mediator. A difference in control between the so-called blush area and the cutaneous vascular bed of the extremities has also been reported by other investigators and Burton suggested that the blush area shows a predominance of control by circulating vasoactive agents.

Such a control mechanism would fall in with two phenomena we have sometimes observed to occur. Figure 8 shows that during the final stage of an anaesthetic, when the finger amplitude shows the typical decrease, the ear amplitude occasionally shows a sudden and pronounced rise. This rise in ear amplitude occurs spontaneously or after a mechanical stimulus but without a corresponding further rise in pulse pressure or a significant increase in expiratory CO_2. On the other hand it does seem to be connected with the patient's waking up and with the kind of drugs used for the anaesthetic. Therefore it is tempting to suggest a relationship with the release of some vasoactive agent. A similar sudden and pronounced rise in ear amplitude has occasionally been recorded during surgery (Fig. 9). It has been observed in the ear or finger plethysmogram separately as well as

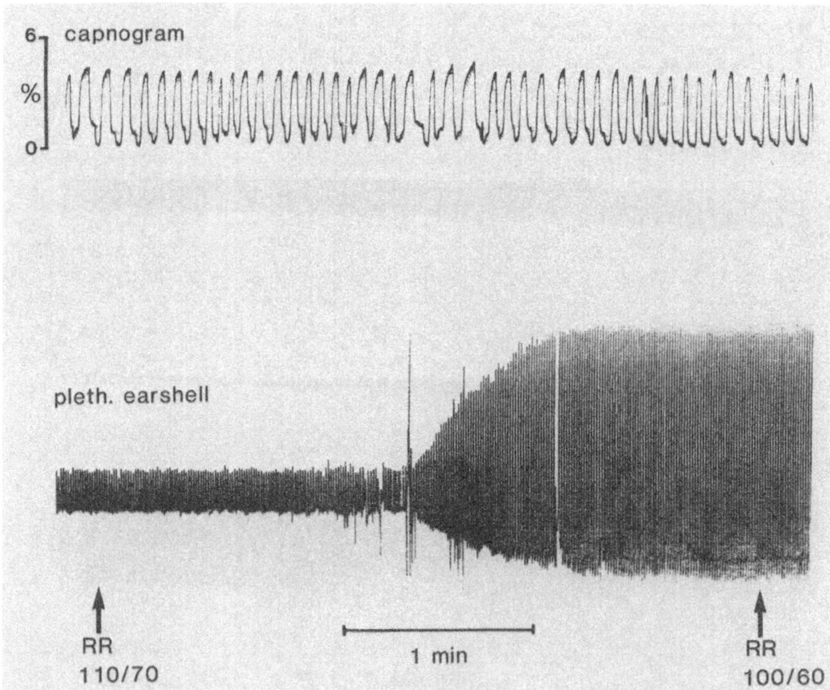

Fig. 9. Sudden and large rise in plethysmographic amplitude in a spontaneously breathing patient during surgery under general anaesthesia

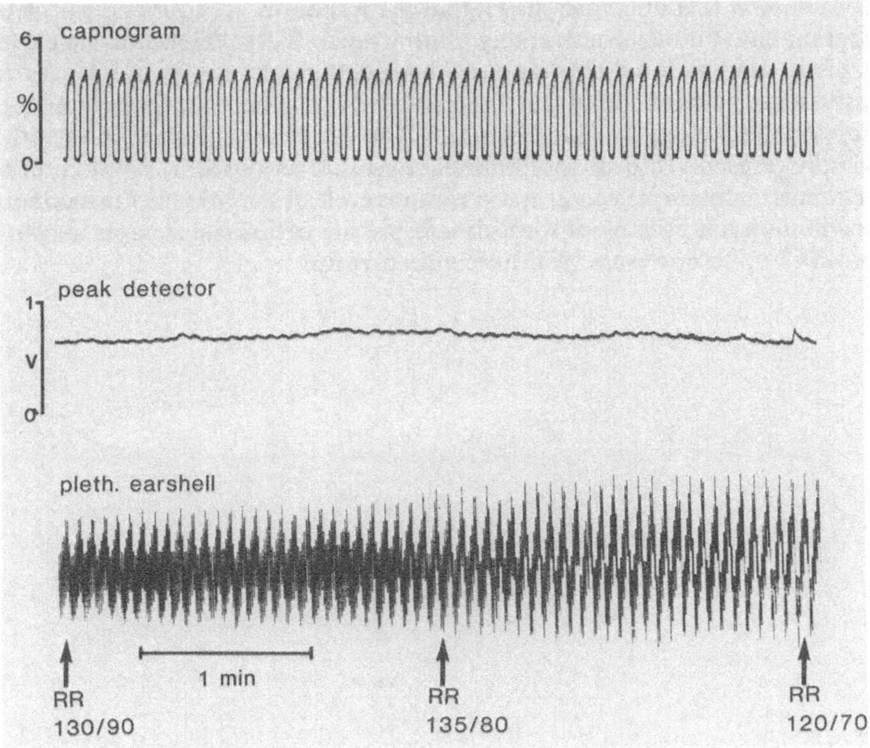

Fig. 10. Increase in height of the ventilatory waves due to the development of hypovolaemia (unchanged ventilation pressures)

in both, and we think it is also of humoral origin, probably as a result of a weak allergic reaction. From some preliminary experiments we have the impression that these humoral reactions in the photoelectric plethysmogram are not accompanied by an equal rise in total finger blood flow or with a rise in pulse pressure. Therefore we think that in these special cases the vasodilatation occurs only in the precapillary arterioles and not in the arteriovenous anastomoses.

Finally changes in the ventilatory waves may also have some diagnostic significance. Figure 10 shows a gradual increase in the height of the ventilatory waves which is due to the development of hypovolaemia. For the explanation it must be remembered that the height of the ventilatory waves depends mainly on the relationship between central venous pressure and the variations in intrathoracic pressure, caused by the ventilation. However, to what extent these pressure variations are reflected in the plethysmogram also depends on the distensibility of the venous walls. Since in hypovolaemia the stretch of the venous walls is decreased, the height of the ventilatory waves will rise despite unchanged ventilation pressures. This may happen independently of eventual changes in arterial pulse amplitude or in expiratory CO_2 level. On account of these considerations an increase in ventilatory waves arising during administration of an anaesthetic with unchanged ventilation pressures is interpreted in our department as a sign of (relative) hypovolaemia.

In conclusion this study has shown that the responses in finger and ear plethysmogram may differ considerably during anaesthesia. Generally speaking changes in amplitude of the finger plethysmogram may be interpreted as responses to sympathetic stimuli but if this reactivity is blocked the finger amplitude will only reflect changes in pulse pressure. The ear plethysmogram on the other hand hardly responds to stressful stimuli but seems very suitable for monitoring the systemic circulation in general and perhaps even stroke volume. Furthermore, a contribution has been made towards interpreting occasional changes in amplitude, which up to now were very difficult to explain.

High-Amplification Electrocardiography [1]

A. Varenne

High-amplification electrocardiography (HA-ECG), which we defined [51] as "the surface recording of the entire electric cardiac activity", started in 1973 with the first non-invasive recordings of His bundle potentials performed quasi-simultaneously by Berbari et al. [2, 3], Flowers et al. [19, 20] and Stopczyk et al. [42], working independently. Then, the same technique was used to detect sinus node activity (Stopczyk et al. [43]) and subsequently the abnormal micropotentials in myocardial ischaemia (Berbari et al. [4]). But the application of HA-ECG is not only limited to recording of cardiac micropotentials; we have demonstrated the advantages of HA-ECG methods in classic electrocardiography (Varenne et al. [50]). Now, 10 years after its introduction, we need to question the present state of HA-ECG, results obtained and expected developments.

Principle and Techniques of HA-ECG

The physiological micropotentials of the conduction system – or the pathological ones issued from the damaged myocardium – cannot be recorded by the classic Einthoven ECG. These very weak signals – of the order of microvolts – are merged into a background noise which is generally ten times greater. This noise – varying with individuals and circumstances – arises from different sources [15]: (1) a physiological noise of about 20 μV caused by muscle activities and respiration movements; (2) an electromagnetic noise related to the alternative current and which is highly variable; in favourable situations, this noise is about 3 μV; and (3) interference signals resulting from the interface skin-electrodes and the amplifier noise; this noise is estimated to be between 1 and 3 μV.

Finally, in favourable measuring conditions, the background noise varies between 10 and 30 μV peak-to-peak. As the His signal has an amplitude of between 1 and 5 μV, its surface recording cannot be obtained just by increasing the amplification gain, but also needs the use of a method to improve the signal-to-noise ratio. The summation-averaging method is used to this end. The fundamental condition for the application of this method is that the expected signal is repetitive

[1] This research was carried out with the collaboration of J. P. Camous, Ph. Blanc and M. Simon and the technical assistance of A. Bally. Grants were received from the "Délégation Générale à la Recherche Scientifique et Technique" (No. 77-7-2028 and 80-7-0397), the "Université de Nicé and the "Association Niçoise pour l'Etude et la Recherche sur les Affections Cardio-vasculaires".

and regular, whereas the noise is variable and at random. In this case, the averaging method will improve the signal-to-noise ratio as the square root of the number of sums. For example, summation of cardiac cycles, identical and strictly synchronized, will allow up to a 5-μV periodic signal to emerge from a 30-μV noise, after a 100-cycle summation-averaging, which, in turn, will increase by 10 the signal-to-noise ratio. Two approaches are possible in the application of the signal averaging method:

1. Sequential averaging, where *n* consecutive cardiac cycles are summed, the signal-to-noise ratio improvement being theoretically proportional to the number of cycles averaged. In practice, and because of slight variations in these biological signals, the optimal number is between 100 and 300 cardiac cycles. This sequential averaging method is today the basis of HA-ECG. It makes possible for statistical studies of the electrical data of cardiac activation.
2. Spatial averaging, which processes the same cardiac cycle recorded from multiple-surface electrodes. Hence, it could allow a beat-to-beat analysis of the cardiac activity and represent the future ideal development of HA-ECG. But it remains a laboratory technique, needing high electromagnetic insulation and sophisticated electronic equipment [21, 31, 44, 56].

All these averaging methods require strict synchronization between the summed signals, which can be obtained by electronic triggering, with a threshold based on the QRS amplitude, or using a pattern recognition method (template matching). Apart from the averaging method, HA-ECG needs other technical conditions: high-gain amplification (1000–10000 times more than the usual ECG gain) using very low noise amplifiers; selective filtering – in order to eliminate undesirable frequencies – like a 50-Hz or 60-Hz noise – whilst respecting the passband of the expected signal; and signal digitization using analog-digital converters. These converters convert the continuous cardiac signal into samples (for example, 1000 μs if the sampling rate is 1000 Hz, 2000 μs if it is 500 Hz) and combine a numerical value (represented by the binary series) with the voltage or electric current of this sample. The higher the resolution power of the converters – expressed in bits – the more precise the conversion will be. Therefore, HA-ECG is sometimes known as high-resolution electrocardiography (HR-ECG). The digital conversion of the cardiac signal permits it to be processed by computers. Hence, most of the HA-ECG devices are microcomputer designed.

The Pancardiograph System and the Recording Procedure

Our first data on His recordings were obtained in 1978 [49] by means of an experimental research system designed in collaboration with Demartini [53]. It was an open, programmable device, microcomputer based, allowing software signal processing and on-line printing of results. Following this experiment, we have contributed to the development of a commercially available HA-ECG system, the "Pancardiograph" (Fig. 1). It is composed of: (1) hardware with: a three-channel amplification system, a 12-bit resolution data logger module, a microcomputer (built-in 2 × 140 K floppy discs, 64 K RAM), and a display console and a plotter;

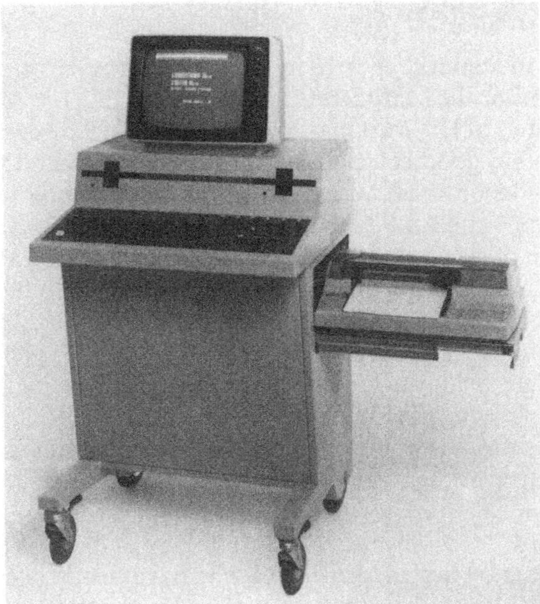

Fig. 1. The Pancardiograph – now produced by ODAM S.A (67160 Wissenbourg, France) – is a three-channel HA-ECG recorder. It is also a multifunction machine for signal processing, software based and directly programmable by the operator. The plotter is mobile and can be pushed back into the basement like a drawer

and (2) software designed to execute a summation-averaging procedure, using signal synchronization, pattern recognition, digital processing and on-line printing of the results. Therefore, it is a conversational data-processing machine, which enables us to choose the cardiac complex (normal or premature) to be introduced into the averaging procedure, to select gains, bandpass filtering, sampling rates, display of signals and selective printing of the three recording leads, or of one of them with a simultaneous normal gain ECG reference. Besides the scalar editions, it makes possible a vectorcardiographic representation of any moment of the cardiac cycle, selected by the operator, using two movable electronic indexes. Other programmes available on magnetic disks give the Pancardiograph a multifunctional capacity and mean that it is the first evolving system in the digital processing of cardiac signals. HA-ECG recordings are performed at the bedside or in a normal examination room, without Faraday's cage. But an excellent earth and the use of short and insulated cables are necessary precautions. Skin impedance is reduced by cleaning and rubbing it, and the patient is invited to relax the muscles. We use prejellified silver/silver chloride ECG electrodes (Red Dots-3M), which are normally positioned according to a three bipolar orthogonal lead system: X the horizontal lead (V6R, negative; V6, positive), Y the frontal lead (nape, negative; epigastrium, positive) and Z the sagittal lead (xyphoid, negative; level of the fifth dorsal vertebra, positive). But the flexibility of the programmes enables the three bipolar leads in other positions to be used, for instance, in a unipolar mode [25] or for intracardiac and surface simultaneous recordings. Save for the choice of the analog high-pass filter (adjustable from 0 to 80 Hz) and of the gains, all the procedures – such as sampling frequency, signal recognition, number of summations, additive digital filters or gains and display of signal or printing are software determined. The signal to be averaged is visually selected by the operator and will serve to pilot the summation-averaging procedure.

Surface Recording of His-Purkinje System Activity

Since the first studies in dogs and in humans reported in 1973, many groups, using either their own laboratory systems or the Marquette high-resolution ECG-MAC I, have published external recordings of His-Purkinje system potentials. However, despite these works and the fact that good correlations have been demonstrated between surface and endocardiac recordings, we have to admit that the non-invasive technique has not yet supplanted the catheter investigation. There are many reasons: (1) The percentage of successful surface recording (70%–85% according to some publications) is less than for the invasive technique, where failures are rare. (2) Intracardiac recordings enable programmed stimulations to be made, considered by some as an indispensable diagnostic tool. (3) The morphology of the surface signal is different from the bundle of His electrogram (Fig. 2) and the timing of the His bundle deflection is more difficult to determine. (4) The features of the surface recordings are not homogeneous in the various publications because of the lack of standardization in the parameters of the cardiac signal processing.

Responses to the two last points – concerning the morphology and the processing of the His signal – were given by Berbari et al. [3–6], who have clearly demonstrated, in remarkable experimental studies, that the surface leads provide an integrated view of the atrioventricular conduction, recording a multiphasic waveform (His-Purkinje system wave, HPS) which is composed of continuous activity from the AV node to the Purkinje cells. This HPS wave – which is reproducible and remains unchanged even in the absence of atrial activity – for instance, after crushing the sinus node – differs from the spike recorded by an intraventricular

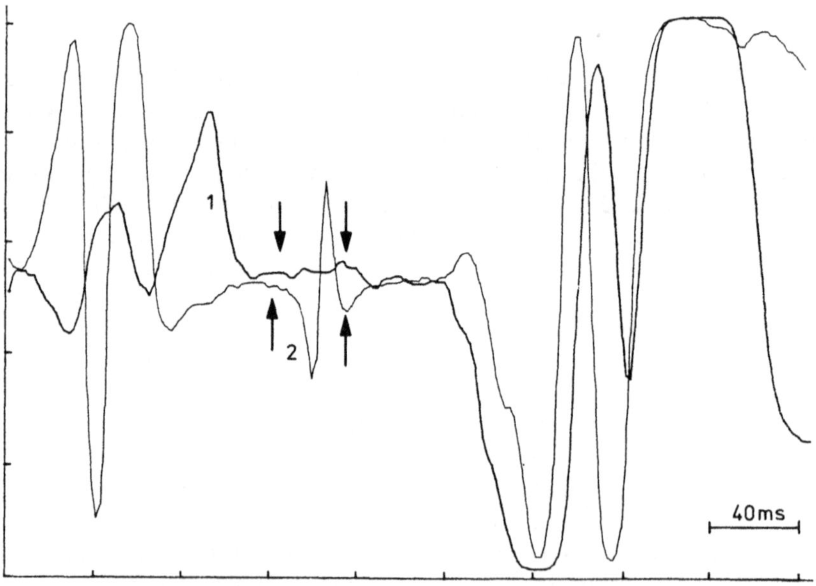

Fig. 2. Simultaneous surface (*trace 1*) and endocardiac (*trace 2*) His recordings, averaging 200 cardiac cycles. Bandwidth is 40–300 Hz. Note the differences between the multiphasic surface waveform and the diphasic endocardiac electrogram. HV is abnormal, 70 ms (divisions are 20 ms on the horizontal scale)

catheter positioned in very close proximity to the His bundle. Secondly, the differences in the recordings published are due to the technique of signal processing and particularly to the filtering. Thus, Berbari et al. [5] have shown that, by using Fourier's analysis in humans, almost 80% of the signals are below 50 Hz. Therefore, a 80- to 300-Hz bandwidth, used to attenuate the overlap of atrial activity, alters their morphology and their chronological relationships. Finally, during the past decade, the various research teams have tried to find, in the choice of filters, the optimal compromise between high-pass filtering (such as 80 Hz or more), which improves His bundle detection but induces some loss of information about physiological data, and filtering at low frequencies (under 20 Hz), which renders detection of the His bundle deflection more difficult and increases the overlap of atrial activity. But it is obvious that the development of HA-ECG will eventually need international standardization of the cardiac signal processing parameters.

In our routine procedure, we record the His bundle, using the 40- to 300-Hz bandwidth filter. Then, we make another edition of this recording increasing the low-frequency cutoff, and with gains to improve the chronological studies (Figs. 3 and 4).

To confirm the signals, we systematically perform two consecutive recordings comprising the same number of cycles (150 or 200 beats), according to the cleanness of the noise, controlled by the screen display, after every 50-beat acquisition. Comparisons of the two recordings enable the reproducibility of the HPS signals to be established – which, because of the residual noise – are similar, but not

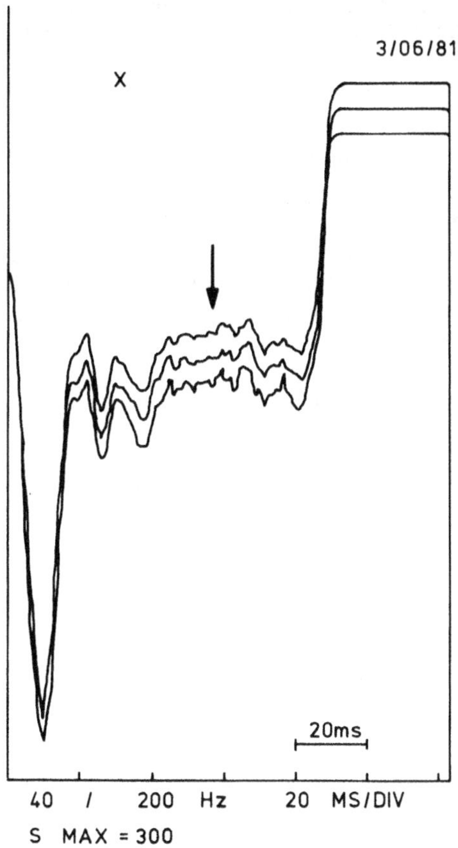

Fig. 3. Averaging procedure (300 beats): X orthogonal lead recording. Bandwidth is 40–200 Hz. Divisions are 20 ms on the horizontal scale. From bottom to top successive traces print each 100-beat acquisition. Noise is progressively attenuated. *Arrow,* His signal with HR = 40 ms

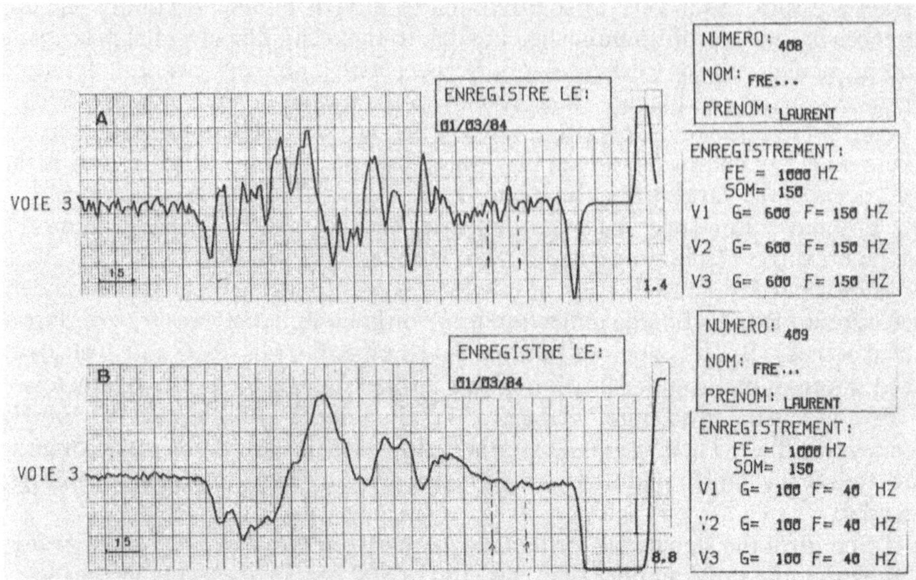

Fig. 4. Effects of gains and filters on the surface His waveform. Two successive recordings in a healthy 23-year-old man. A Very high amplification gain (vertical scale: 1 cm = 1.4 μV) and 150- to 300-Hz bandwidth. B Usual gain (vertical scale: 1 cm = 8.8 μV) and usual filter 40- to 300-Hz bandwidth). Changes in His signal morphology are seen. Timing of the His wave is easier to measure in A than in B. HV is normal at 37 ms (horizontal scale = 15 ms/division)

strictly identical. Intravenous drugs – such as verapamil or ajmaline – have been proposed for confirmation of the His surface recording, but their use is not free from risk of acute problems of conduction. The existence of a short PR interval (less than 0.12 s) makes the His surface recording difficult because of the overlap of atrial activity. Other difficulties or failures in the His surface recording can also be due to excessive muscular noise, electromagnetic interferences or some abnormal conditions such as short PR, atrial fibrillation, flutter or unstable disturbances in atrioventricular conduction. But using an automated discrimination circuit, Takeda et al. [46] were able to obtain successful recordings even in patients with complete atrioventricular blocks.

Our experience – which includes a study of more than 250 patients in the past 5 years – leads us to conclude that:

1. Using an HA-ECG system, which is progressively improving due to more sophisticated algorithms, we can now obtain non-invasive recordings of the His-Purkinje system in about 85% of patients with a normal sinus rhythm or prolonged PR interval. The vector-cardiographic approach – using the Frank system or, more simply, three orthogonal leads – increases the successful recordings and enables the collected signals to be correlated [33, 47, 51].
2. HA-ECG His recording can be used to detect conduction troubles below the level of the bundle of His and to select the litigious cases which justify an endocardiac investigation. Because it is a non-invasive examination, it can be easily used in cardiopaediatry [18, 38]. Above all, it enables repetitive record-

ings to be made in patients with an atrioventricular conduction borderline and who need antiarrhythmic drugs. Therefore, the technique provides for the safety and comfort of the patient and reduces the economical cost.

3. The surface signal is richer in information than the His bundle electrogram. Unfortunately, we are not yet able to give a complete interpretation of it. So, using standardized signal processing parameters, we must now describe a new semeiology, founded on numerous and careful correlations with the histological and clinical data.

Surface Recording of the Sinus Node

The first recording of pre-P electrical activity was performed in dogs by Stopczyk et al. [43], using prememorized signal averaging, and showed a good correlation with the intra-atrial recordings. In man, Stopczyk recorded a pre-P wave in 50% of cases but wondered about its possible origin from a muscular ring at the superior vena cava to the right atrial junction. Others [27, 32, 57] have reported non-invasive pre-P-wave recordings, with dissimilar results, especially in their duration and their relationship to the atrial activity. In fact, several reasons make the problem complex:

1. The physiological values of the sinus node potentials in humans are not well documented, because direct recordings – by epicardiac or endocardiac electrodes – are rare and difficult.
2. There are physiological fluctuations in the PR interval [36] and, probably, in the sinoatrial interval, which result in inadequate use of sequential averaging founded on QRS synchronization.
3. The sinus node activation is mainly a low-frequency phenomenon which can be distorted and even obliterated by filtering.
4. It can be difficult to establish the beginning of the atrial activation, in a one-lead recording, and here too the advantages of a vectorcardiographic approach (Fig. 5) are obvious.

The next decisive steps in non-invasive sinus node recordings would need beat-to-beat detection and P-wave synchronization. P-wave synchronization can be obtained by using an oesophageal lead, but the method is not totally non-invasive. Another way – in which we are engaged – is the direct recognition of P-wave by means of new algorithms.

Non-invasive Recording of Pathological Micropotentials

In fact, the ever-increasing interest in HA-ECG is principally related to the non-invasive recording of pathological cardiac micropotentials. In 1973, Boineau and Cox [7] demonstrated that fractionated and delayed electrical activities can be recorded from an ischaemic area. They suggested these potentials could induce – by intraventricular re-entry mechanisms – deleterious arrhythmias, and this hypothesis was confirmed later by El-Sherif et al. [16, 17]. First studied by epicardial or endocardial electrodes, these delayed potentials can easily be recorded by HA-ECG as demonstrated in dogs by Berbari et al. [4] and in man by Fontaine et al.

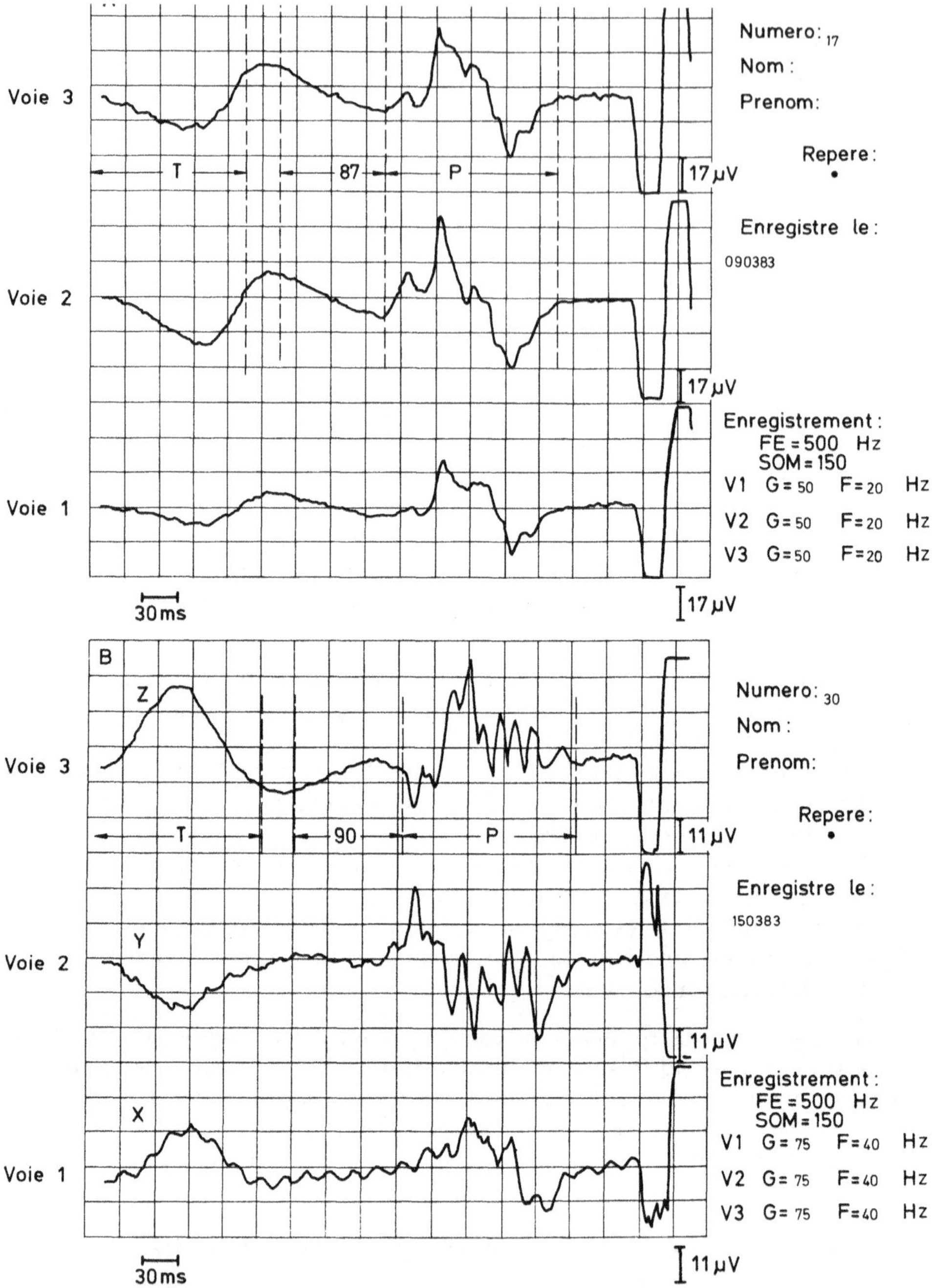

Fig. 5. Recording of pre-P-wave electrical activities. A shows three parallel precordial leads, with the electrode positioned in close vicinity: in VI–V4; 150 beat averaged. Bandwidth, 20–300 Hz; vertical scale, 17 µV/division; horizontal scale, 30 ms/division. The end of the T-wave is followed by an 87-ms-duration slope (1), then by a fast wave of 27 µs duration (2 a) and finally by the whole atrial activation (2 b). In B, preatrial activity is recorded in an another patient, but with a three-orthogonal system (X and Y leads are contaminated with 50-Hz noise); 150 beats averaged; bandwidth, 40–300 Hz; vertical scale, 11 µV/division; horizontal scale, 30 ms/division. The same phenomena are recorded, but it is obvious that the 2 a accident belongs to the atrial activity. Here too, a slow slope (1) of 90 ms duration precedes the P-wave. Its origin from the sinus node is not proven but possible

[22, 23]. These potentials can affect the atrial activation, can induce atrial rhythm troubles and can be superimposed onto the His-Purkinje activation, which renders their identification difficult. But because of the severity of the rhythm problems they can produce – tachycardia or fibrillation – ventricular abnormal potentials become the main concern. These potentials represent low, fragmented activity, issued from the damaged ischaemic area, and of variable duration. To be recorded on the surface by HA-ECG they must overstep the QRS complex and must therefore take place inside the ST segment. They have various names: postexcitation potentials, delayed potentials, late potentials or after- or postpotentials (which is in principle a term reserved for cellular activation). Their characteristics are dependent on the equipment used and the parameters of the recordings, and especially the filtering bandwidth. Hence their descriptions and their prevalence rates differ. For instance, amplitude can vary from 2 to 25 μV and duration from 10 to 70 ms. An unsolved problem is the quantification of their relationship with the end of the QRS complex. For the limit of the QRS complex is difficult to establish and so far no method is foolproof. Rozanski et al. [37] – like the other teams using the high-resolution ECG recorder Marquette Mac I – proposed recognizing as a normal end of the QRS complex the termination of ventricular activity in the simultaneous normal gain ECG; and delayed potentials are described as 4- or 7-μV potentials that reach an average of 70 ms according to this guide line and that exist on different recordings made with 20, 40, 80 and 300 bandpass filterings. For Breithart et al. [8, 9], the limit of the QRS complex is the isoelectric section between the QRS complex and the late potentials – the bandwidth analog filter being 100–300 Hz; and they consider as late potentials the low-amplitude post-QRS signals exceeding threefold the noise level. An original approach is proposed by Simson et al. [39–41]: three filtered orthogonal leads X, Y, Z (25–250 Hz) are combined into a vector expression $\sqrt{X^2+Y^2+Z^2}$ and the high-frequency information thus summed defines a filtered complex, the end of which is determined by a computer algorithm. A late potential is defined as "a low-amplitude signal (25 μV) in the last 40 ms of the filtered QRS complex". This interesting technique, adopted by other teams, has the merit of giving attention to the totality of the ventricular depolarization. But the presence of bundle-branch blocks limits this method. Using the three orthogonal system described previously, we determined the end of the QRS complex by correlations between the three leads and comparison between two different filterings (20–300 Hz and 100–300 Hz). This subjective measurement is completed by the easier quantification of the whole ventricular depolarization (from the onset of the QRS complex to the termination of the last low-level deflection). Therefore, correlations can be made between the respective durations of QRS and late potentials (Figs. 6–8).

The clinical significance of these late potentials is not yet clearly defined, because of the lack of extensive and homogeneous statistics. Less than 20 teams are working on this new application of HA-ECG and only several hundred patients have been examined, as we saw, with no comparable methods. Despite these facts, and until a wide and well-controlled multicentre study provides documented data collected with homogeneous systems and identical parameter recordings, some proposals can be given:

1. Abnormally low level potentials can be recorded by HA-ECG on the ST segment. They can differ according to the substratum of the damaged myocar-

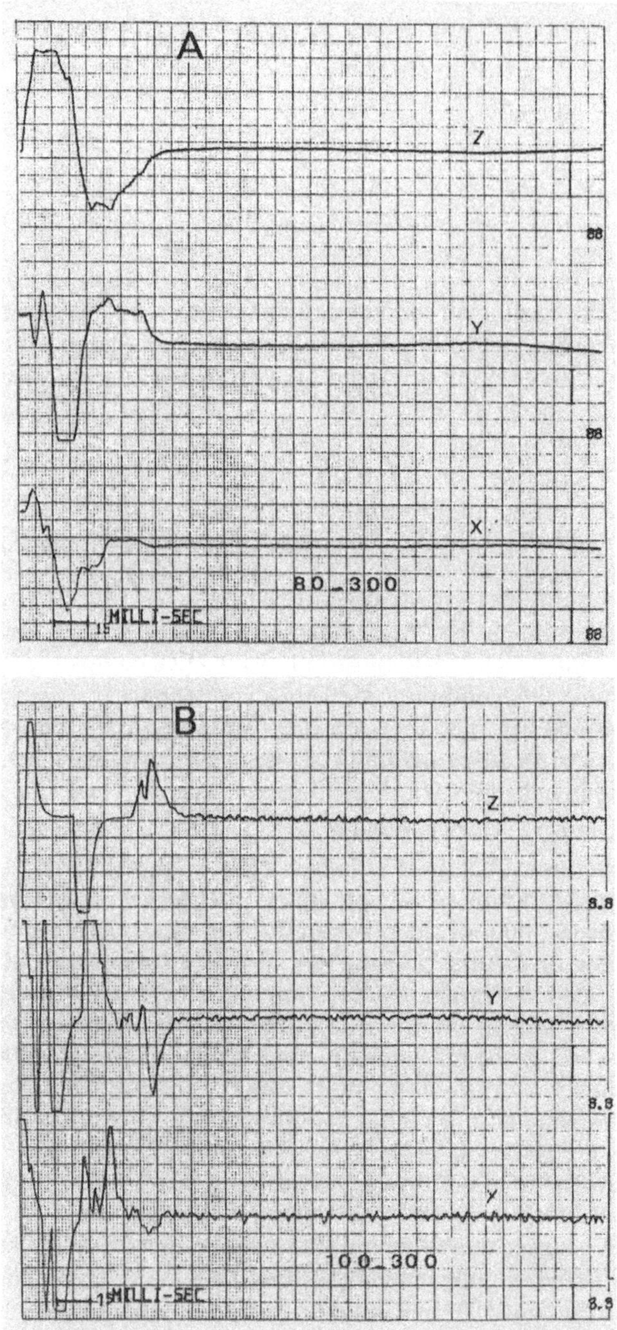

Fig. 6. Normal averaged ST segment in a 23-year-old healthy woman – using different gains and filters. A Vertical scale, 88 μV/division; bandwidth, 80–300 Hz. B Vertical scale 8-8 μV/division: bandwidth, 100–300 Hz. Horizontal scale in A and B = 15 ms/division. Demonstrations (a) of the possible pitfalls due to signal processing (15). A normal S-wave presents a multiphasic feature after increasing gain and low cutoff. (b) The usefulness of the vectorcardiographic recording enables comparisons to be made between the three leads

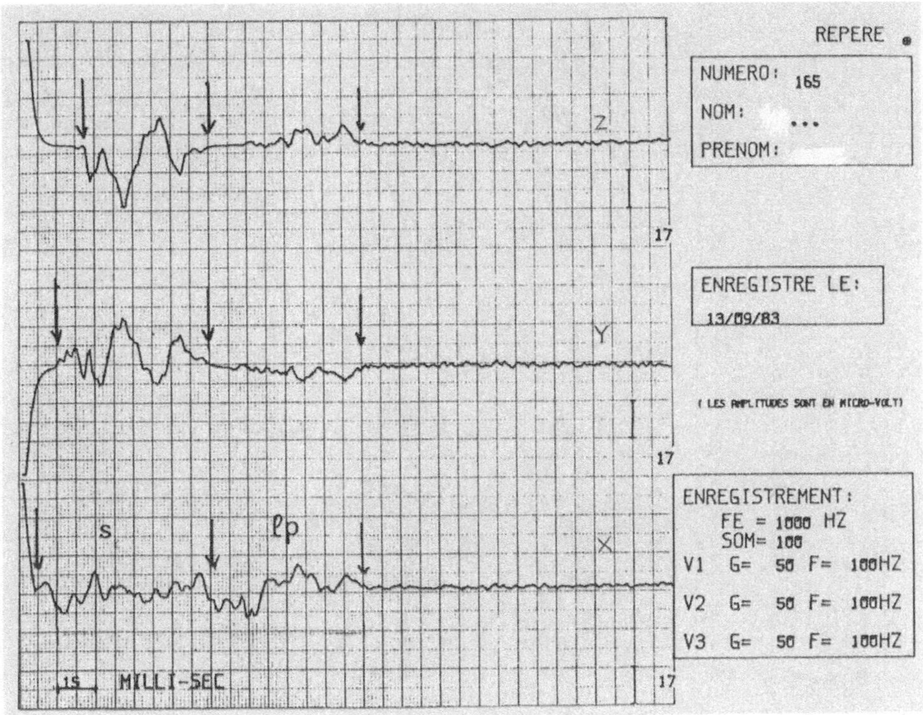

Fig. 7. In a 75-year-old patient with coronary disease, right bundle branch block and left anterior hemi-block, there is long-duration (127 ms in the X lead) multiphasic activity. The first part (*S*) is an S-wave (70 ms) with fragmented activity; the second part (*R*) can be considered as late potentials (57 ms). Note the difficulty – due to saturation of the S-wave in the Y and Z leads – in defining the beginning of the phenomenon

dium. For instance, there are differences of patterns and durations between the generally monophasic potential resulting from right ventricular dysplasia [22] or other congenital diseases and the multiple polyphasic micropotentials which overlap the terminal deflection of QRS [24] in coronary diseases.

2. These potentials are considered as the expression of delayed ventricular depolarization. However, the hypothesis can be suggested that some low-frequency potentials could be induced by inhomogeneous repolarization phenomena [56]. Consequently, it must be kept in mind that filtering can suppress important information (Fig. 6). In the same way, it is useful to adopt the vectorcardiographic approach with three orthogonal leads, which increases the changes of successful recordings [48].
3. The rate frequency of these potentials after myocardial infarction has to be evaluated according to the delay of the recordings. But opinions remain different, i.e. Breithart et al. [10, 11] find positive recordings in 51% of 160 patients after acute recent myocardial infarction, and only 34% in 146 patients with stable coronary artery diseases. In the follow-up of patients they notice a rate frequency of late potentials decreasing with time. On the other hand, Höpp et al. [28–30] reported an augmentation of late potentials (from 25% in the acute period to 60% 2 or 3 months later).

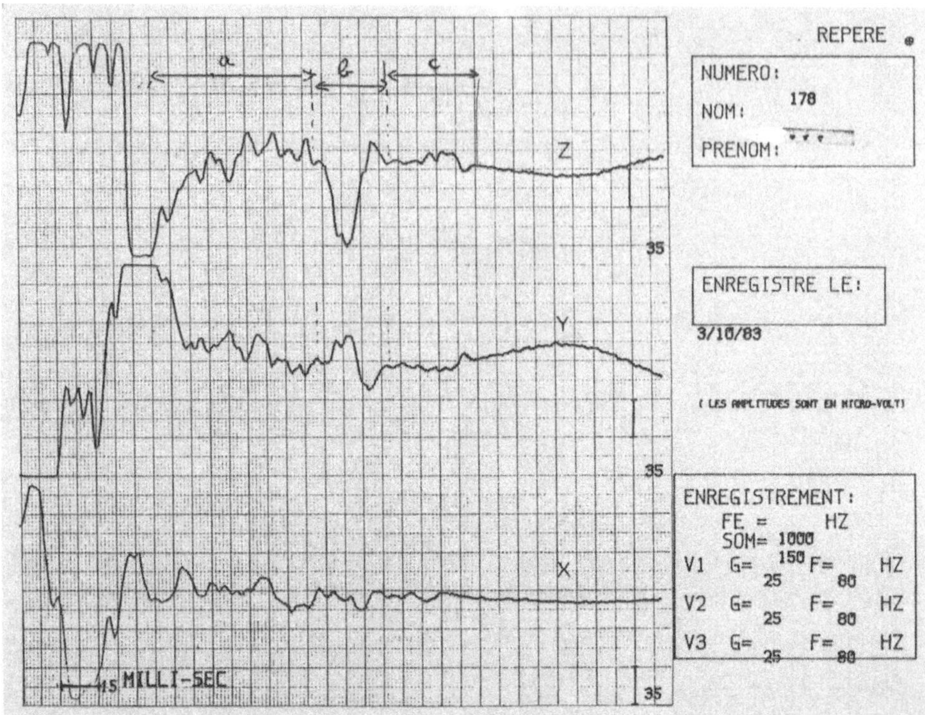

Fig. 8. Late potentials in a 74-year-old patient with anterior myocardial infarction in 1955 and major aneurysm of the left anterior wall. In August 1983, ventricular failure and ventricular tachycardia occurred. HA-ECG is recorded 1 month later; three orthogonal leads, 150 averaged; Bandwidth, 80–300 Hz; vertical scale, 35 μV/division; horizontal scale, 15 ms/division. Note the presence of abnormal potentials of very long duration: (a) fragmented low electrical activation (about 20 μV) of 60 ms duration: (b) a "giant" abnormal repolarization wave of 70 μV amplitude and 28 ms duration: (c) a terminal low-level fragmented activity of about 10 μV and 36 ms duration. It is difficult to realize that all these potentials are late or delayed depolarization potentials. Inhomogeneous repolarization phenomena can also be discussed. On the other hand, we considered – with reservations until statistical confirmation – that the giant abnormal repolarization wave could be the pattern of a major aneurysm

4. The prevalence of late potentials in patients with ventricular tachycardia is remarkable, being more than 70% [10, 26, 27, 40]. In a recent group of 15 patients who presented with ventricular tachycardia after myocardial infarction, we found significant late potentials more than 40 ms in duration in 12 of them (80%). But prevalence does not mean a direct relationship. In our 15 patients, we also noted an increase in QRS complex duration (mean value, 117 ms; control group of 10 normal subjects, 102.5 ms) and of P-wave duration (mean value, 130.8 ms; same control group, 109.6 ms). Of course, all these findings are due to the severity of the myocardial damages, and previous work has shown correlations between late potentials and anatomical lesions such as ventricular aneurism [1, 37] and with a haemodynamic situation.

Hence, it is still not known whether these late potentials are able to induce problems of rhythm. The fact that their duration could not be modified by antiarrhythmic drugs (Fig. 12) is not in favour of a direct relationship and, moreover, the possibility that they could remain after surgery whilst the problems of rhythm have disappeared.

So, we must keep in mind that today we are studying only the statistical features of these late potentials and not their dynamic behaviour. It is possible that they vary in duration or in amplitude from one cycle to another under the influence of interfering factors and, hence, the only verification of this hypothesis would result from a beat-to-beat recording [34].

Nevertheless, late potentials have to be considered as useful indicators of patients exposed to ventricular rhythm problems, and therefore their detection by HA-ECG will probably have a promising place in the routine examinations of coronary patients.

Applications of High-Amplification Electrocardiography Methods to Classic Electrocardiography

In 1979, we presented initial data which demonstrated that high gains, an averaging method and signal digitization used in HA-ECG could also be applied to the classic ECG [50]. With examples we emphasized the perspectives provided by this technique in taking a new look at atrial and ventricular electrical signals and in performing automatic quantification of ECG intervals or surfaces.

Thus we proposed to call the computerized quantification of ECG waves or VCG loops "automatic electrocardioplanimetry" or "automatic vectorcardioplanimetry", and we suggested that this new approach could be superior to thoracic mapping to follow the electric evolution of myocardial infarction (Fig. 9).

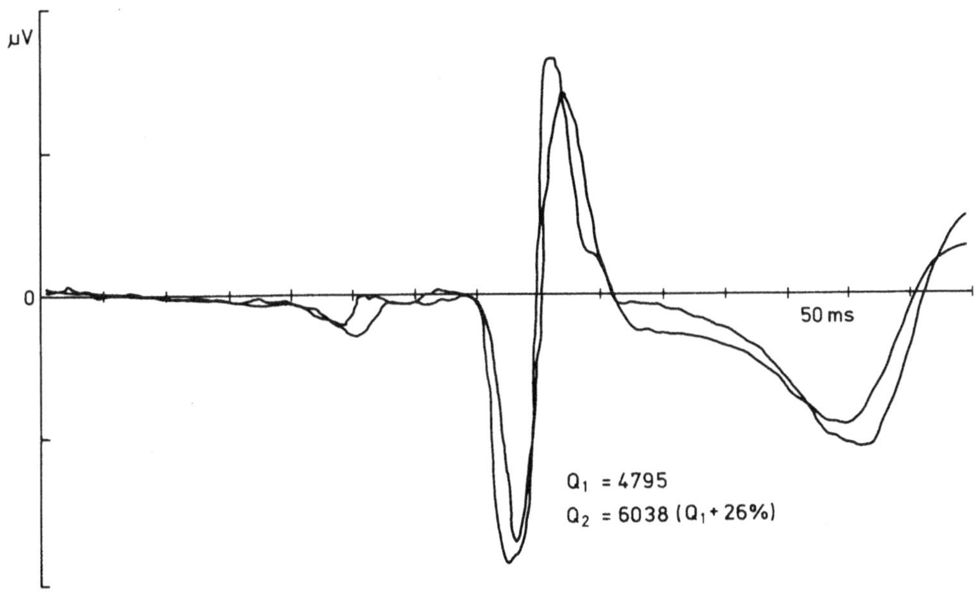

Fig. 9. Comparative electrocardioplanimetry between two Q-waves in a case of posterior myocardial necrosis (*thin line*, 18 May 1979; thick line 22 May 1979). Same Z component; same number of summations (100 complexes). Results, Q area increased 26% (4.795-6.098); sampling frequency, 400 Hz

In 1979 we also developed – under the name of "automatic electrocardiochronography" (ECCG) – a computerized method for on-line quantification of the average values of RR, PR and RT intervals in samples of cardiac cycles. The programme – which eliminates and counts premature beats – statistically processes *n* cardiac cycles, thus defining an "average cardiac cycle" (ACC), using PR, RR and RT values of this ACC and their standard deviations. The effect of a chronotropic drug on these parameters can be easily quantified, when comparing the ACC values before and after its administration. So, automatic electrocardiochronography has a specific place between normal ECG and Holter's long duration recording: it provides on-line data, high precision and objectivity in measurements and, as we have demonstrated it in the study of a beta-blocker [54] (Fig. 10), it is especially adapted to acute or pharmacological studies. It can also be used to detect undesirable chronotropic actions of antiarrhythmic drugs or of digitalis. We also think that ECCG will refine our knowledge of the normal cardiac rhythm and the physiological and reciprocal variations of PR, RT and RR intervals, and could open the way for automatic His bundle chronology either in intracardiac investigations or in HA-ECG surface recordings.

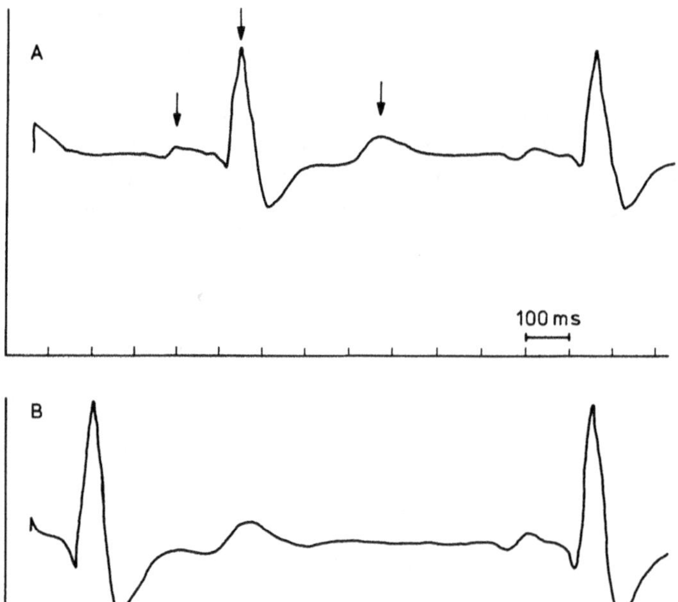

Fig. 10. Automatic electrocardiochronography (ECCG) in a 73-year-old patient with hypertension. A before, B, after timolol (oral administration of 10 mg/day for 5 days). Comparisons of the two average cardiac cycles (each one three samples of 100 successive beats). Intervals are on line calculated from the top of P-, R- and T-waves as indicated by *arrows*. Results show an increase of RR (+34.5%), PR (+0.06%), RT (+12.42%) and corrected RT (−3.98%). The procedure enables us to quantify objectively and on line the bradycardia and demonstrates the lack of significant effects of the beta-blocker on the atrioventricular activation and on the repolarization

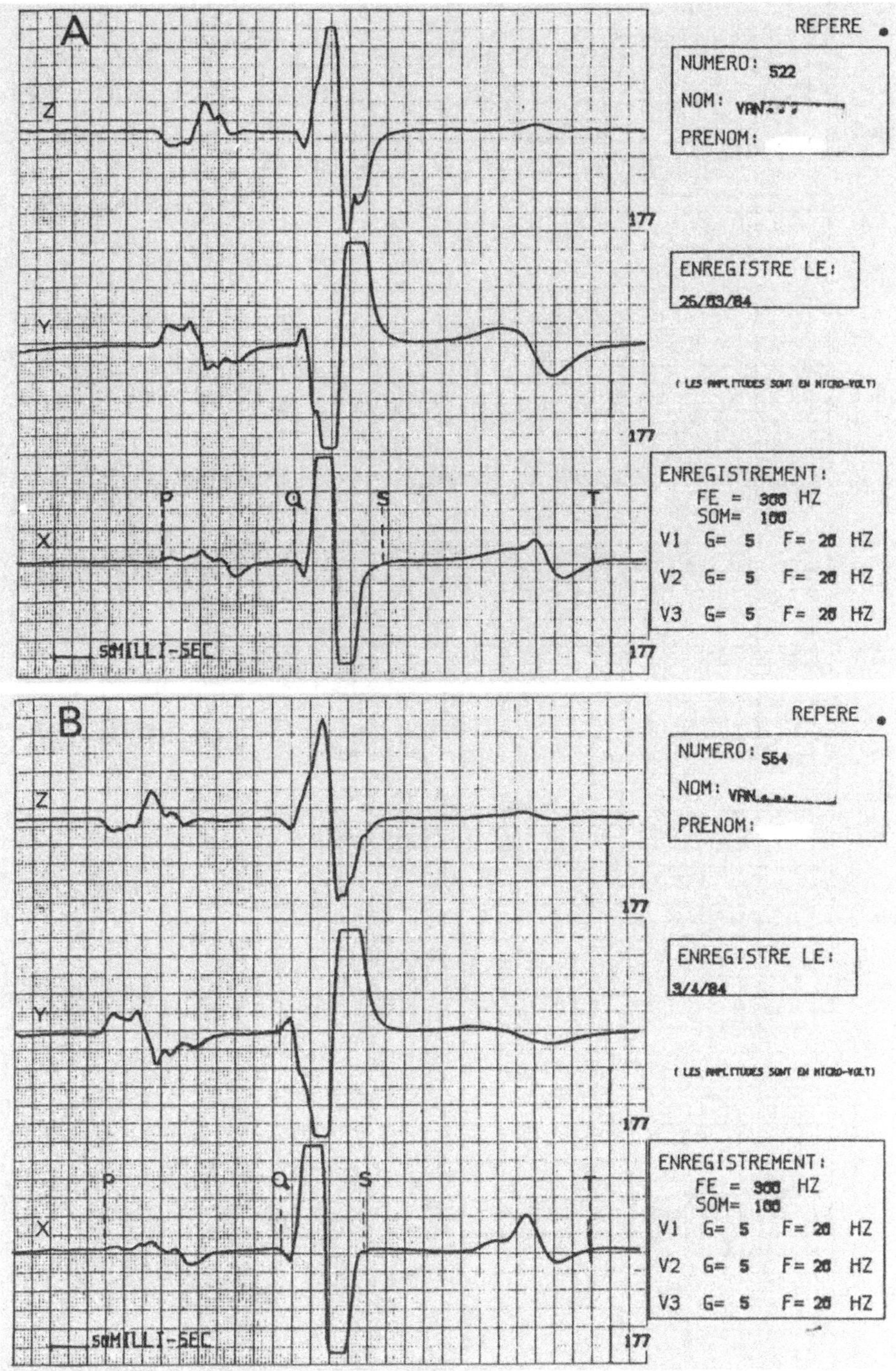

Fig. 11. Effects of Propafenone on the average cardiac complex (ACC) in a 71-year-old patient with coronary disease, averaging 100 beats. Three orthogonal lead (X, Y, Z) recordings. Bandwidth, 20–30 Hz; vertical scale, 177 μV/division; horizontal scale, 50 ms/division. A, before treatment; B, after 6-day treatment (600 mg/day). Measurement of the ACC intervals are dependent on the operator's choice. PQ increases from 185 to 235 ms (27%), QRS from 125 to 135 ms (8%) and ST from 275 ms (7.2%)

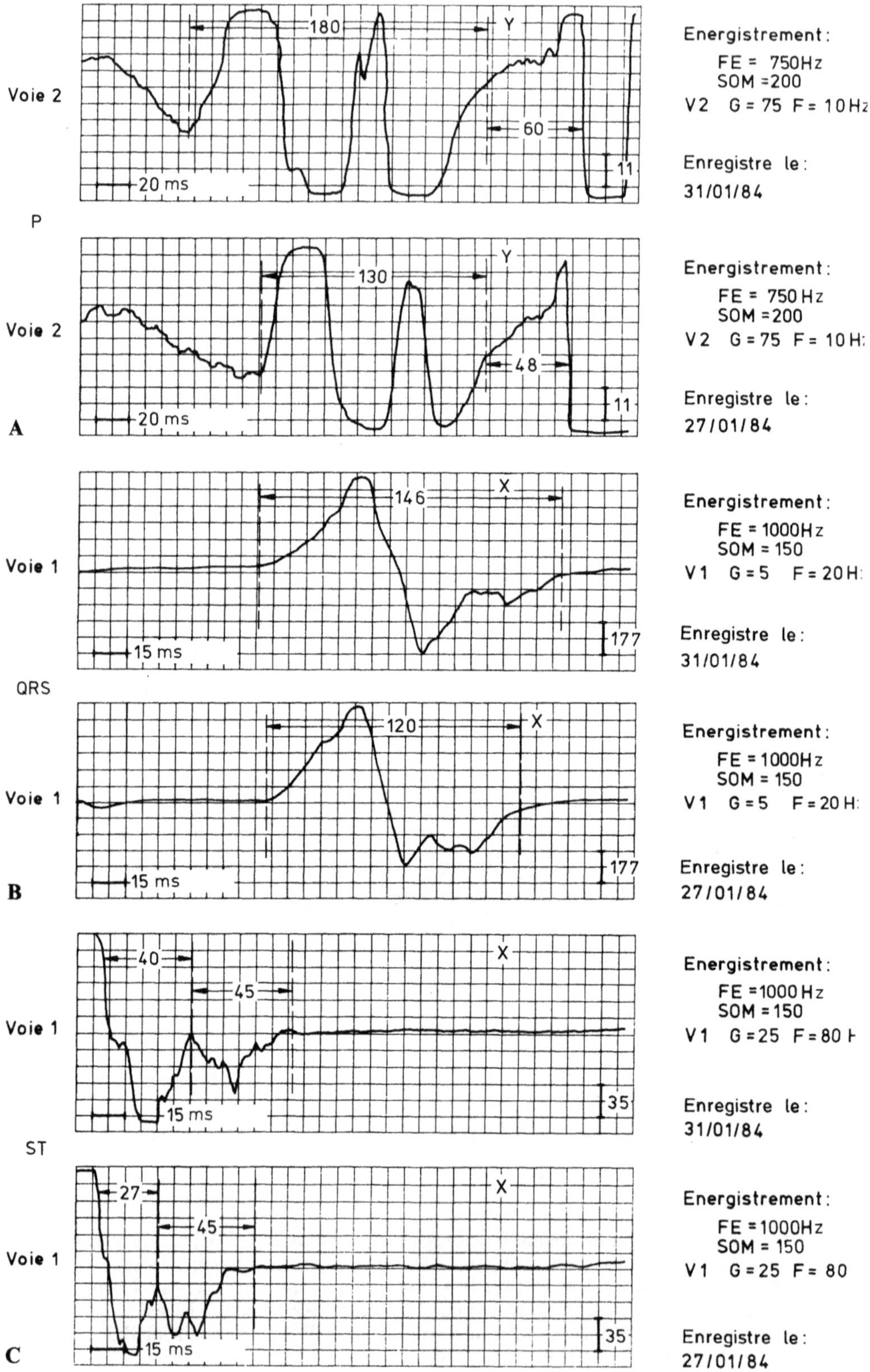

Voie 2
180
Y
60
11
20 ms
Energistrement:
FE = 750Hz
SOM = 200
V2 G = 75 F = 10 Hz
Enregistre le:
31/01/84
P
Voie 2
130
Y
48
11
20 ms
Energistrement:
FE = 750 Hz
SOM = 200
V2 G = 75 F = 10 H:
Enregistre le:
27/01/84
A
Voie 1
146
X
177
15 ms
Energistrement:
FE = 1000Hz
SOM = 150
V1 G = 5 F = 20 H:
Enregistre le:
31/01/84
QRS
Voie 1
120
X
177
15 ms
Energistrement:
FE = 1000Hz
SOM = 150
V1 G = 5 F = 20 H:
Enregistre le:
27/01/84
B
Voie 1
40
45
X
35
15 ms
Energistrement:
FE = 1000 Hz
SOM = 150
V1 G = 25 F = 80 H
Enregistre le:
31/01/84
ST
Voie 1
27
45
X
35
15 ms
Energistrement:
FE = 1000Hz
SOM = 150
V1 G = 25 F = 80
Enregistre le:
27/01/84
C

Another programme, called "semiautomatic electrocardiochronography", is adapted to study the time constants of an average cardiac complex obtained in HA-ECG recordings. The operator – by moving two electronic indexes – chooses the interval to be measured and can therefore obtain numerical data on P and QRS durations and the timing of the His signal or late potentials (Fig. 11).

Atrial electrical activity is represented in a standard ECG by the P-wave, which has too weak an amplitude and duration to enable all the auricular activation problems to be evaluated exactly. This P-wave is very useful in the diagnosis of rhythm problems, but only major modifications in its activation, such as left, right or combined atrial strains, are visible and it is in fact difficult to identify ischaemic lesions or intra-atrial conduction disorders.

The auriculogram obtained by HA-ECG reveals a new morphology – with notches, previously described by Brody et al. [12] – and its semeiological analysis will need much work. It also offers a new model for the study of the effects of antiarrhythmic drugs on atrial activation (Fig. 12).

The analysis of the ventricular depolarization – the QRS complex – can be improved by HA-ECG which, for instance, increases the detection of low delta waves in Wolff-Parkinson-White syndromes. It also reveals abnormal details which fragment the upward and downward deflections of the R-wave and which represent delays in the depolarization. In the S-wave, they are difficult to distinguish from late potentials. Moreover, the modifications in the duration of high-gain QRS complexes enable the effects of drugs on the ventricular depolarization to be appreciated. And if we have until now largely demonstrated the new aspects of the ST segment revealed by HA-ECG, we would add that summation is also helpful in the analysis of the U-wave.

Perspectives and Conclusion

For a long time HA-ECG has been limited to the research laboratory because of the high cost of equipment. Now all the new possibilities offered by the impressive advances in microcomputers and software signal processing have made possible commercially available HA-ECG systems which today are proposed for bedside use.

Therefore non-invasive recording of the physiological low potentials of the conduction system is possible. Of course, we must keep in mind that the sequen-

Fig. 12. Effects of Propafenone on the ACC in an 84-year-old woman with coronary disease and rhythm ventricular troubles. Three different HA-ECG recordings (P wave, QRS complex and ST segment) are made before (*A*) and after (*B*) 4 days of oral administration of 600 mg/day Propafenone. A P-wave, y lead recording, average of 200 beats; bandwidth, 10–300 Hz; vertical scale, 11 μV/division; horizontal scale, 20 ms/division. The P-wave increases from 130 to 180 ms (38.4%) and the end P-V interval from 48 to 60 ms (25%). B QRS complex, X lead recording; average of 150 beats; bandwidth, 10–300 Hz; vertical scale, 177 μV/division; horizontal scale, 15 ms/division. QRS increases from 120 to 146 ms (21%). C ST segment, X lead recording; average of 150 beats; bandwidth, 80–300 Hz; vertical scale, 35 μV/division; horizontal scale, 15 ms/division. Increase of the S-wave from 27 to 40 ms (48.1%). The duration of the fragmented activity following the S-wave remains the same (45 ms), but with some morphological changes. In conclusion, Propafenone induces important lengthenings in atrial and ventricular conduction, and also in AV conduction, but does not modify the late potential duration. This example shows the new possibilities in non-invasive electrophysiological studies offered by HA-ECG

tial averaging method used provides only statistical data and that, consequently, HA-ECG still does not eliminate the usefulness of intracardiac electrophysiological investigations. Hence, it is obvious that the next and decisive step in the development of this new electrocardiology will result in beat-to-beat micropotential recordings: something that was a challenge yesterday, and which is today a promising research field with already some positive experimental results. Refinement of this technique using spatial averaging and including an improvement in the quality of electronics, selective filterings and new pattern recognition algorithms, and perhaps directional electrodes [45], is still necessary and a lot of work must be done before bedside use is a possibility. But we have no doubt personally that the future digitized ECG will enable on-line surface recording to be performed of the entire electrical cardiac activity. Therefore, endocardial investigations will be limited to their therapeutical applications. However, in its present state HA-ECG gives a new impetus to electrophysiology, making possible by repetitive examinations an approach to the natural history of cardiac conduction system diseases. In practice, HA-ECG, because it is comfortable for the patient and not expensive, will soon take a more important place in the monitoring of cardiac conduction in acute cardiac situations or in the follow-up of chronic conduction disorders.

HA-ECG will probably also soon help in the evaluation of the real relationships between late potentials and the risks of sudden cardiac death. If they are only indicators of risks, they can be of useful predictive value. But if their close relationship with the development of ventricular arrhythmias is recognized, in that case we will be induced to take positive action, such as surgery, drugs or specific electrical treatment, that will change the prognosis. Finally, the new possibilities offered by computerized cardiac signal processing introduced 20 years ago by Pipberger [35] and Caceres [13] should not be underestimated. Whereas the physiological and pathological micropotentials still need a lot of work in semeiology and experimental procedures, immediate applications of HA-ECG methods are possible in the study of atrial and ventricular signals, and promise a rebirth of classical electrocardiography.

References

Collective Books (Symposia)

A. Varenne A (ed) (1980) High amplification electrocardiography. In: 1st International symposium on high amplification electrocardiography. Crenaf, Nice (distributed by libraine des Facultés, 174 Bd Saint-Germain, 75006 Paris)

B. Hombach W, Hilger HH (eds) (1981) International Symposium on signal averaging technique in clinical cardiology. Schattauer, Stuttgart

C. Varenne A (ed) (1981) 2nd Symposium on high amplification electrocardiography (Abstracts). OPFMN, Nice

Articles

1. Abboud S, Behlassen B, Laniado S, Sadem D (1983) Non-invasive recording of late ventricular activity using an advanced method in patients with a damaged mass of ventricular tissue. J Electrocardiol 16(3):245–251

2. Berbari EJ, Lazzara R, Scherlag BJ (1973) Surface recording technique for detecting electrical activity during the PR segment. Am J Cardiol 31:120 (Abstract)
3. Berbari EJ, Lazzara R, Samet P, Scherlag BJ (1973) Non-invasive technique for detection of electrical activity during the PR segment. Circulation 48:1005–1013
4. Berbari EJ, Scherlag BJ, Hope RR, Lazzara R (1978) Recording from the body surface of arrhythmogenic ventricular activity during the ST segment. Am J Cardiol 41:697–702
5. Berbari EJ, Lazzara R, Scherlag BJ (1979) The effects of filtering the His Purkinje system electrocardiogram. EEE Trans Biol Med Eng 26/2:82
6. Berbari EJ, Scherlag BJ, Lazzara R, Collins S (1979) The His Purkinje system electrocardiogram. In: Varenne A (ed) 1st International symposium on high amplification electrocardiography. Crenaf, Nice, pp 94–121
7. Boineau JP, Cox JL (1973) Slow ventricular activation in acute myocardial infarction. A source of reentrant premature ventricular contractions. Circulation 48:702–713
8. Breithardt G, Becker R, Seipel L (1980) Non-invasive recording of late ventricular activation in man. Circulation [Suppl 3] 62:320
9. Breithardt G, Becker R, Seipel L, Abendroth RR, Ostermeyer J (1981) Non-invasive detection of late potentials in man. A new marker for ventricular tachycardia. Eur Heart J 2:1–11
10. Breithardt G, Borggrefe M, Karbenn U, Abendroth RR, Yeh HL, Seipel L (1982) Prevalence of late potentials in patients with an without ventricular tachycardia – correlation to angiographic findings. Am J Cardiol 49:1932–1937
11. Breithardt G, Borggrefe M, Karbenn U, Haerten K, Ostermeyer J, Seipel L (1983) The possible relevance of late potentials for the identification of patients needing antiarrhythmic treatment. In: Schlepper M, Olson B (eds) Cardiac arrhythmias: Proceedings of the 1st international Rythmonorm-congress. Springer, Berlin Heidelberg New York, pp 37–52
12. Brody DA, Arzbaecher RC, Woolsey MD, Sato T (1967) The normal atrial electrocardiogram morphology and quantitative variability in bipolar extremity leads. Am Heart J 1:4–12
13. Caceres CA (1963) Electrocardiographic analysis by a computer system. Arch Int Med 111:114–120
14. Demartini J (1979) Les bases physiques du traitement du signal. In: Varenne A (ed) 1st International symposium on high amplification electrocardiography. Crenaf, Nice, pp 38–61
15. Demartini J (1981) Rappel des bases théoriques et techniques du recueil des bas potentiels cardiaques. In: Varenne A (ed) 2nd symposium on high amplification electrocardiography (Abstracts). OPFMN, Nice, pp 4–5
16. El-Sherif N, Scherlag BJ, Lazzara R, Hope RR (1977) Reentrant ventricular arrhythmias in the late myocardial infarction period I conduction characteristics in the infarction zone. Circulation 55:686
17. El-Sherif N, Scherlag B, Lazzara R, Hope R (1977) Reentrant ventricular arrhythmias in the late myocardial infarction period II patterns of initiation and termination of reentry. Circulation 55:702
18. Faugère G, Sans P, Levy S, Gérard R (1982) Etude de corrélation entre dépolarisation du système de His Purkinje enregistré par ECF HA et par voie endocavitaire. In: Varenne A (ed) 2nd symposium on high amplification electrocardiography (Abstract). OPFMN, Nice, pp 6–7
19. Flowers NC, Horan LG (1973) His bundle and bundle branch recordings from the body surface. Circulation 48 [Suppl 4]:102 (Abstract)
20. Flowers NC, Hand CR, Orander PC, Miller CB, Alden MO, Horan LG (1974) Surface recording of electrical activity from the region of the bundle of His. Am J Cardiol 33:384
21. Flowers NC, Shvartsman V, Kennelly B, Sohi GS, Horan LG (1981) Surface recording of His Purkinje activity on an every beat basis without digital averaging. Circulation 63:948–952
22. Fontaine G, Frank R, Gallais-Hamonno F, Allali I, Phan-Thuc H, Grosgogeat Y (1978) Electrocardiographie des potentiels tardifs du syndrome de post-excitation. Arch Mal Coeur 71:854–864

23. Fontaine G, Guiraudon G, Frank R (1978) Intramyocardial conduction defects in patients prone to ventricular tachycardia. III. The post-excitation syndrome in ventricular tachycardia. In: Sandoe E, Julian DG, Bell JW (eds) Management of ventricular tachycardia role of Mexiletine. Excerpta Medica, Amsterdam, pp 67–69
24. Fontaine G, Gallais-Hamonno F, Frank R, Fillette F, Malkawi K, Grosgogeat Y (1979) High amplification electrocardiography in cardiac arrhythmias and conduction defects. In: Varenne A (ed) 1st International symposium on high amplification electrocardiography. Crenaf, Nice, pp 226–301
25. Feron F, Mialet G, Schuller CH, Breton D, Perrin J, Degeorges M (1979) Recueil et traitement des signaux d'activité électrique des voies de conduction spécifiques chez l'homme. Arch Mal Coeur 72:48
26. Hombach V, Höpp HW, Braun V, Behrenbeck DW, Tauchert M, Hilger HH (1980) Die Bedeutung von Nachpotentialen innerhalb des ST Segments im Oberflächen-EKG bei Patienten mit koronarer Herzkrankheit. Dtsch Med Wochenschr 105:1457–1462
27. Hombach V, Höpp MW, Braun V, Hilger HH (1981) The signal averaged high gain amplified electrocardiogram. Technical aspects and clinical applications. In: Varenne A (ed) 2nd Symposium on high amplification electrocardiography. OPFMN, Nice, pp 12–13
28. Höpp HW, Hombach V, Braun V, Behrenbeck DW, Tauchert M, Hilger HH (1981) Kammerarrhythmien und ventrikuläre Spätdepolarisationen bei akutem Myokardinfarkt. Z Kardiol 70:319
29. Hopp HW, Hombach V, Braun V, Hilger HH (1982) Prognostic significance of ventricular late potentials in patients with chronic coronary heart disease. Circulation 66:4–42 (Abstract)
30. Höpp H, Hombach V, Osterspey A, Deutsch M, Winter V, Hilger HH (1983) Diagnostic and pronostic significance of ventricular late potentials complex ventricular arrhythmias and repetitive ventricular response in patients with ventricular tachycardia/fibrillation. Circulation 68:4–1688 (Abstract)
31. Kepski R, Plucinski Z, Walczac F (1982) Non invasive recording of His Purkinje system (HPS) activity in man on beat to beat basis. Pace 3:586
32. Mackintosh AF, English MJ, Vincent R, Woollons DJ, Chamberlain DA (1979) Low voltage electrical activity preceding right atrial depolarisation in man. Br Heart J 42:117–123
33. Mehra R, Kelen G, Zeiler R, Zephiran D, Fried P, Gomes JA, El-Sherif N (1982) Non-invasive His bundle electrogram value of three vector lead recording. Am J Cardiol 49:344–348
34. Oeff M, Leitner ER, Schröder R, Erné SN, Lehmann HP, Fenici RR (1983) Failure of signal averaging technique to record arrhythmogenic diastolic potentials: advantage of non invasive beat for beat recording. Circulation 68 [Suppl 3]:218, no. 872 (Abstract)
35. Pipberger HV (1962) Use of computer in interpretation of electrocardiograms. Circ Res 11:555–579
36. Ros HH, Van Den Akker TJ, Karreman AJP, Eisses JC (1979) Non-invasive bundle of His detection based on interval fluctuation properties in the ECG. In: Varenne A (ed) 1st International symposium on high amplification electrocardiography. Crenaf, Paris, p 123
37. Rozanski JJ, Mortara D, Myerburg RJ, Castellanos A (1981) Body surface detection of delayed depolarizations in patients with recurrent ventricular tachycardia and left ventricular aneurysm. Circulation 63:1172–1178
38. Siegel L, Murphy GW, Manning JA (1976) Conduction electrocardiography. Non-invasive recording from the human bundle of His. Circulation 54 [Suppl 2]:184
39. Simson MB, Euler D, Michelson EL, Falcone RA, Spear JF, Moore EN (1981) Detection of delayed ventricular activation on the body surface in dogs. Am J Physiol 241:363–369
40. Simson MB (1981) Use of signals in the terminal QRS complex to identify patients with ventricular tachycardia after myocardial infarction. Circulation 64:235–242
41. Simson MB, Euler DE, Michelson EL, Falcone R, Spear JF, Moore N (1981) Confirmation of a new technique for detecting slow ventricular activation on the body surface. Am J Cardiol 47:488

42. Stopczyk MJ, Kope J, Zochowski RJ, Pienieak M (1973) Surface recording of electrical heart activity during the PR segment in man by a computer averaging technique. IRCS 2:3–17
43. Stopczyk MJ, Palko T, Peczalski K, Wajszczuk W (1979) Recording sino-atrial node activity by prememorized signal averaging. In: Varenne A (ed) 1st International symposium on high amplification electrocardiography. Crenaf. Nice, pp 80–93
44. Stopczyk MJ, Walczak F, Kepski R, Plucinski Z, Peczalski K (1981) The history of non-invasive His bundle recording from averaging to continuous record. In: Hombach W, Hilger HH (eds) (1981) International symposium on signal averaging technique in clinical cardiology. Schattauer, Stuttgart, pp 283–289
45. Stopczyk MJ (1981) La dérivation locale son intérêt en électrocardiographie à haute amplification. In: Varenne A (ed) 2nd Symposium on high amplification electrocardiography. OPFMN, Nice, pp 30–31
46. Takeda H, Kitamura K, Hishimoto Y (1979) Non-invasive recording of His Purkinje activity in patients with complete atrioventricular block. Circulation 68:421–426
47. Trethewie ER (1981) Surface His bundle potentials by ABC electrocardiography. In: Hombach W, Hilger HH (eds) International symposium signal averaging technique in clinical cardiology. Schattauer, Stuttgart, pp 275–282
48. Uther JB, Dennett CJ, Tan A (1978) The detection of delayed activation signals of low amplitude in the vectorcardiogram of patients with recurrent ventricular tachycardia by signal averaging. In: Sandoe E, Julian DG, Bell JW (eds) Managagement of ventricular tachycardia. Role of Mexiletine. Excerpta Medica, Amsterdam, pp 80–82
49. Varenne A, Demartini J (1979) Application d'une chaîne d'acquisition ultra-rapide de signaux transitoires au traitement de l'activité électrique cardiaque. Colloque Images Bio-Médicales Iries Edit Beynes, pp 15–21
50. Varenne A, Demartini J, Hugues JP (1979) Application of high amplification electrocardiography methods to classic electrocardiography. In: Varenne A (ed) 1st International symposium on high amplification electrocardiography. Crenaf, Nice, p 303
51. Varenne A, Boudouy M, Camous JP, Guarino L, Demartini J, Guiran JB (1979) Vectorcardiographic approach of non-invasive His Purkinje system. In: Varenne A (ed) 1st International symposium on high amplification electrocardiography. Crenaf, Nice, pp 212–225
52. Varenne A (1979) Introduction to high amplification electrocardiography. In: Varenne A (ed) 1st International symposium on high amplification electrocardiography. Crenaf, Nice, pp 18–29
53. Varenne A, Demartini J (1979) High amplification electrocardiography unit. In: Varenne A (ed) 1st International symposium on high amplification electrocardiography. Crenaf, Nice, p 163
54. Varenne A (1983) Automatic electrocardiochronography, a new method to quantify chronotropic effects of drugs. In: Levy S, Libbey J et al. (eds) Recent advances in cardiac arrhythmias. Wiley, London, pp 105–110
55. Varenne A, Blanc PH, Bally A (1983) Recueil par électrodes de surface des micro-potentiels anormaux post-QRS. Arch Mal Coeur 76 [Suppl 68]:9
56. Wajszczuk W, Palko T, Bauld T, Przbylski J, Rubenfire M (1981) Signal processing and current status of non-invasive recording of the cardiac conduction system activity on a beat to beat basis. In: Varenne A (ed) 2nd Symposium on high amplification electrocardiography. OPFMN, Nice, pp 37–38
57. Wajszczuk WJ, Palko T, Przybylski J, Stopczyk MJ, Bauld TJ, Rubenfire M (1981) External recording of sinus node region activity in animals and in man by signal averaging. In: Varenne A (ed) 2nd Symposium on high amplification electrocardiography. OPFMN, Nice, pp 65–79

An Electronic Procedure and Device for Determining the Position of a Catheter or a Probe

S. Kunke and V. Schulz

In the past years many different electronic systems and apparatuses have been introduced in medical technology and diagnosis; however, most of them are based on well-known technology, are very complicated and are expensive. So we welcome the opportunity to present a new system which is uncomplicated to handle, cheap and useable in a large number of clinical patients. The physical characteristics of the system presented are basically new and absolutely innocuous for the patient and medical personnel.

With anaesthesia, internal medecine and surgery a large number of patients have to be supplied with venous catheters or stomach probes for diagnostic reasons or for therapy, e.g. for enteral or parenteral nutrition or pressure measurements in central vessels. In all cases it is absolutely necessary to control the position of the incorporated tubes, which is done by X-ray methods. X-ray control burdens the patient and medical personnel; it also increases cost and leads to delays in medical treatment.

So we have developed a new system for the localization of catheters or other incorporated tubes by using electromagnetic waves in the range of radiofrequencies. The system consists of a small battery-driven transmitter which is moved outside the body; a receiver is tuned to the frequency of the transmitter (e.g. 100 kHz) and uses the catheter or the probe as an antenna for the oscillation,

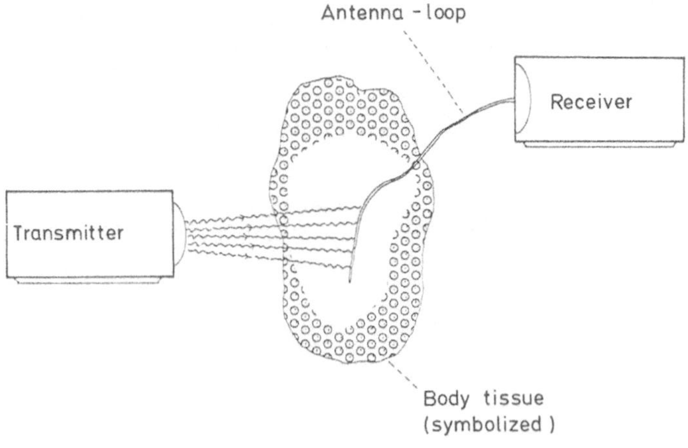

Fig. 1. The transmitted electromagnetic waves pass through the body tissue and reach the antenna loop (catheter). The signal is received and indicated (receiver)

which is transmitted from the surface of the body. The principle of this system is shown in Fig. 1, where it can be seen the transmitted waves pass through the human tissue, reaching the probe without any interference. The antenna loop is coupled to the receiver-input by inductivity, so that the magnetic component of the electromagnetic waves is used. This type of inductive coupling is necessary, because body fluids are conductive and would disturb the accuracy of the localization.

The power level which is received and is amplified is a function of the distance between the transmitter and antenna, which in this case means the incorporated catheter. In this way it is possible to detect the catheter's projection on the body's surface, because the volume received increases if the transmitter comes closer to the catheter. The point on the body's surface which relates to the highest received volume marks the shortest distance to the catheter, i.e. the catheter's position is just underneath this point, which can be marked from outside.

Design of an Electronic System

The receiver works by the superheterodyne principle, which is tuned to 100 kHz. The transmitter is a simple transistorized oscillator connected to a ferrit coil, tuned to the transmitting frequency. Both the right transmitter and left receiver are shown in Fig. 2. The receiver includes an adjustment for desired sensitivity and

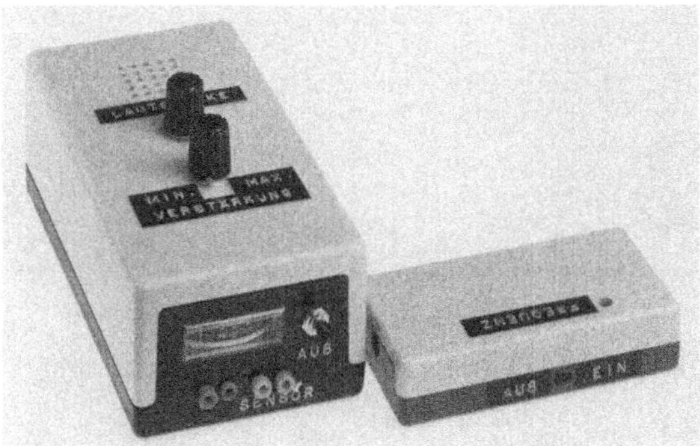

Fig. 2. Receiver (*left*) and transmitter (*right*)

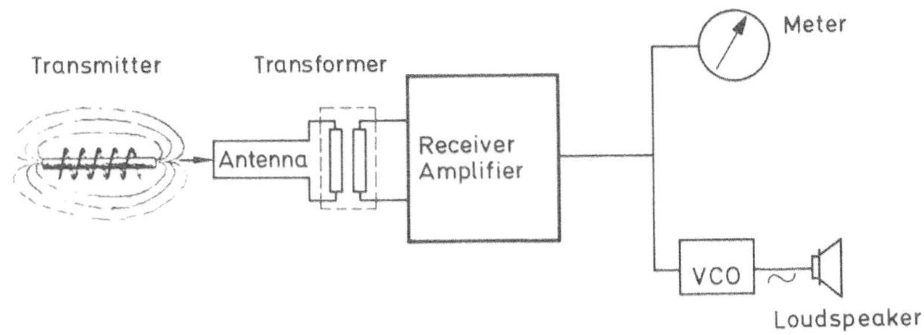

Fig. 3. Schematic of the whole system: transmitter with ferrit coil (*left*); probe with antenna loop; transformer and filter; receiver and amplifier; and optical and acoustic (via *V*oltage *C*ontrolled *O*scillator) indicators

two indicators for the received volume. One indicator works from a DC meter, which shows the level of received signal; the second works from a built-in loudspeaker. The loudspeaker is connected to a voltage-controlled oscillator which generates a sound frequency dependent on the level of the received signal: the highest sound frequency will indicate the smallest distance between the transmitter and catheter, so that *simple* and *fast* catheter localization is possible.

Figure 3 is a simplified shematic of the whole system: the transmitting ferrit coil is shown on the left side, followed by the antenna loop in the catheter and a transformer arrangement, which adapts the impedance of the antenna to the receiver's input. The receiver output is controlled by means of DC voltage and the optical (meter) and acoustical (loudspeaker) indicators. The system has a working distance of between 2 and 60 cm in relation to the chosen sensitivity.

Special Types of Plastic Tubes for Electronic Localization

As shown above,it is necessary to use two wires inside the catheter or the probe to close the antenna loop. These two wires or conducters have to be connected together at the tip, as shown in Fig. 4. In this case the whole length of the catheter may be localized.

Figure 5 shows a catheter whose antenna wires form a small coil at the tip. This type reacts with a higher sensitivity in the region of the tip, so that a distinction between the catheter's tip and the rest of its length through the body is possible.

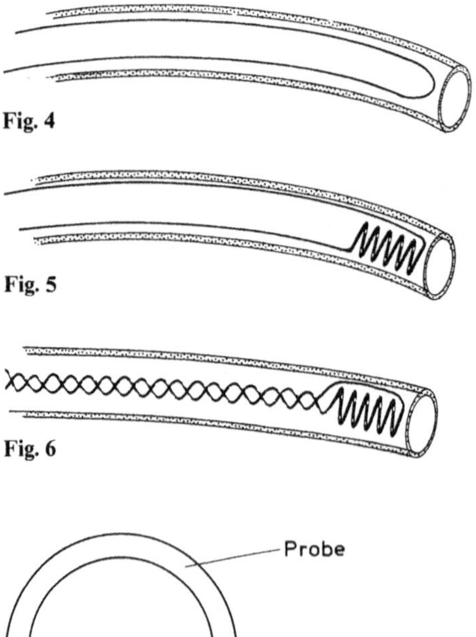

Fig. 4

Fig. 5

Fig. 6

Figs. 4, 5, 6. Different types of catheter (see text)

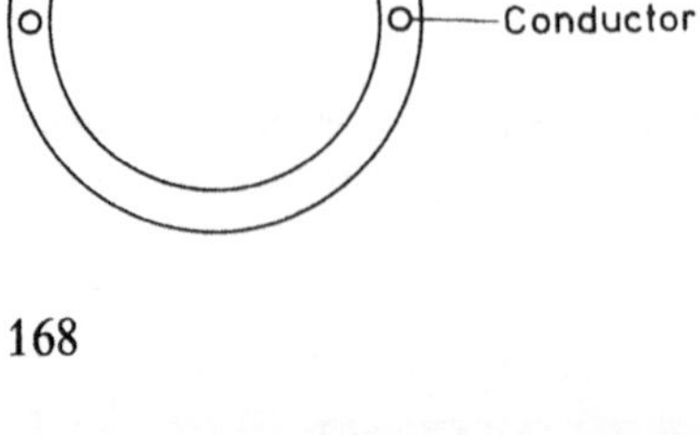

Fig. 7. Diameter of a probe. The conductors are inside the plastic body of the probe

Another form is shown in Fig. 6, where the two wires are twisted, forming a coil at the tip. In this case only the tip gives a strong signal, but the rest of the catheter's length will be *"silent"*, because of the shielding effect of the twisted wires. In these examples the conductors are inside the catheter; it is also possible to produce catheters whose conducting lengths are positioned inside the catheter's walls (Fig. 7). The material forming the conductors or the coil do not have to consist of metal; all other conducting products can be used, e.g. conducting materials or conducting resins. For industrial production the easiest way would be to extrude two non-metallic liners inside the catheter's wall.

Results and Clinical Application

The new localization system has been tested successfully in many patients. Mostly we used stomach probes which could be localized easily in the oesophagus, stomach or duodenum. Before application, normal stomach probes were prepared by pulling twisted copper wires inside, with a small coil at the probe's tip. The different points where the probe was localized could be marked with a pencil, so that the probe's position in the body could be seen from outside (Fig. 8). An X-ray control of the probe's position gave identical results: there was almost no difference between the X-ray and electronic position control. Since the application of self-prepared vena cava catheters was too dangerous (contamination, pyrogen reactions), the vena cava catheter was also supplied with thin copper wires and fixed on the backside of the patient's thorax, so that the normal length of a vena cava catheter was simulated. The catheter was electronically localized from the frontside and painted on the thorax; X-ray controls confirmed exactly the results of electronic localization (Fig. 9). All position controls could easily be performed in less than 1 min, even by personnel using this system for the first time. All apparatuses are battery driven with a low power consumption, are cheap and are

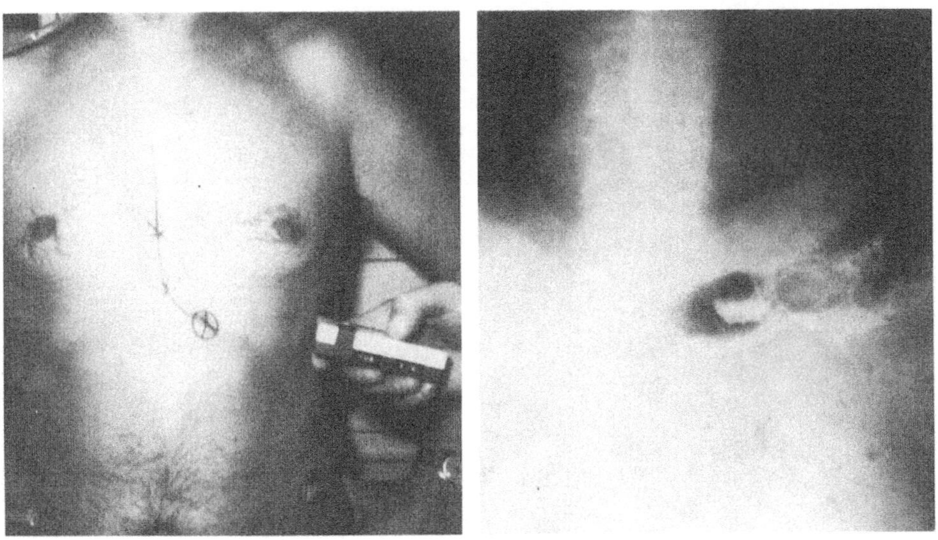

Fig. 8. Electronic localization of a stomach probe (*right*) and X-ray (*left*)

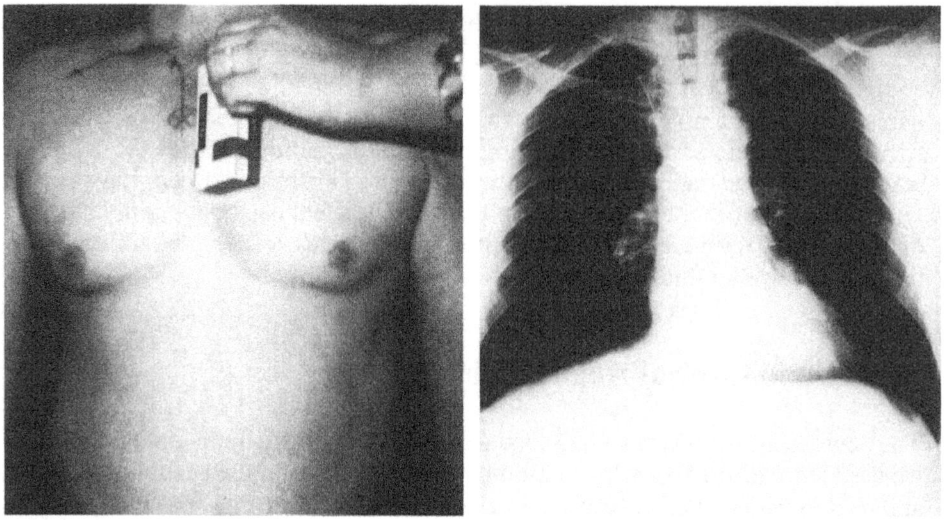

Fig. 9. Electronic localization of a vena cava catheter (fixed on the back side of the thorax and X-ray)

easy to produce. Their use is definitely *not dangerous,* because no X-rays or direct electrical connections to patients are necessary. Also the production of catheters or probes equipped with conducting plastics should be possible at a moderate price. We think this system should be developed to a new standard method in intensive care.

New Aspects of Respiration Physiology and Circulation

Effect of Different Ventilator Settings and Surfactant Replacement on Lung Function in Severe Respiratory Insufficiency

B. Lachmann

Introduction

The therapeutic goal in severe respiratory insufficiency [acute respiratory failure (ARF), respiratory distress syndrome (RDS)] consists of attempting to overcome hypoxaemia as well as metabolic and respiratory acidosis by means of respiratory therapy, increased inspiratory oxygen concentration and infusion of buffer solution. Some patients who showed no improvement from this therapeutic regime were treated with extracorporeal membrane oxygenation [43] or with extracorporeal elimination of CO_2 in combination with low-frequency ventilation [14]. Although the first of these methods has resulted in clinical failure [21], extracorporeal elimination of CO_2 together with low-frequency ventilation seems more promising [14]. But the last-mentioned method will be hampered by personal and technical prerequisites. Lung transplantation as a therapeutic measure has no clinical importance at present, due to the immunological problems involved [36].

The aim of ventilatory therapy in respiratory insufficiency is to maintain the gas exchange in the lung by opening and stabilizing closed units with a minimal depression of the heart function and circulation. This is not easily achieved, because lungs from patients with a surfactant deficiency have an extreme tendency towards collapse of the alveoli during expiration. Therefore numerous clinical and experimental studies were performed to investigate the influence of continuous positive airway pressure (*CPAP*), positive end-expiratory pressure (*PEEP*), inspirator/expiratory ratio (*I/E* ratio), frequency, inspiratory flow, end-inspiratory pause (*EIP*) and intermittent mandatory ventilation (*IMV*) on gas exchange of severely damaged lungs [25].

Influence of Inspiratory/Expiratory Ratio (I/E ratio) on Gas Exchange

In clinical investigations of newborn infants with RDS [34, 35] and in experimental studies of animals with surfactant-deficient lungs we were able to show that a prolonged pressure-generated insufflation followed by a short expiration with low or no *PEEP* was advantageous to all other known patterns of ventilation for the improvement of lung mechanics and gas exchange [23–25]. The greatest improvement of lung thorax compliance (Fig. 1) and PaO_2 (Fig. 2) were found when inspiration time was prolonged to cover 80% of the respiratory cycle. However,

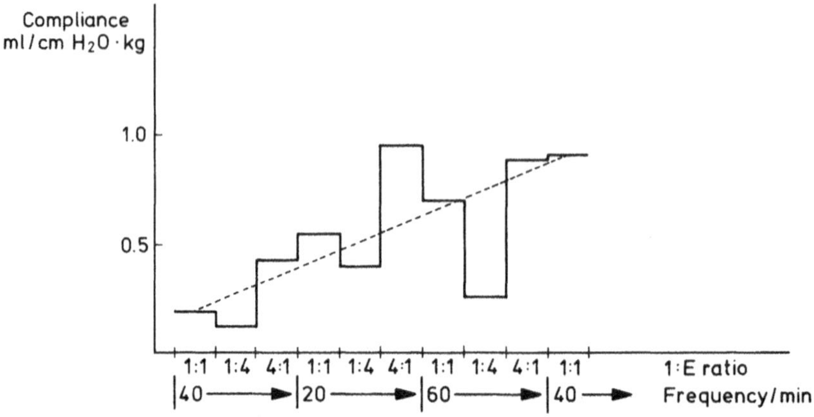

Fig. 1. Variations in lung-thorax compliance at different frequencies and inspiration: expiration ratios (I:E) (mean values) from immature rabbit fetuses. *Arrow,* onset of artificial ventilation, each I/E ratio period at the abscissa corresponding to approximately 2 min. There is a gradual "baseline drift" towards improved compliance, as indicted by the *broken lines.* (Lachmann et al. [23])

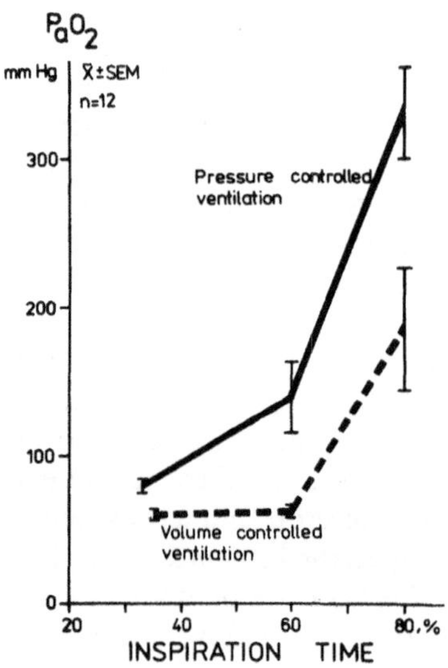

Fig. 2. PaO_2 in beagle dogs with severe ARDS, induced by repeated lung lavage. The animals were treated with pressure- or volume-controlled ventilation at a frequency of 40/min and varying inspiration time. Note the poor oxygenation during ventilation with a short inspiration time, especially in animals treated with volume-controlled ventilation. (Lachmann et al. [25])

prolongation of inspiratory time to 80% of the cycle led to an increase of mean airway pressure, which caused a decrease in cardiac output (33% in pressure-controlled ventilation; 45% in volume-controlled ventilation) and led also to a decrease in oxygen transport and systemic pressure as well as to an increase in pulmonary artery pressure and pulmonary vascular resistance. But the negative cardiocirculatory consequences were less influenced by a high *I/E* ratio with pressure-controlled ventilation than with volume-controlled ventilation with high *PEEP* values.

In theoretical, experimental and clinical investigations other authors have also shown the superiority of pressure-controlled ventilation with a long inspiration time over volume-controlled ventilation, especially for ventilation of so-called stiff lungs with surfactant deficiency [16, 30].

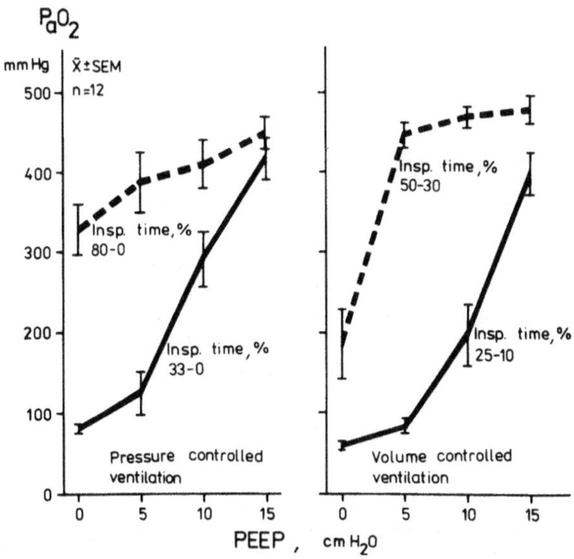

Fig. 3. Effects of variations in *PEEP* and inspiration time on PaO_2 during pressure- and volume-controlled ventilation. Figures for inspiration time represent the duration of insufflation and end-inspiratory pause, respectively (same animals as in Fig. 2). (Lachmann et al. [25], with permission)

Long Inspiration Time Versus *PEEP* Ventilation

On the basis of the favourable results with pressure-controlled ventilation with an inspiratory time of 80%, it must be asked what adventages this ventilation pattern has in contrast to other ventilation patterns that have successfully been clinically applied in connection with *PEEP*. Investigations on our rabbit RDS model showed that also by pressure-controlled ventilation with an *I*/*E* ratio of only 1:2 (frequency of 40/min) in combination with high *PEEP* values of 16 cm H_2O an oxygenation could be reached similar to that with an *I*/*E* ratio of 4:1 and a *PEEP* of zero [24]. However, in these experiments *PEEP* had the disadvantage in comparison with a high *I*/*E* ratio that ventilation decreased to less than 50% and therefore $PaCO_2$ increased to more than 90 mm Hg.

At volume-controlled ventilation, $PaCO_2$ could also effectively be increased with *PEEP*. The drawback of *PEEP* at volume-controlled ventilation was, however, that very high peak airway pressures appeared (higher than 60 cm H_2O) which led to bronchopleural fistulae in many animals. These results were confirmed by findings in beagle dogs with severe RDS [25] (Fig. 31). Starting from the PaO_2 tension at pressure-controlled ventilation with an *I*/*E* ratio of 4:1 and a *PEEP* of zero, and searching for other ventilation patterns in combination with *PEEP* which produce the same degree of oxygenation, all such patterns led to a lower cardiac output and a lower oxygen transport in beagle dogs with severe respiratory insufficiency [25].

Pressure-Controlled Ventilation with an *I*/*E* Ratio of 4:1 in ARDS Patients

Patients who could not be sufficiently ventilated by common ventilation patterns including *PEEP* and an F_IO_2 of 1 were pressure-controlled ventilated with an *I*/*E* ratio of 4:1 [25]. This ventilation pattern led to a drastic improvement of gas ex-

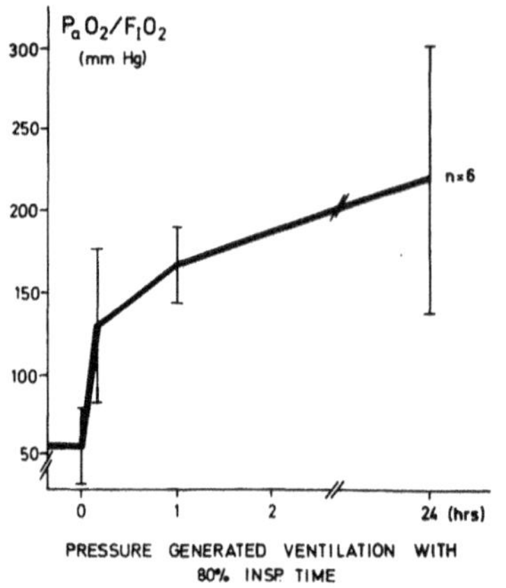

Fig. 4. Variations in the quotient PaO_2/F_IO_2 in six patients with severe ARDS, after a change of ventilator settings from volume-controlled ventilation with I/E ratio 1:2 or 1:1, to pressure-controlled ventilation with I/E ratio 4:1. Values are given as mean ± SD. If the values for each patient after 24 h are compared with the values for the same patient at 0 h, the differences for the whole group are statistically significant ($P<0.01$). (Lachmann et al. [25])

change within a short time. Arterial oxygen tension increased significantly within 10 min and increased further in the following 23 h (Fig. 4) despite a lowering of the ventilation pressure from 44 to 33 cm H_2O. F_IO_2 could simultaneously be reduced from 1 to 0.65 in the same time.

The arterial-to-end expiratory CO_2 gradient was about 40 mm Hg before starting this special ventilation pattern. Normalization to 4 mm Hg could be observed within 24 h. The thorax-lung compliance improved very little within the 1st hour but showed a significant improvement after 24 h.

Rationale of Pressure-Controlled Ventilation with Long Inspiration Time

Considering the impressive experimental and clinical results by application of pressure-controlled ventilation with a high *I/E* ratio in severe acute respiratory distress syndrome (ARDS), it seems that this form of ventilator therapy is superior to others. For optimal ventilation this ventilation pattern requires that:

1. Insufflation pressure must overcome a critical opening pressure during inspiration.
2. Inspiration must be maintained for a sufficiently long period to overcome the viscosity of the alveolar fluid as well as the adhesive forces of collapsed airways and alveoli.
3. During expiration no critical time that would allow closure of lung units should pass.

The critical opening pressure is necessary to overcome forces related to surface tension, e.g. adhesive forces of collapsed alveoli and terminal bronchioli and capillary forces in the small fluid-filled airways, so that air can reach the alveoli. The height of the critical opening pressure is a function of the content of surface-active phospholipids in the lungs of patients with RDS. A varying content of surface-active material in different lung areas could also explain the apparent paradox that a large shunt can exist even with high *PEEP* and with a pressure which exceeds critical opening pressure. In such cases lung units with a very low content of surfactant will collapse when expiration is too long and/or when the counter-pressure induced by *PEEP* is not high enough to prevent collapses in these regions.

A sufficiently long application of the critical opening pressure is necessary to ventilate all the alveoli despite different retraction forces in the alveoli. An intrapulmonary pressure that balances closing pressure must be maintained for most of the respiratory cycle. Even a slightly lower pressure will lead to collapse of lung units and to an increase of the intrapulmonary shunt. This was illustrated in dogs with severe respiratory insufficiency ventilated with pressure-generated ventilation [25].

Each dog was ventilated with two patterns at two frequencies. In one pattern, the pressure was applied during the whole inspiratory phase. In the other, insufflation was followed by a pause during which both inspiratory and expiratory lines of the ventilator were shut. Such a pause allows some stress relaxation to occur – particularly at low frequencies when each phase is longer. Although the airway pressure never fell more than 3 cm H_2O during the pause, this fall was sufficient to cause a pronounced drop of PaO_2 at the lower frequency (Fig. 5). This reflects the delicate balance between closing and opening forces acting within the terminal lung units with surfactant deficiency. The large increase of the intrapulmonal right-to-left shunt especially during a frequency of 20/min can further be explained by the fact that blood flow through alveoli which collapse due to surfactant deficiency increases manyfold [6, 31]. This supports the fact how important it is to apply a ventilation pattern which enables the opening of all alveoli to reduce the blood flow through non-aerated alveoli as much as possible in lungs with a surfactant deficiency.

The expiration should ideally be interrupted as soon as the expiratory flow has fallen to low values. Monitoring of expiratory flow at the airway opening may

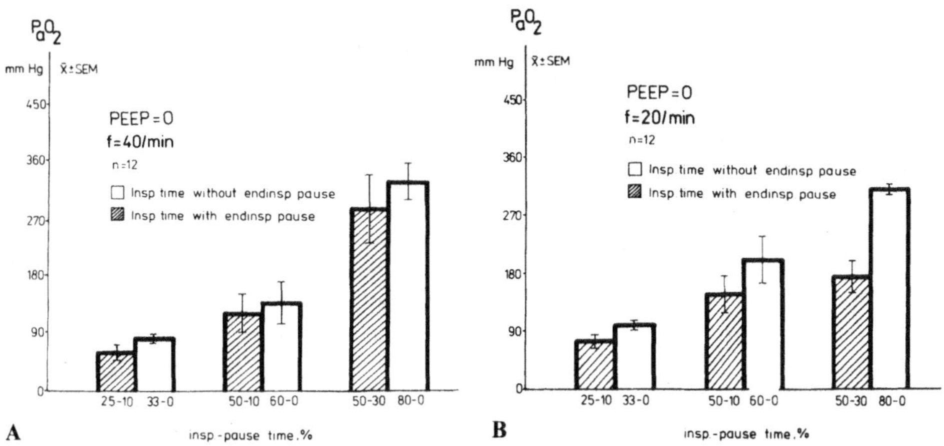

Fig. 5 A, B. PaO_2 in adult beagle dogs subjected to repeated lung lavage. Values obtained during pressure-controlled ventilation with a frequency of 40/min **A** and 20/min **B** are shown in relation to the duration of inspiration. Figures for inspiration time represent duration of insufflation and end-inspiratory pause, respectively. At a frequency of 20/min, there is a striking difference in PaO_2 between animals ventilated with 50% inspiration time plus 30% end-inspiratory pause time, and those ventilated with 80% inspiration time without end-inspiratory pause. During the pause time, intrapulmonary pressure fell by only 2–3 cm H_2O. (Lachmann et al. [25])

be valuable in this regard. It is, however, possible that some units have collapsed even before the total flow has ceased. It may be so that *PEEP* has a value as an adjuvant to the high *I/E* ratio with severe RDS, particularly when very short pulmonary time constants warrant frequencies higher than 20/min.

During ventilation of surfactant-deficient lungs it is more rational to control pressure than volume, since the physical and therapeutic effects are closely linked to positive airway pressure. Adequate ventilation is then produced by releasing this pressure for periods that are long enough to allow the escape of a proper tidal volume, but shorter than the time needed for closure of lung units. This concept implies that insufflation pressure is responsible for stabilization of lung units and that the expiration phase is responsible for ventilation. It is contrary to basic principles for volume-controlled ventilation with *PEEP*, in which insufflated tidal volumes maintain ventilation, whereas *PEEP* is applied to prevent alveolar collapse. A major influence on pulmonary circulation is not to be expected as long as the applied pressure is precisely adjusted to balance alveolar surface tension. If so, the applied pressure is not transmitted to the vascular bed.

Indications for Pressure-Controlled Ventilation with an *I/E* Ratio of 4:1

The most important clinical consequence is that in therapy of the most severe forms of respiratory distress syndrome, pressure-controlled ventilation with decelerating flow and an *I/E* ratio of 4:1 should be applied to improve gas exchange. This ventilator setting leads furthermore to less structural damage and less marked cardiorespiratory impairments in contrast to volume-controlled ventilation and *PEEP* [25]. We therefore propose in RDS patients the use of the ventilator pattern mentioned above if the PaO_2/F_IO_2 is below 100 mm Hg, peak airway pressure at volume-controlled ventilation with *I/E* ratio of 1:1 is higher than 35 cm H_2O and *PEEP* exceeds 8 cm H_2O.

When the necessary *PEEP* cannot be attained in some patients due to grave defects in the lung parenchyma leading to excessive gas leakage to the pleural space, pressure-controlled ventilation with a very long inspiration time is besides high-frequency ventilation the only possibility of maintaining the gas exchange. The critical opening pressure leading to a sudden improvement of the oxygenation must be searched for by repeated or preferably continuous determination of arterial blood gases. This pressure is different in each patient with RDS. Monitoring of expiratory flow helps identify a frequency at which the end-expiratory flow remains above zero. If this frequency is even higher than 20/min, one may apply a *PEEP* of 5–10 cm H_2O instead of increasing frequency. When a clear improvement of gas exchange has occurred, inspiratory pressure is first lowered. This measure is urgent because, in our opinion, pressure constitutes the most important aetiological factor for lung lesions induced by artificial ventilation. F_IO_2 is reduced later on. Inspiratory time must be shortened when, due to improved surfactant, the airway pressure becomes increasingly transmitted to the capillary bed. This situation is recognized by a considerable improvement of lung compliance, increased mean pulmonary arterial pressure and decreased pressure gradient between airway and oesophagus.

High-Frequency Ventilation

Artificial ventilation by high-frequency ventilation has recently been shown to be a useful form of respiratory support in humans with pulmonary diseases [8, 9] and in animal models of acute pulmonary injury [7, 40]. Since the tidal volumes employed during high-frequency ventilation are smaller than during conventional artificial ventilation, peak airway pressures and tidal fluctuations in alveolar volume and pressure should be reduced proportionately [7, 18, 40]. This potential advantage of high-frequency ventilation suggests that it may be associated with a lower incidence of pulmonary barotrauma than conventional artificial ventilation. High-frequency ventilation could also prevent excessive depletion of surface-active material during conventional artificial ventilation with large tidal volumes. Several authors have shown that an exceptionally high consumption of surfactant develops when a rhythmic change of the alveolar volume beyond the static surface tension occurs [2, 3, 11, 39, 42]. In severely damaged lungs with a decreased functional residual capacity a very strong compression of the alveolar surfactant film below the level of the static surface tension may occur, and displaces some portions of the surface-active material into the bronchial system. This means that an optimal ventilation for most severely damaged lungs is characterized by a nearly constant static surface tension to prevent an additional consumption of surface-active material by the artificial ventilation itself. Its level is about 50%–60% of the vital capacity and may contribute to a decrease of surfactant consumption. That means that high-frequency ventilation (HFV) could be an alternative method to low-frequency ventilation with extracorporeal CO_2 removal. This concept is confirmed by experimental results of Hamilton et al. [15], who used our lung lavage model to produce an acute respiratory insufficiency. They investigated the influence of conventional artificial ventilation as well as high-frequency ventilation on gas exchange and morphological changes of the lungs by the same mean airway pressure. Animals ventilated with HFV showed a marked improvement in oxygenation of 400 mm Hg (conventional ventilated animals, 100 mm Hg) and they also showed significantly less hyaline membrane formation, and only a few bronchiolar epithelial lesions. This study demonstrates not only that high-frequency ventilation improves gas exchange in the acutely injured lung, but also that the large phasic pressure/volume fluctuations associated with conventional mechanical ventilation induce per se pulmonary damage and that avoidance of these fluctuations by the use of high-frequency ventilation results in reduced pulmonary damage [15]. Less morphological damage during high-frequency ventilation were also experimentally demonstrated by other authors in sick and normal lungs [12, 13, 15, 20].

High-frequency ventilation results in a continuous distending airway pressure, therefore preventing the closure of the alveoli. This distending pressure acts as a super *PEEP*, or *CPAP*, in combination with a method for CO_2 removal by high-frequency ventilation. With this background it is clear that the same principal concept can also be reached by pressure-controlled ventilation with an *I*/*E* ratio of 4:1. A complete collapse of alveoli is prevented during the expiration phase in this special ventilation pattern.

It was experimentally proved that both ventilation patterns lead only to minimal morphological damages of the lungs in comparison with conventional artificial ventilation [15, 24, 25], while comparable improvements of gas exchange in the same model occurred.

The resulting question of which ventilation pattern leads to less mechanical depletion of the surfactant system, or which form of ventilation should be performed during surfactant replacement therapy still cannot be answered. If one compares the volume changes during a ventilation pattern characterized by an *I/E* ratio of 4 : 1, a frequency of 40/min and *PEEP* of 5 cm H_2O (about 10 ml/kg) with the volume changes by high-frequency jet ventilation (9–6 ml) measured by Carlon et al. [10], it can be said that fluent transitions exist. But when frequency is increased, the pulse volumes will be smaller and are on average only 2–4 ml/kg at 15 Hz.

Findings during high-frequency ventilation on cardiocirculatory parameters were not uniform. Some authors who found improvements of gas exchange, however, were not able to demonstrate any advantages of high-frequency ventilation in comparison to conventional mechanical ventilation in damaged lungs with regard to improvements of cardiocirculatory parameters [1, 38, 40]. However, when for prevention of an alveolar collapse in lungs with surfactant deficiency an adequate counterpressure during high-frequency ventilation must be implemented by *PEEP*, which leads to the same cardiocirculatory depression as in conventional ventilation, an important advantage is that high peak airway pressure which destroys the lung does not occur.

It must be stressed that mean airway pressure values measured by many authors during high-frequency ventilation do not reflect the real pressure conditions in the lung, because intratracheal airway pressure measurements were made nearly beyond the tip of the tracheal tube. We found in pressure measurements with a tip catheter pressure transducer that at a distance of 5–6 cm from the jet origin and with a flow rate of 2–5 litres/s during the pulse a short-term subatmospheric pressure of −35 up to −51 cm H_2O appeared. Measurements of the lung pressure in left lower lobe bronchi with a diameter of less than 1.5 mm by a retrograde catheter technique developed from Macklem and Mead [29] and Hughes et al. [17] showed mean pressure differences between central and peripheral bronchi of up to 20 cm H_2O (unpublished observations from Lachmann, Jonson, and Danzmann). These findings are in contrast to many data in the literature, but in

Table 1. Effects of frequency (*F*), pulse volume (*PV*) and *PEEP* on PaO_2 and $PaCO_2$ in four beagle dogs with severe ARDS ($F_IO_2 = 1$)

	Dog 1/83			*Dog 2/83*			
F (Hz)	4	15	15	4	4	15	15
PEEP (cm H_2O)	10	0	10	0	10	0	10
PV (ml)	109	31	25	132	88	38	27
PaO_2 (mm Hg)	365	325	350	350	350	390	375
$PaCO_2$ (mm Hg)	6	30	50	7	10	27	55
	Dog 3/83			*Dog 4/83*			
F (Hz)	4	4	15	5	10	15	
PEEP (cm H_2O)	0	10	10	15	10	10	
PV (ml)	155	117	29	73	35	26	
PaO_2 (mm Hg)	390	375	430	385	380	380	
$PaCO_2$ (mm Hg)	6.5	10	46	22	46	57	

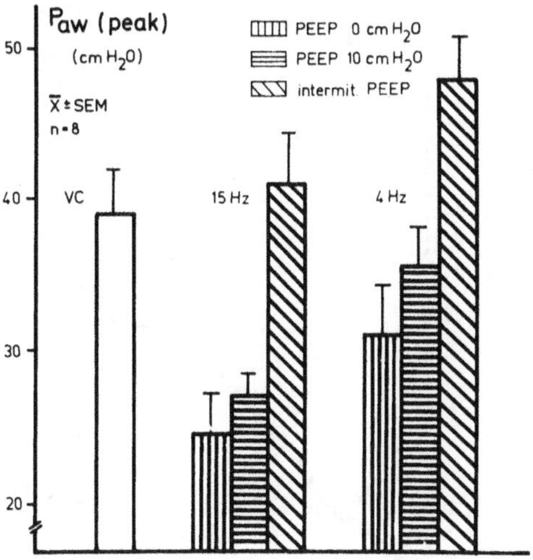

	VC	15 Hz			4 Hz		
V_T (ml)	200	33	28	33	127	107	118
P_aO_2 (mm Hg)	335	358	373	375	348	346	378
P_aCO_2 (mm Hg)	30	31	40	24	7.5	9	9

Fig. 6. Influence of PEEP and pulse volume during volume-controlled ventilation (VC) and high-frequency ventilation (15 and 4 Hz) on intrapulmonary peak pressure [P_{aw} (peak)] and arterial CO_2 tension ($PaCO_2$) in eight beagle dogs with severe ARDS. Despite there being nearly the same degree of oxygenation there are big differences in $PaCO_2$ during different ventilator settings

accordance with the clinical feature of an overinflated lung. Only when pressure measurements during high-frequency ventilation take place at least 12 cm distally from the catheter tip where pulses are released, can true pressure within the lung be recorded.

When a high *PEEP* level is applied as compensation for surfactant deficiency, CO_2 removal is usually hampered [3]. However, we showed that in animals with severely damaged lungs where *PEEP* values of 20 cm H_2O on average were needed for sufficient oxygenation, with a frequency of 4 Hz and *I*/*E* ratios of between 1:5 and 1:1, an arterial CO_2 tension of 22–34 mm Hg resulted [18]. Furthermore, in recent studies in our laboratory we showed in dogs with severe ARDS that by variations of *PEEP* as well as by changes of frequency from 4 to 15 Hz and by changes of pulse volume and flow rate, arterial CO_2 tension could be adjusted precisely within wide ranges while oxygenation was sufficient (Table 1, Fig. 6).

Prophylaxis of ARDS by Early Ventilator Therapy

Several authors [37, 41] have reported that patients identified as being at risk for development of ARDS do not develop it if they breath spontaneously during *CPAP* or were early ventilated with *IPPV* and *PEEP*. Therefore it was recommended for all patients with polytrauma. The clinical results obtained by Wolff (210) are very impressive. In 250 cases of polytrauma, only seven succumbed from respiratory insufficiency caused by ARDS. Consequent application of ventilation has shown that ARDS can in some cases be prevented. This form of therapy probably prevents the start of the vicious circle of permeability disturbance of the alveolar-capillary membrane, surfactant inactivation, washout of surfactant into

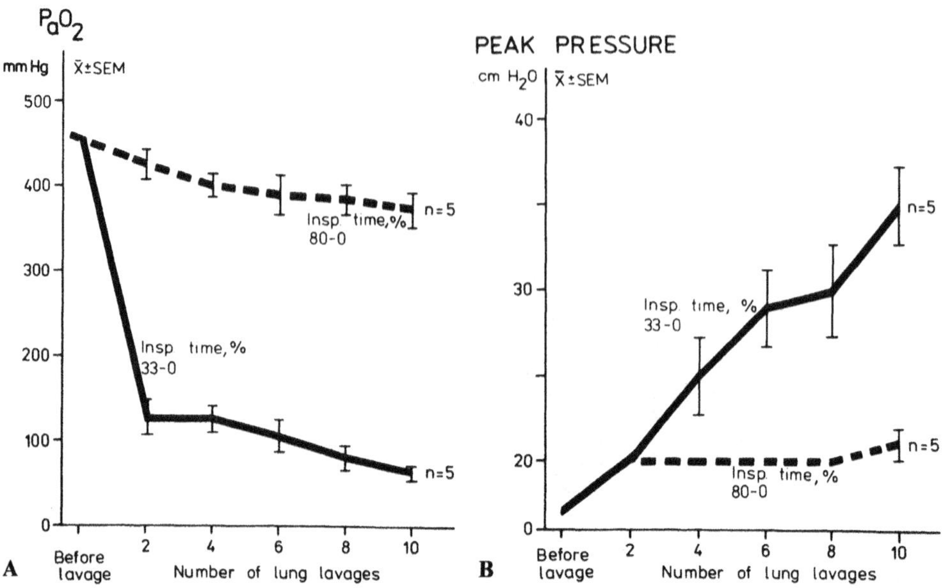

Fig. 7 A, B. Course of PaO_2 **A** and peak insufflation pressure **B** with pressure-controlled ventilation in relation to the number of lung lavages with different durations of inspiration. (Lachmann et al. [25])

the bloodstream, decreased functional residual capacity and compliance, inhibition of surfactant synthesis by hypoxia and acidosis etc., which plays an important role in the pathogenesis of ARDS. This hypothesis was tested in a series of dogs after inducing a surfactant deficiency by bronchial lavage. The dogs were divided into two groups. One group was ventilated prior to lavage with an *I/E* ratio of 4:1 and the other group with an *I/E* ratio of 1:2. Both groups received pressure-controlled ventilation using an F_IO_2 of 1. Ventilation pressure was increased when arterial oxygenation fell below 70 mm Hg after lung lavage. The group ventilated with an *I/E* ratio of 4:1 showed only a small decrease of oxygen tension that was dependent on the number of lavages given (Fig. 7 a). Other cardiocirculatory parameters that were studied also showed only slight deterioration due to the number of lavages given. The animals with an *I/E* ratio of 1:2 had decreased arterial oxygenation of about 300 mm Hg already at the first lavage. The ventilation pressure (Fig. 7 b) had to be raised after each lavage in order to prevent excessive hypoxaemia. Lung lavages in this group also led to a higher decrease in compliance, cardiac output and oxygen transport.

It can be assumed that the progress of functional impairment due to disturbances in the surfactant system can be compensated for by use of the ventilation pattern described above, which gives the lung a chance to maintain its normal function. These findings and earlier clinical results [5, 37, 41] have convinced us that there are strong indications for artificial ventilation with *PEEP* or with a long inspiratory time or high-frequency ventilation in patients with acute respiratory failure following severe trauma, extensive shock, burns, etc., especially during the latent period and even when functional lung parameters at this early stage do not seem to require artificial ventilation. *CPAP* may be a rational alternative at an early stage of RDS.

Surfactant Replacement Therapy in RDS

While many experimental and clinical observations show that a surfactant deficiency in premature and newborn infants can be compensated for by tracheal instillation of surfactant, there are only single in vivo investigations about surfactant replacement in the RDS of the adult [4, 19, 22, 26, 27, 33]. Recent investigations with the lung lavage model in adults show that also in the ARDS model a massive improvement of the gas exchange is possible by tracheal instillation of surfactant. A striking improvement of oxygenation (Fig. 8 a) as well as a decrease

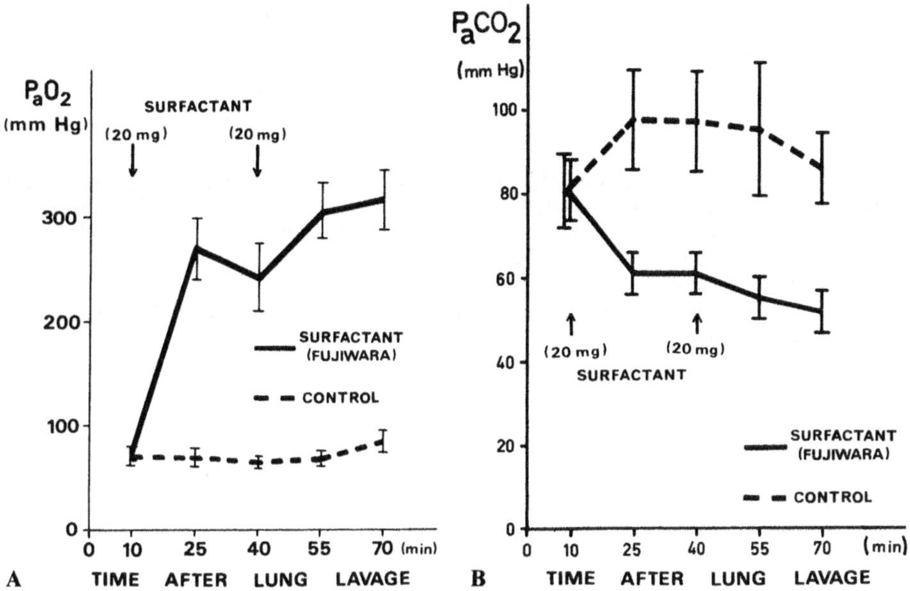

Fig. 8 A, B. Effect of surfactant replacement on PaO_2 **A** and $PaCO_2$ **B** in guinea pigs with severe ARDS induced by repeated lung lavage. The animals were ventilated with pressure-controlled ventilation, 100% oxygen, I/E ratio, 1:1; frequency, 20/min; insufflation pressure, 28 cm H_2O; and *PEEP*, 5 cm H_2O. Surfactant was administered twice via the tracheal cannula (*arrows*). Values are given as mean ± SD. (Lachmann et al. [**A**, 22; **B**, 26])

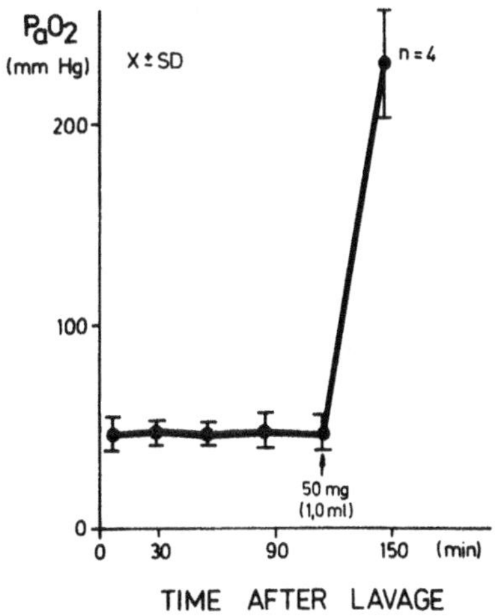

Fig. 9. Course of PaO_2 in guinea pigs with severe ARDS. Surfactant was instilled 2 h after the lavage period

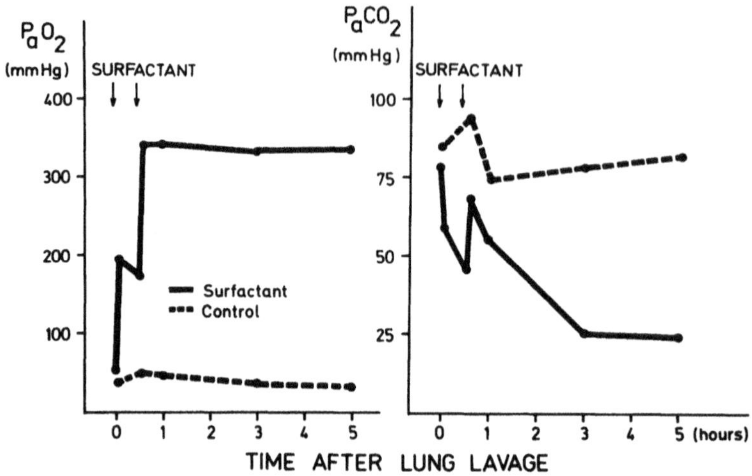

Fig. 10. Sequential recordings of *Pa*O_2 and *Pa*CO_2 in two adult guinea pigs subjected to repeated lung lavage, followed by ventilation for 5 h with pressure-controlled ventilation; 100% oxygen; I/E ratio, 1:2; frequency, 30/min; insufflation pressure, 28 cm H_2O; and *PEEP*, 6 cm H_2O. One animal received two tracheal instillations of natural surfactant (each dose 50 mg), 5 and 30 min after lavage (*arrows*). The improved blood gases, recorded after surfactant replacement, are stable throughout the period of observation (Lachmann and Danzmann [28])

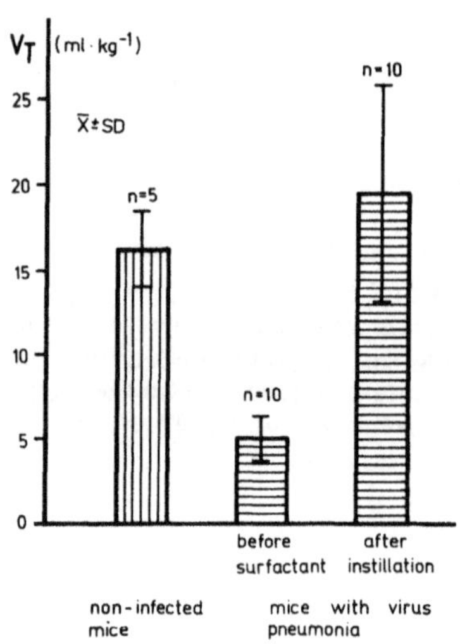

Fig. 11. Tidal volumes in mice with viral pneumonia before and 10 min after tracheal instillation of surfactant. *On the left* is the tidal volume of noninfected mice

in arterial CO_2 tension (Fig. 8 b) occurred in comparison with the controls, even if the treatment is given 2 h after the lavage procedure (Fig. 9). Other experiments have documented that in animals receiving surfactant the improved blood gases are stable for at least 5 h, whereas *Pa*O_2 in control animals remains low despite ventilation with *PEEP* and pure oxygen (Fig. 10).

We have also found that surfactant replacement is an effective therapeutic measure in experimental viral pneumonia [28]. In these studies mice were infected with influenza virus [32] and lung mechanics were investigated 6 days later before and after tracheal instillation of surfactant. The course of compliance or augmentation of tidal volumes revealed that before surfactant instillation lungs could not be sufficiently ventilated at a peak pressure of 25 cm H_2O, while after instillation of surfactant aeration with the same peak pressure was possible (Fig. 11).

Concluding Remarks

If it becomes possible in the near future to control mechanisms of blood coagulation and complement release as well as to prevent or delay toxic influence of high oxygen concentration and free oxygen radicals by specific agents and if on the other hand early damage in the surfactant system of the lung can be prevented by surfactant replacement combined with "non-traumatic" artificial ventilation, the high mortality of the respiratory distress syndrome can probably be reduced.

References

1. Auffant RA, Shuptrine JR, Hotchkiss RS, Maffeo CJ (1982) Effects of HFV vs IPPV on cerebral perfusion pressure and cardiopulmonary function. Anaesthesiology 57:88 (Abstract)
2. Benzer H (1969) Respiratorbeatmung und Oberflächenspannung in der Lunge. Springer, Berlin Heidelberg New York
3. Benzer H, Coraim F, Mutz N, Geyer A, Pauser G (1979) Probleme der respiratorischen Beatmung bei der Schocklunge. In: Mayrhofer-Krammel O, Schlag G, Stoeckel H (Hrsg) Acute respiratory failure. Thieme, Stuttgart, S 263–270
4. Berggren P, Curstedt T, Grossman G, Lachmann B, Robertson B (1983) Surfactant replacement in experimental respiratory distress induced by repeated lung lavage. IRCS Med Sci 11:787–788
5. Blaisdell FW, Lewis FR Jr (1977) Respiratory distress syndrome of shock and trauma: post-traumatic respiratory failure. In: Ebert PA (ed) Major problems in clinical surgery. Saunders, Philadelphia, pp 9–132
6. Bredenberg CE (1982) Surface tension and alveolar changes during ventilation. In: Prakash O (ed) Applied physiology in clinical respiratory care. Nijhoff, The Hague, pp 191–206
7. Bohn DJ, Miyasaka K, Marchak BE, Thompson WK, Froese AB, Bryan AC (1980) Ventilation by high frequency oscillation. J Appl Physiol 48:710–716
8. Gallagher TJ, Klain MM, Carlon GC (1982) Present status of high frequency ventilation. Crit Care Med 10:613–617
9. Derderian SS, Rajogopal KR, Albrecht PH, Bennett LL, Doplar DD, Hunt KK (1982) High frequency positive pressure jet ventilation in bilateral bronchopleural fistulae. Crit Care Med 10:119–121
10. Carlon GC, Kahn RC, Howland WS, Ray C, Turnbull AD (1981) Clinical experience with high frequency jet ventilation. Crit Care Med 9:1–6
11. Faridy EE, Permutt S, Riley RL (1966) Effect of ventilation of surface forces in excised dogs lungs. J Appl Physiol 21:1453–1462
12. Frank I, Noack W, Lunkenheimer PP, Ising H, Keller H, Dickhuth HH, Rafflenbeul W, Jacobson M (1975) Light and electron microscopic investigations of pulmonary tissue after high frequency positive pressure ventilation (HFPPV). Anaesthesist 24:171–176
13. Frey DJM, Beller U, Eiermann T, Deilmann M, Lesch R (1981) Injekt-Beatmung, Hochfrequenz-Oszillations-Injekt-Beatmung und Respirator-Beatmung – tierexperimentelle Studie im Langzeitversuch. Prax Klin Pneumol 35:641–648
14. Gattinoni L, Pesenti A, Rossi GP, Vesconi S, Fox U, Kolobow T, Agostini A, Pelizzola A, Langer M, Uziel L, Longoni F, Damia G (1980) Treatment of acute respiratory failure with low frequency positive-pressure ventilation and extracorporeal removal of CO_2. Lancet 2:292–294

15. Hamilton PP, Onayemi A, Smyth JA, Gillan JA, Cutz E, Froese AB, Bryan AC (1983) A comparison of conventional and high frequency ventilation: oxygenation and lung pathology. J Appl Physiol 55:131–138
16. Herman S, Reynolds EOR (1973) Methods for improving oxygenation in infants mechanically ventilated for severe hyaline memebrane disease. Arch Dis Childh 48:612–617
17. Hughes JMB, Jones HA, Wilson AG, Grant BJB, Pride NB (1974) Stability of intrapulmonary bronchial dimensions during expiratory flow in excised lungs. J Appl Physiol 37:684–694
18. Jibelian G, Lachmann B (1984) Gas exchange during conventional and high-frequency pulse ventilation in the surfactant-deficient lung: influence of positive end-expiratory pressure. Crit Care Med 12:769–773
19. Kataoka H, Takada Y, Kobayashi T, Murakami S, Kobuko M (1982) Effects of surfactant supplementation following lung lavage on rabbits.In: Proceedings of the 14th scientific meeting of Japanese medical society for biological interface, Niigata City, pp 26–27
20. Keszler M, Klein R, McClellan L, Nelson D, Platt M (1982) Effects of conventional and high frequency jet ventilation on lung parenchyma. Crit Care Med 10:514–516
21. Kolobow T, Solca M, Gattinoni L, Pesenti A (1981) Adults respiratory distress syndrome (ARDS): why did ECMO fail? Int J Artif Organs 4:58–59
22. Lachmann B, Fujiwara T, Chida S, Morita T, Konishi M, Nakamura K, Maeta H (1981 a) Improved gas exchange after tracheal instillation of surfactant in the experimental adult respiratory distress syndrome. Crit Care Med 9:158
23. Lachmann B, Grossmann G, Freyse J, Robertson B (1981 b) Lung-thorax compliance in the artificially ventilated premature rabbit neonate in relation to variations in inspiration/expiration ratio. Pediatr Res 15:833–838
24. Lachmann B, Jonson B, Lindroth M, Robertson B (1982 a) Modes of artificial ventilation in severe respiratory distress syndrome. Lung function and morphology studied in rabbits after wash-out of alveolar surfactant. Crit Care Med 10:724–732
25. Lachmann B, Danzmann E, Haendly B, Jonson B (1982 b) Ventilator settings and gas exchange in respiratory distress syndrome. In: Prakash O (ed) Applied physiology in clinical respiratory care. Martinus Nijhoff, The Hague, pp 141–176
26. Lachmann B, Fujiwara T, Chida S, Morita T, Konishi M, Nakamura K, Maeta H (1983) Surfactant replacement therapy in the experimental adult respiratory distress syndrome (ARDS). In: Cosmi EV, Scarpelli EM (eds) Pulmonary surfactant system. Elsevier, Amsterdam, pp 231–235
27. Lachmann B, Berggren P, Curstedt T, Grossman G, Robertson B (1984) Surfactant replacement in experimental respiratory distress syndrome induced by lung lavage. In: von Wichert P (ed) Current concepts in surfactant research. (Progress in Respiration Research) Karger, Basel, pp 251–256
28. Lachmann B, Danzmann E (1984) Adult respiratory distress syndrome. In: Robertson B, van Golde ME, Batenburg F (eds) Pulmonary surfactant. Elsevier, Amsterdam, pp 505–548
29. Macklem PT, Mead J (1967) Resistance of central and peripheral airways measured by retrograde catheter. J Appl Physiol 22:395–401
30. Manginello FP, Grassi AE, Schechner S, Krauss AN, Auld PAM (1978) Evaluation of methods of assisted ventilation in hyaline membrane disease. Arch Dis Child 53:878–881
31. Niemann GF, Bredenberg CE, Clark WR (1981) Alveolar function following surfactant deactivation. J Appl Physiol 51:895–904
32. Noack K, Bergmann KC, Eckert H, Luther P, Tischner H, Pohl W.D. (1982) Tierexperimentelles Modell einer aerogenen Influenzainfektion. Z Erkrank Atmungsorgane 159:155–165
33. Obladen M, Stevens P, Girndt R, Zimmermann I, Lachmann B (1984) Substitution spreitfähiger Phospholipid-Vesikel beim experimentellen Atemnotsyndrom der Ratte. Atemw Lungenkrankh 10:360–363
34. Reynolds EOR (1971) Effect of alterations in mechanical ventilator settings on pulmonary gas exchange in hyaline membrane disease. Arch Dis Child 46:152–159
35. Reynolds EOR (1974) Pressure waveform and ventilator setting for mechanical ventilation in severe hyaline membrane disease. Int Anesthesiol Clin 12:259–280

36. Skoskiewicz MJ (1976) Role of pulmonary transplantation in patients with acute respiratory failure. In: Zapol WM, Quist J (eds) Artificial lungs for acute respiratory failure. Hemisphere/Academic, Washington,pp 438–488
37. Schmidt GB, Parulkar DS, Brennan T, Feder J (1977) EPAP without intubation. Crit Care Med 5:207–209
38. Schuster DP, Snyder JV, Klain M (1982) Comparison of venous admixture during high frequency ventilation and conventional ventilation in oleic acid-induced pulmonary edema in dogs. Anesth Analg Curr Res 61:735–740
39. Thet LA, Alvarez H (1982) Effect of hyperventilation and starvation on rat lung mechanics and surfactant. Am Rev Respir Dis 126:286–290
40. Thompson WK, Marchak BE, Froese AB, Bryan AC (1982) High frequency oscillation compared with standard ventilation in pulmonary injury model. J Appl Physiol 52:543–548
41. Wolff G (1980) Was ist die akute respiratorische Insuffizienz? In: Peter K (Hrsg) Akute respiratorische Insuffizienz. (Anaesthesiology and intensive care medicine, vol 131) Springer, Berlin Heidelberg New York, pp 21–59
42. Wyszogrodski I, Kyei-Aboagye K, Taeusch HW Jr, Avery ME (1975) Surfactant inactivation by hyperventilation: conservation by end-expiratory pressure. J Appl Physiol 38:461–466
43. Zapol WM, Snider M, Hill JD (1979) Extracorporeal membrane oxygenation in severe acute respiratory failure. J Am Med Assoc 242:2193–2196

Microphysiological Studies on Oxygenation of Normal or Ischaemic Myocardium

N. S. Faithfull, W. Erdmann, M. Fennema, A. Kok, and C. E. Essed

This paper contains some observations on the state of oxygenation of myocardial tissue that were obtained during studies on the collateral supply of oxygen during haemodilution and during the production of myocardial infarction [4]. It was possible to obtain on-line partial pressures of oxygen (PO_2) from the myocardium for extended periods, and very high fidelity recordings were produced. It was thus possible to make accurate observations of myocardial oxygenation in relation to flow in the main coronary arteries and in relation to areas of ischaemic hypoxia.

Materials and Methods

Electrode Systems

The measurement of myocardial PO_2 was accomplished with the use of four steel-protected gold microelectrodes (Clark Electromedical Instruments) and a silver/silver chloride reference electrode. The gold microelectrodes, 200 µm in diameter, were embedded in a thin flexible plastic plate ±5 cm × 2 cm, which was sewn onto the epicardium. The distance between the electrodes was 1 cm and they protruded 3 mm into the left ventricular wall to ensure contact with the myocardium. When the gold electrodes are negatively polarized, oxygen is reduced, causing a current to flow to replenish the electrons used up in the process. At a voltage of −800 mV, this current is directly proportional to the oxygen concentration. To ensure partial pressure measurement, the electrode tips are covered with a plastic membrane, which also prevents protein poisoning and minimizes convestion dependency. Because the currents are so small (1–20 nA) measurements must be performed in an isolated Faraday cage [3]. Before starting the experiment, the electrodes were calibrated in a 37 °C saline solution, through which gases of known oxygen partial pressure were bubbled for equilibration. After the experiments, the electrodes were again calibrated to ensure reliability and to estimate any drift that had taken place.

Anaesthesia and Monitoring

Juvenile female Yorkshire pigs were used in this investigation, in which anaesthesia was induced with an intraperitoneal injection of sodium thiopentone (30 mg/kg bodyweight). After intubation with a cuffed endotracheal tube, the animals were ventilated with 33% oxygen in nitrous oxide or, in some cases, 0.5%

fluothane in 100% oxygen using a Minivent ventilator adjusted to maintain the arterial PCO_2 at between 35 and 45 mm Hg. Pancuronium bromide was used to maintain muscle relaxation and this was administered intravenously, using a Braun Melsungen Perfuser, adjusted to administer the drug at a rate of approximately 0.5 mg/kg per hour.

Through an incision in the groin, an arterial catheter was introduced into the femoral artery and advanced into the aorta. A venous catheter was introduced into the femoral vein and advanced into the inferior vena cava. A seven french gauge KMA thermodilution catheter was introduced into the other femoral vein and advanced under pressure monitoring into the pulmonary artery. The arterial line was connected to a Gould Statham P231ID pressure transducer, and the pulmonary artery line of the Swan Ganz and the central venous pressure line were connected to Gould Statham P23DC transducers. These, together with a Millar microtip pressure transducer PC470, which was introduced into the left ventricle via the carotid artery in the neck, were fed into a 12-channel Grass 7D polygraph and recorded on paper using a Grass ink-writing oscillograph.

Using the above instrumentation, the following parameters were monitored: systemic and pulmonary artery pressure, central venous pressure, pulmonary capillary wedge pressure, left ventricular pressure and left ventricular *dp*/*dt*. Cardiac output was determined by thermodilution using a KMA thermodilution cardiac output computer model 3500. Arterial blood was withdrawn at regular intervals for blood gas analysis using a Radiometer ALB1 acid base laboratory. Haemoglobin was estimated using a Radiometer OSM2 haemoxymeter. The thorax of the animal was opened using a sternal splitting technique, and the pericardium was then also opened. The pig was moved into a Siemens electrically isolated Faraday cage to minimize noise interference and all lines were led outside, via the grill "windows", to transducers and recording apparatus. The pig lay on a warming mattress through which water was pumped by a GRI aquamatic K heater circulator module. The PO_2 microelectrodes protruding through the plastic plate,

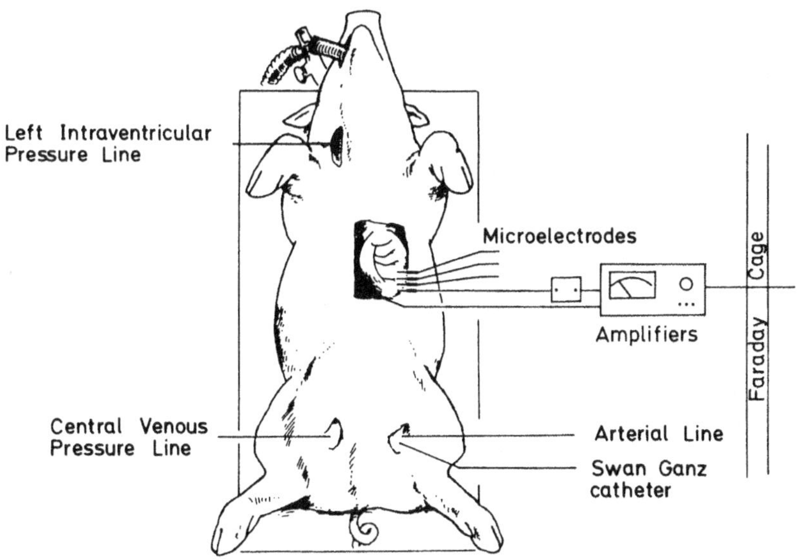

Fig. 1. Diagrammatic representation of the experimental setup

as described above, were sutured onto the epicardium after the electrodes had been placed in position in the expected area of distribution of the chosen branch of the left anterior descending coronary artery (LAD). This is a branch that was constantly observed, issuing laterally and to the left from the LAD about 2–3 cm above the apex of the heart. The electrical output from the electrodes was amplified by DC amplifiers inside the Faraday cage and the resulting signals were fed into a Rikadenki electronic recorder model KA60. The experimental arrangement is demonstrated in Fig. 1.

Results

Normal Oxygenation of the Myocardium

The oxygen partial pressures measured at the tip of the microelectrodes showed considerable variation between different electrodes. Swings in oxygen tension, coinciding with heart beat, were constantly observed. In general, the greater the myocardial oxygen tension measured, the greater the variation in tension throughout the heart cycle.

The variations seen in the electrode were constant in relation to the phase of the cardiac cycle. In Fig. 2, electrodes 1 and 3 show that maximum values are reached about 200 m/s after aortic valve closure and maximum coronary flow in the LAD. In Fig. 3 this pattern is repeated in electrodes 3 and 4, but peak oxygen values in electrodes 1 and 2 are reached during the ventricular systole. In this figure it can also be seen that the amplitude of the PO_2 variation is proportional to the mean myocardial tension at that particular point. These variations in the timing and amplitude of PO_2 variations were very commonly observed.

In addition to the above-mentioned changes in PO_2 dependent on the cardiac cycle, swings in oxygen concentrations could be observed coinciding with differ-

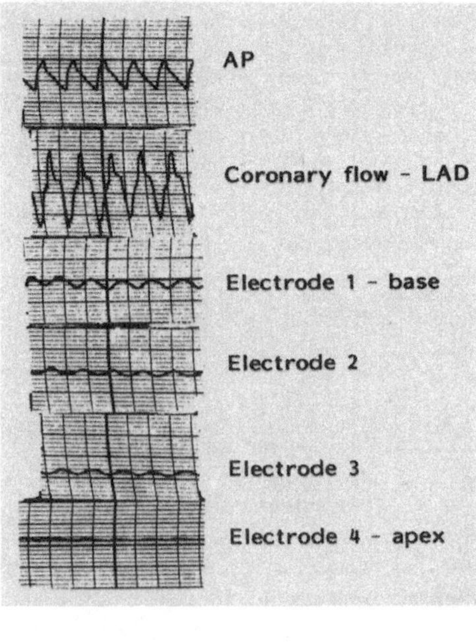

Fig. 2. Relationship between myocardial oxygen tension and coronary artery flow

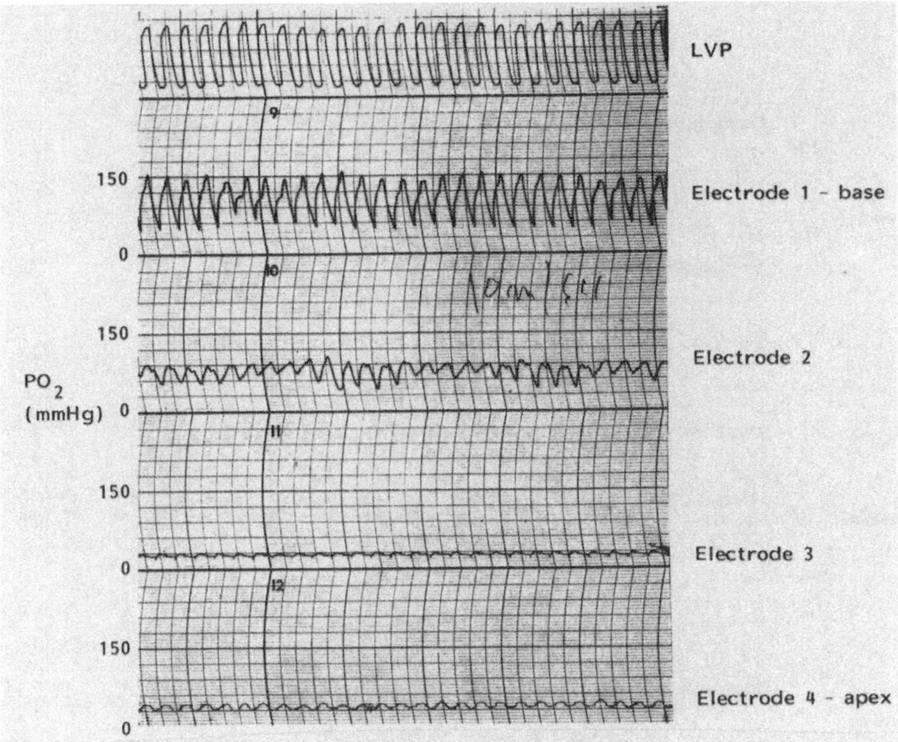

Fig. 3. Myocardial oxygen tension and left intraventricular pressure

ent phases of ventilation. These swings were sometimes very large and, superimposed on the cardiac swings already mentioned, caused variation of up to 10% in measured oxygen concentrations. In Fig. 4, the large downward deflections, caused by the intermittent positive pressure ventilation (IPPV), can be seen to coincide with inspiration and hence increased intravascular pressure caused by the IPPV. As can be seen the down swing of the oxygen concentration coincides with a rise of CVP (central venous pressure), PAP (pulmonary arterial pressure) and AP (aortal pressure). Inflation of the lungs, by causing increased flow of blood into the left heart, increases left ventricular fibre length and hence force of contraction – oxygen consumption is therefore raised and oxygen concentration falls. The direction of respiratory swings observed were always the same, though slope of the downward oxygen curve varied from electrode to electrode. The correlation coefficient between the total variations observed in the oxygen tension was: 0.77 (SE = 0.11) and the regression equation was: total oxygen variation $= 0.243 \times PO_2 + 0.17$.

Electrical Activity

In general the amplitude of electrical activity measured at the tips of the electrode was proportional to the maximum oxygen concentration. There appeared to be a critical oxygen concentration below which the amplitude of this activity was

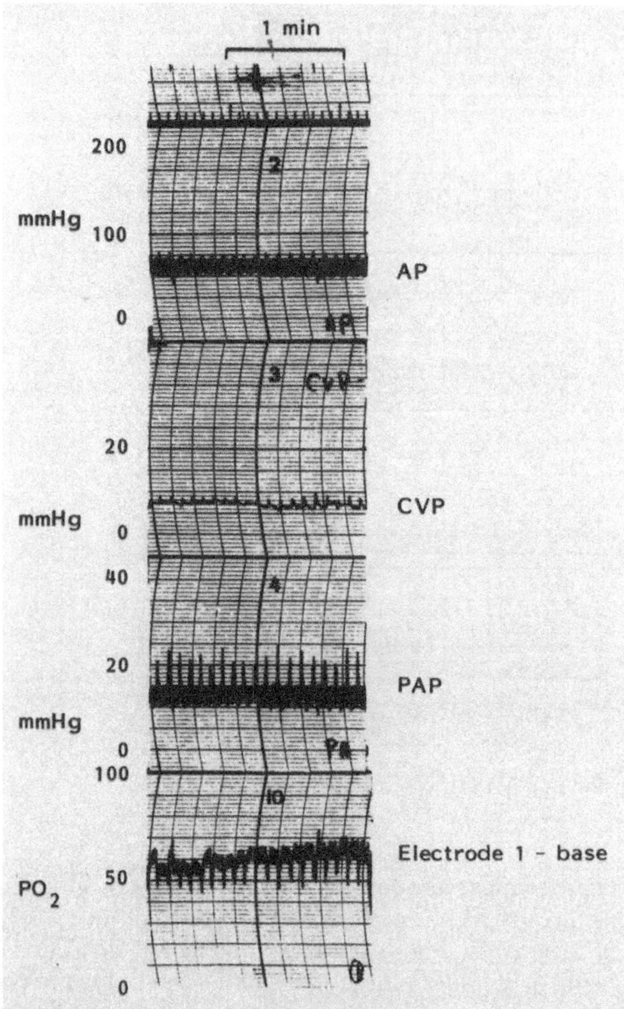

Fig. 4. The effect of intermittent positive pressure ventilation on myocardial oxygen tension and various cardiovascular parameters. *AP*, systemic arterial pressure; *PAP*, pulmonary artery pressure; *CVP*, central venous pressure

very low. These effects are demonstrated in Fig. 5, which shows the marked changes in electrical activity in electrode 4 related to changes in PO_2. However, this type of response was not always seen and in some cases decreasing PO_2 was accompanied by a rise in the amplitude of the electrical signals.

Effect of Cross-Clamping of the LAD Branch

Figure 6 demonstrates what may be considered a "classical" response to clamping as described by Reves et al. [8]. Electrodes 1 and 2 might be considered to be in non-ischaemic areas. Electrode 3, which shows a marked and immediate decrease in myocardial oxygen tension as the vessel is clamped, would be in the ischaemic areas and the subsequent rises in PO_2 indicated in electrode 4 would indicate an

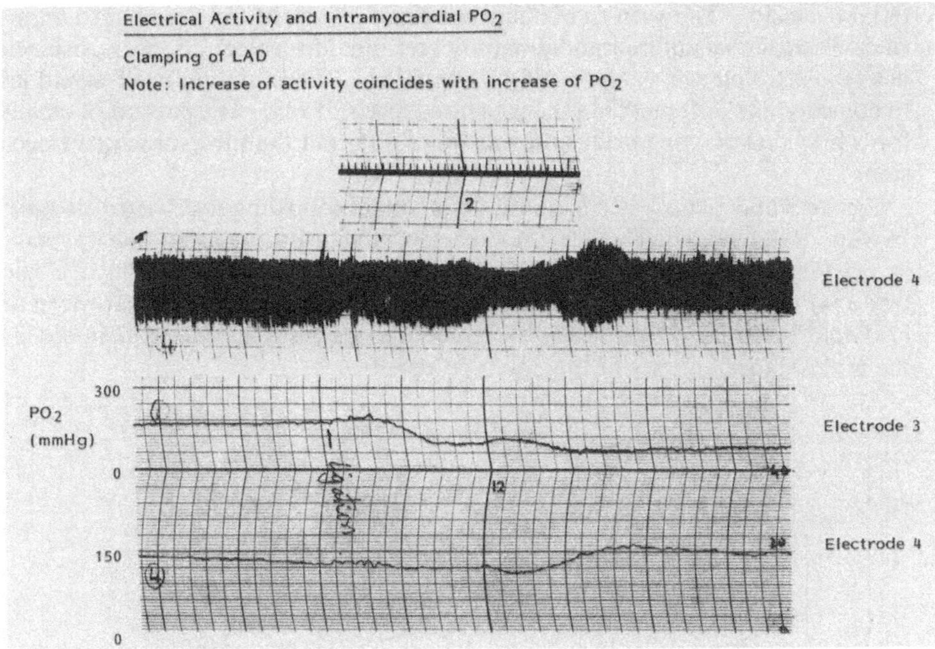

Fig. 5. The relationship between myocardial oxygen tension and the amplitude of myocardial electrical activity

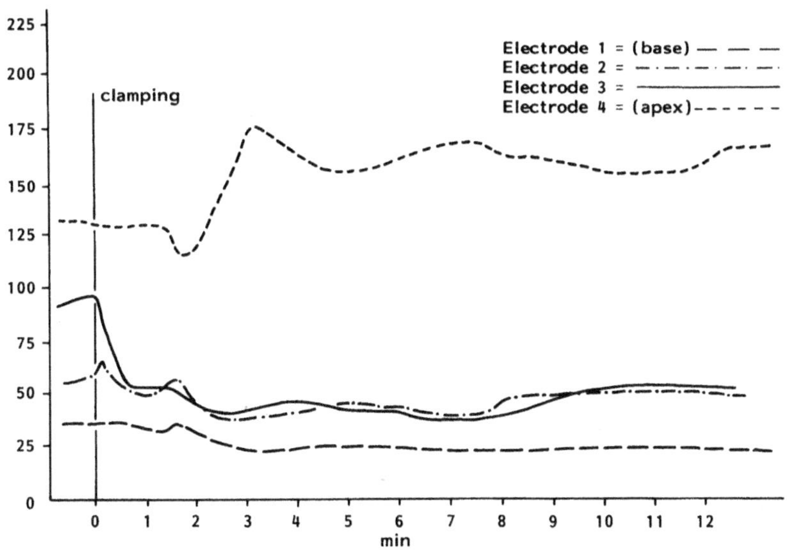

Fig. 6. "Classical" changes of myocardial PO_2 following clamping of a terminal branch of the LAD

autoregulatory increase in oxygen flux occurring in the partially ischaemic "border" area.

In view of the random placement of the electrode over the expected area of supply of the chosen branch of the LAD, it was almost impossible to predict the degree or direction of changes occurring at individual electrodes following arterial occlusion. The pattern of changes occurring varied from animal to animal. In addition, it was quite impossible to determine if an electrode was positioned near the arteriolar or venular end of a capillary – a fact that in itself would lead to considerable differences in the measured levels of PO_2. The pattern of changes for a first short-lasting occlusion was quite different than for subsequent occlusions.

Figure 7 and 8 show two examples of changes following short-term clamping. In Fig. 7, the two electrodes that reacted slowly during clamping (1 and 3) showed marked rebound on release of the occlusion while the most "active" electrode (4) hardly altered. In Fig. 7, similarly "inexplicable" changes are seen and it should be stressed that it was extremely difficult logically to explain some of the multifactorial causes of the observed results.

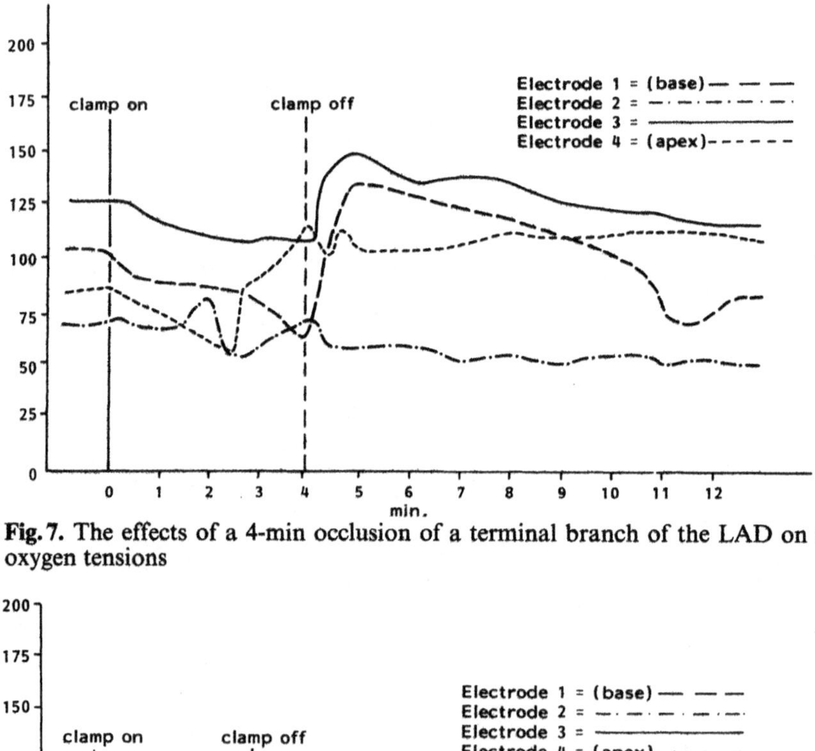

Fig. 7. The effects of a 4-min occlusion of a terminal branch of the LAD on myocardial oxygen tensions

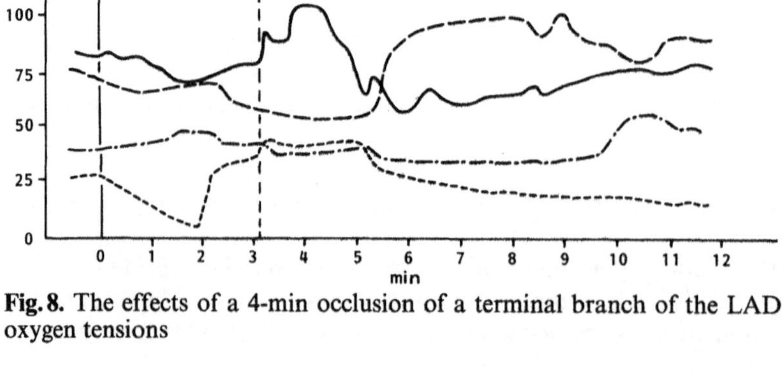

Fig. 8. The effects of a 4-min occlusion of a terminal branch of the LAD on myocardial oxygen tensions

Discussion

We have demonstrated that the arrival of oxygen at the myocardial tissues does not always occur during diastole. Coronary artery blood flow to the left ventricle was first shown by Marston et al. [7] to occur predominantly during diastole during the period immediately following closure of aortic valve and coincident with the dicrotic notch of aortic pulse wave. However, systolic extravascular compression of the coronary vessels as they course through the myocardium may cause a small back flow in the artery at the beginning of systole [5] – this effect is also seen in Fig. 2. Whereas flow in the main coronary arteries of the left ventricle is greater in diastole than in systole, the reverse is true for the right ventricle, in which flow during systole is not greatly opposed by the much smaller intramural tension generated in this chamber. Hence in the right ventricle the flow is greatest during systole.

The above statements are true for the major coronary arteries, though they obviously do not apply in the microcirculation. Tillmans et al. [10] using high-speed cinematography with transillumination of the left ventricle have studied flow in arterioles, capillaries and venules in turtle and dog hearts. They demonstrated that there is a transition of flow pattern from predominantly diastolic flow to predominantly systolic flow at the region of the arteriolar-capillary junction. Hence it is reasonable to conclude that the maximum oxygenation measured in microelectrodes would vary, depending on their positioning. For instance, if situated near an arteriole, maximum oxygenation would occur in diastole and it would be seen during systole if measurements were made in the vicinity of a capillary or venule.

The situation is further complicated by the spread of contraction through the ventricles. The spread of activation of contraction throughout the left ventricle begins in the intraventricular septum and at the atrial ventricular region. Spread through the ventricular walls is from endocardium to epicardium and Harris [6] has shown that the last portion of the ventricle to be activated is the apex. Hence, in some parts of the ventricle, blood would be squeezed onwards by extravascular compression during systole slightly earlier than in other parts. This would cause further variation in the precise timing of the arrival of maximal oxygen flux in the myocardium during systole.

Reves et al. [8] have presented results of cross-clamping of the LAD of dogs using 300-μm oxygen electrodes and have described a myocardial "steal" effect, in which PO_2 in normal areas of the myocardium was decreased. This they attributed to shunting of blood via collaterals into hypoxic border areas – in which autoregulation had resulted in decreased coronary vascular resistance.

In some recordings, we were able to observe biphasic myocardial PO_2 curves occurring over a period of 20–30 s. This would indicate that the initial changes caused by decreased oxygen supply due to impaired myocardial circulation are in some cases very rapidly compensated for by autoregulation and opening of channels of collateral supply. The existence of these channels has been postulated by many authors and Stam and de Jong [9] produced embolization of the coronary arteries of isolated perfused rat hearts using 20- to 80-μm diameter microspheres. Coronary blood flow decreased rapidly following microsphere injection but then increased again to reach a constant rate after 10 min. At this time the flows were significantly more than observed 2 min after embolization.

Berne and Rubio [1] have stated that adenosine is the only substance that can account for the entire coronary dilation observed in myocardial ischaemia and Stam and de Jong [9] noted that no rise in coronary flow following microembolisation occurred if the perfusate contained this substance, which is one of the breakdown products of ATP, produced by dephosphorylation of AMP. De Jong and Goldstein [2], working with pigs, studied the effects of ischaemic hypoxia on the release of inosine, hypoxanthine and lactate from the myocardium. They found very significant increases in levels of these substances over a 6-min period following 72% occlusion of the LAD.

The local release of ATP breakdown products may well be fast enough and of great enough magnitude to account for the extremely rapid increases in myocardial PO_2 that we observed. Indeed, Thompson et al. [11] have seen cyclical changes in adenosine during the cardiac cycle, with increases occurring during each systolic contraction of the myocardium. It may equally be argued that they are caused by acute local haemodynamic changes in the microcirculation causing increased local perfusion in certain areas.

The results obtained by the present authors do not tend to agree with the classical results of Reves et al. [8], in which they describe clear-cut ischaemic border and normal results. This may be due to two reasons. Firstly, their electrodes were distributed very widely over the left ventricle and hence they were certain to have at least one electrode measuring in the "normal" area of the myocardium – this was not so in the present study in which all four electrodes were positioned over a length of 3 cm. Secondly, their studies were not performed in a Faraday cage (Erdmann 1983, personal communication) and hence it was necessary, in order to filter out extraneous electrical "noise", to work with electrically damped signals. This would prevent their measuring some of the extremely rapid biphasic changes that were seen in these records.

In conclusion we have demonstrated that considerable variation in myocardial oxygen tension may be measured throughout the cardiac cycle and that these are a net result of the supply/demand situation in the tissues. Oxygenation of the myocardium in the normally functioning heart is not uniform but varies considerably over relatively short distances – this, we would suggest, is governed by the relationship to different vascular structures. Rapid and unpredictable changes may occur in myocardial PO_2 as a result of occlusion of terminal branches of the coronary arteries.

References

1. Berne RM, Rubio R (1969) Acute coronary occlusion: early changes that induce coronary dilation and the development of collateral circulation. Am J Cardiol 24:766
2. De Jong JW, Goldstein S (1974) Changes in coronary venous inosine concentration and myocardial wall thickening during regional ischemia in the pig. Circ Res 35:111
3. Erdmann W (1980) Continuous on-line acquisition of tissue PO_2, tissue perfusion, oxygen diffusion parameters and neuronal activity. In: Kimmich HP (ed) Monitoring of vital parameters during extra-corporeal circulation. Karger, Basel, p 73
4. Faithfull NS, Fennema M, Essed CE, Erdmann W, Jeekel H, Lapin R (1983) Collateral oxygenation of the ischemic myocardium – the effect of viscosity and oxygen carrying fluorocarbons. In: Bolin RB, Geyer RP, Nemo GJ (eds) Advances in blood substitute research. Liss, New York, p 229

5. Gregg DE (1963) Physiology of the coronary circulation. The George E Brown memorial lecture. Circulation 27:1128
6. Harris SA (1941) The spread of excitation in turtle, dog, cat and monkey ventricles. Am J Physiol 134:319
7. Marston EL, Barefoot CA, Spencer MP (1959) Non-cannulating measurements of coronary blood flow. Surg Forum 10:336
8. Reves JG, Erdmann W, Mardis M, Karp RB, King M, Lell WA (1978) Evidence for existence of myocardial steal. In: Silver IA et al. (eds) Oxygen transport to tissue, III. Plenum, New York, p 755
9. Stam H, de Jong JW (1977) Sephadex-induced reduction of coronary flow in the isolated rat heart: a model for ischemic heart disease. J Mol Cell Cardiol 9:633
10. Tillmans H, Ikeda S, Hansen H, Sarma JSM, Fauvel JM, Bing RJ (1974) Microcirculation in the ventricle of the dog and turtle. Circ Res 34:561
11. Thompson CI, Rubio R, Berne RM (1980) Changes in adenosine and glycogen phosphorylase activity during the cardiac cycle. Am J Physiol 238:H389

Autotransfusion in Surgical Practice: An Update

R. Lapin, F. Garcia, M. Zia, and C. Wright

Introduction

The increasing demand for homologous blood for major surgical procedures has strained the available sources of the blood banks. The increased number of patients being operated on, coupled with decreased donation, has created new problems for both anaesthesiologists and surgeons for which a solution must be found in order to keep operating rooms functioning at a high efficiency level. Current measures to reduce the number of homologous transfusions for patients undergoing emergency or elective procedures has resulted in the utilization of various blood-saving apparatuses and systems. In the past 15 years, intraoperative reinfusion of blood shed during surgery has been utilized for many reasons. The advantages of this approach have been to reduce the need for banked blood as well as avoid problems of transmittable diseases. The purpose of this manuscript is to outline our extensive experience with this technique in patients who refuse blood transfusions on religious grounds, as well as analyse the current state of the art of this concept. The authors hope that this information will serve only as a preliminary guideline for further research and development in this field.

Material and Methods

From January 1977 until Juli 1984, 1397 patients were operated on using an autotransfusion device. We have not used preoperative blood banking techniques on any of these patients. In all but 107 cases, the Haemonetics Cell Saver I was used. The patients ranged from 3 to 94 years of age. The breakdown of the numbers of patients, the surgical procedure, the intraoperative blood loss as well as the amount reinfused are given in Table 1. The hematological and biochemical changes which occurred following reinfusion are listed in Table 2.

We have encountered no mechanical failure of any of the autotransfusion devices listed in Table 3 used. None of the patients developed any transmittable disease following the reinfusion; furthermore, no cases of DIC (disseminated intravascular coagulopathy) were observed. The seven deaths that have occurred were related primarily to the advanced disease of the patients and not to the fact that they underwent autotransfusion.

Table 1. Experience with reinfusion techniques from 1977 to 1984

Procedure	Number of patients	Average blood loss (ml)	Average RBC suspension returned to patient (ml)	Complications
Orthopedic				
Total hip replacement	185	350	200	None
Harrington rod	83	675	350	None
Laminectomy, fusion	92	450	240	None
Open reduction	56	475	275	None
Aneurysmal bone cyst	4	550	300	None
Transthoracic spinal stabilization	6	600	325	None
Cardiothoracic				
Lobectomy	38	425	250	None
Pneumonectomy	11	400	230	None
Closed chest injury	36	900	500	None
Pulmonary decortication	8	1200	700	None
CABG	520	450	250	None
Valve replacement	32	500	285	2 deaths
Transposition	2	650	350	None
ASD	4	400	200	None
VSD	7	475	300	None
Vascular				
Abdominal aneurysmectomy	43	750	400	4 deaths
Lower extremity reconstruction	16	350	160	None
General, gynaecological and urology				
Splenectomy	23	650	375	None
Liver and pancreatic resection	5	1300	730	None
Hysterectomy	64	520	280	None
Ectopic pregnancy	14	1350	800	None
Abdominal trauma	24	1400	900	1 death
Open prostatectomy	28	450	200	None
Abdominal perineal resection	98	225	0	None
Total	1397			
Average blood loss	646 ml			
Average reinfusion	358 ml			

The Systems

Receptal – Sorenson Research Company, Inc., Salt Lake City, Utah, United States

This system is by far the least expensive and simplest to use, is extremely light and compact but is very effective for rapid reinfusion of whole blood in a patient experiencing exsanguinating haemorrhage.

The heart of the system is a gas-sterilized disposable flexible plastic bag with 1900 ml capacity which allows for uninterrupted collection of shed blood. This inner liner is placed in a reusable rigid plastic canister. The liner, which as of yet

Table 2. Haematological changes in patients following reinfusion

	Preop.	Day 1	Day 3	Day 7
Haemoglobin (g%)	9.6	10.8 mg%	11.0	11.4
Haematocrit (%)	29.8	29.6	31.5	32.0
Red blood cells (mm^3)	3.2	3.9	4.2	4.9
White blood cells (mm^3)	7.3	4.9	10.6	8.3
Total serum protein (%)	6.4	5.3	5.9	6.5
Platelets (mm^3)	153 000	68 000	93 000	140 000
Fibrinogen (mg/100 ml)	250	195	240	365
Fibrin-split product	Normal	Normal	Normal	Normal
PTT (s)	27	23	32	30
Plasma-free haemoglobin (mg/100 ml)	0.0	0.10	0.0	0.0
Urine haemoglobin (mg/100 ml)	0.0	0.10	0.0	0.0
Bacterial culture				
Staphylococcus epidermitis		3	Negative	Negative
E. coli		2	Negative	Negative
Klebsiella		1	Negative	Negative
2,3-DPG (mol/ml)	2.6	2.3	2.5	2.6
pH	7.35	7.49	7.41	7.36
Total bilirubin (mg)	0.5	1.3	1.1	0.9
BUN (mg/100 ml)	17	23	21	21
SGOT (IU/litre)	31	45	43	40

is not adaptable for use with an external pressure cuff because of its large size, welded plastic seams and friction-sealed inlet port, is equipped with a coarse 170-μm filter and a reinfusion intravenous port. This size filter is commonly applied to normally used blood administration bags and is adequate for removing blood clots, tissue debris, bony fragments and foreign bodies from the shed blood prior to entering the bag. When the bag is full or when a decision is made to reinfuse, further blood harvesting can continue by switching automatically to another lined canister. The liner containing the filtered blood is removed from its container. An intravenous administration set is connected directly to the port at the bottom of the liner. Active suction is required to speed up the collection of shed blood from the injured area. Adequate drainage can be achieved through a tube thoracostomy by employing 15–25 torr suction to the system, while 35–45 torr level is sufficient for aspiration from an open surgical field. Care must be taken to keep the suction pressure as low as possible so as to avoid damage to the erythrocytes.

The system is anticoagulated by the use of citrate-phosphate-dextrose (CPD) solution which is provided in a glass bottle as part of the entire system. The CPD solution enters the system at the inlet port. A volume control device is available in order to regulate the amount of CPD which is deemed necessary by the physician up to 240 ml for the 1900-ml liner.

There is still controversy as to whether anticoagulation is indeed necessary for blood harvested from chest injuries. It is generally accepted that blood which has been in contact with serous surfaces does not clot [1], and that platelets and fibrinogen levels are depressed [2]. Broadie has shown that fibrinolysis causes defibrination rather than the mechanical action of the cardiopulmonary system. Some authorities believe, therefore, that additional anticoagulation is unnecessary [3, 4], while others believe that it is mandatory [5, 6]. We believe, however, that sys-

Table 3. Autotransfusion devices

	Didelo-electromedics autotransfuser BT 7958	Haemonetics cellsaver I	IBM blood cell processor model 2991	Bentley ATS 100	Sorenson research Co. receptal ATS truma
Construction	Metal body construction. Metal i.v. pole stands. Large rubber wheels. Low centre of gravity. Internal cooling fan. Weight, 158 kg	Fibreglass body construction. Small rubber wheels. High centre of gravity. Internal cooling fan. Weight, 104 kg	Metal and plastic construction. Large rubber wheels. High centre of gravity. Weight, 161–195 kg	Metal housing using a metal roller pump head. Weight, 136 kg	Two plastic canisters, pole or roller mounted in brackets
Operation	Horizontal working surface. Power tubing clamps. Safety latch prevents exposure to spinning bowl. Single cam chuck. Non-O-ring seal in centrifuge. Large pump head roller. High-side-mounted drainage bag. Built in aspiration	Vertical working surface. Manual tubing clamps. Safety switch in lid must align before and during operation. Three cam chucks. O-ring seal. Small pump head roller. Low front-mounted drainage bag. Exterior aspiration	Horizontal and vertical working surface. Pegboard controls with timer dials to programme each run. External suction. Uses doughnut plastic spinning ring. Finished product displaced by pumping hydraulic fluid under centrifuge surface to flatten doughnut sending cells to reservoir bag	Roller head provides suction to reservoir from pump head. Returned to patient via gravity	Sterile line is placed into canister vacuum. External regulation of negative pressure is advised
Processing	Pump speed, 0–300 ml/min with faster manual override. 2-min setup. Processing time, 6–9 min. Variable speed centrifuge, 0–4800 ± 200 rpm. Wash solution, 0.9% NaCl	Pump speed, 0–300 ml/min. No manual override. 3-min setup. Processing time, 7–10 min. Single speed centrifuge, 0–4600 ± 200 rpm. Wash solution, 0.9% NaCl	Processing time up to 20 min depending on programming. Centrifuge is agitated during wash cycle	Processing is continuous once blood is sequestered. No wash cycle	Dependent on rate of blood loss. 1900 ml total. Includes anticoagulant. No wash cycle

(continued)

Table 3 (continued)

	Didelo-electromedics autotransfuser BT 7958	Haemonetics cellsaver I	IBM blood cell processor model 2991	Bentley ATS 100	Sorenson research Co. receptal ATS truma
Blood component returned	Packed washed cells. Anticoagulant washed away.[a] Amount varies with bowl size (125, 225, 350)	Packed washed cells. Anticoagulant washed away.[a] Amount varies with bowl size (125, 225, 350)	Packed washed cells. Anticoagulant washed away.[a]	Whole blood, operative site aspirate and anticoagulant	Whole blood with component, operative site or trauma site aspirates and anticoagulant
Anticoagulant	Heparin 30000 U/litre dripped down field suction tubing, 60/100 ml/h	Heparin 30000 U/litre dripped down field suction tubing, 60/100 ml/h	Heparin 30000 U/litre CPD 30–60 ml/h dripped down suction line	Regional heparinization 2 mg/kg	CPD 30–60 ml/h dripped into sterile reservoir
Blood reservoir	Cardiotomy	Cardiotomy or clam shell reservoir	Cardiotomy or Sorenson ATS trauma set	Cardiotomy incorporated in system	Incorporated
Unit cost	$ 16200 with reservoir	$ 13900	$ 23000 Model 1 $ 13750 Model 2	Approx. $ 3500	Free with use of liners
Software	Autotransfusion pack, $ 64.50. Cardiotomy, $ 45.00. Suction tubing, $ 17.00	Autotransfusion pack, $ 65.00. Cardiotomy, $ 45.00. Clam shell liner, $ 27.00. Suction tubing, $ 17.50	Processing unit $ 13.35 (good for 400 cc/pcs). Suction tubing, $ 17.00. Citrate, $ 7.92. Note: Rights have been sold to Cobe Medical	A200 software, $ 150.00–$ 200.00. No longer in production	Liners, $ 20.92. Suction, $ 17.80. Citrate, $ 7.92 for 500 ml

[a] 1000 ml wash solution

temic anticoagulation should be avoided at all cost when harvesting blood for the purpose of reinfusion from a patient suffering from multiple trauma so as to avoid increased bleeding in the brain, abdomen, pelvis and lungs. If the physician chooses to use heparin instead of CPD, this can be accomplished by using heparinized Ringers' lactate, connecting it to the inlet port. The activated clotting time should be measured and kept at greater than 200 s. The clotting time can be easily measured in the operating room by the use of a Hemochron (blood coagulation timing system, International Technidyne, Metuchen, New York).

Most authorities in this field agree that reinfusion of shed blood can be safely accomplished without great concern for the problem of major coagulopathy as long as the reinfused volume is not greater than 3000 ml [2, 7–9].

The Sorenson system employs only a 170-micron coarse filter which may not always be adequate to protect the patient from the risk of pulmonary insufficiency resulting from infused lysed erythrocytes, fat, fibrin or other foreign bodies. We would recommend incorporating a second-in-line microfilter into the system with a pore size of between 20 and 40 mm in order to reduce the possibility of microaggregate reinfusion and also reduce the absolute bacterial count in final infusion. We realize, however, that the second filter may also trap a large number of valuable platelets and leucocytes as well as increase the overall processing time.

The system is easily adaptable to postoperative continuous harvesting of shed blood, especially from the thorax. This is accomplished by connecting the chest tubes through an underwater seal to the container and periodically reinfusing the collected material.

The system is extremely cost effective when compared with the use of homologous banked blood, which costs approximately $ 80.00 per unit. Two units of reinfused blood from a trauma patient cost $ 25.00 while 2 units of mediastinal blood reinfused postoperatively cost $ 30.00.

To date, over 10000 patients have benefited from the use of this system, with few complications.

Bentley Autotransfusion System (ATS 100-209) Bentley Laboratories, Irvine, California, United States

This intraoperative reinfusion apparatus is manufactured by Bentley Laboratories of Irvine, California. This device, which was designed by Klebanoff in 1970 [29] using adapted components of a pump oxygenator, is capable of aspirating blood from the wound at a rate of several litres per minute. This system has inaugurated the modern era of autotransfusion with its successful use in battlefield medicine during the Vietnam conflict. The system consists of two main components: a permanent single-roller head pump and frame assembly with a sensor device designed to minimize the possibility of air embolization; a disposable plastic reservoir and tubing for aspiration and reinfusion. Negative-pressure aspiration is created by the roller-head pump, which totally occludes the tubing with the rollers. The blood passes to the cardiotomy-type collection reservoir, where it passes through a coarse nylon pad and a 170-micron macrofilter. Blood which is collected in the reservoir may be reinfused through two intravenous lines at a rate of 1000–2000 ml/min. Reinfusion rate is limited only by the size of the intravenous lines in the recipient. Flow dynamics through small tubes is proportional to the 4th power of the diameter of the tube; therefore, doubling the size of the tube increases flow rate 16-fold. When rapid reinfusion is anticipated to be life saving, a No. 8 Fr. catheter can be placed in the pulmonary artery to serve such a purpose. Three methods of anticoagulation have been employed: (1) systemic heparin (2–3 mg/kg), (2) regional heparinization and (3) titration of CPD into the collected blood with Venturi suction allowing mixing with the blood at a 7:1 ratio.

A modification of the system was made at Indiana University, where one outflow line from the reservoir was connected to another roller pump with calibration of the tubing for the amount of blood pumped by one revolution. A rotameter was connected to the pump head, which allowed for direct reading of the exact amount of blood infused. This modification enabled the operator to retroinfuse under pressure, by gravity, or both [10].

The cost of the disposable plastic ware is approximately $150.00–$200.00.

The problems associated with the use of this system have been related to pump-induced mechanical trauma to blood components as well as massive and fatal air embolization to the patient caused by operator error. Because of these problems, Bentley Laboratories voluntarily withdrew this system from the market in 1981. These devices are still in use both in the United States and internationally because of the availability of the software.

IBM Cell Processor Model 2991, IBM Corporation, Princeton, New Jersey, United States

As an outgrowth of cell-washing technology from blood banking, IBM, Corporation of Princeton, New Jersey, has manufactured this device since 1974. This system is by far the most expensive, least mobile, as well as the most difficult to operate. It has both horizontal and vertical working surfaces and relies on a complicated pegboard control system with timer dials to program each run. This apparatus is designed to wash collected whole blood with saline solution and remove all unwanted material from it. At the present time, the device does not contain a reservoir in order to remove blood from the surgical field prior to washing. The Sorenson disposable liner and aspiration system are suited for this purpose at a cost of $50.00. The centrifuge is designed with a hydraulic shim which permits the processing of variable amounts of erythrocytes suspension within the same bag. Because the functional volume of the systems is variable, the wash provides a high-quality red cell suspension free of WBC, platelets and clotting factors. The concentration and purification is performed inside a disposable plastic doughnut-shaped liner with 600-ml capacity which costs $13.00. The washing bag can also serve as a transfusion bag. The collected blood is usually regionally anticoagulated with heparin or CPD.

The system can be programmed early to wash the blood once or many times depending on the quality of the collected material.

The washed red cells are suspended in saline before reinfusion begins. These cells have a normal 2,3-diphosphoglycerate (2,3-DPG) level and are considerably more resistent to osmotic lysis. The half-life of autotransfused cells is equal to that of homologous cells. It must be kept in mind that in such a mode of reinfusion technique, no clotting factors, platelets or WBCs are returned to the patients and, as such, fresh frozen plasma and platelets may be needed to augment the loss especially if more than 2500 ml is reinfused.

The serious disadvantages of the IBM cell processor are its lack of collection system, lack of mobility due to its bulky size, complicated mode of programming, and the fact that the collected blood and the wash phase are not done simultaneously in the operating room, thus allowing for potential error if more than one patient is undergoing a blood harvesting process.

Haemonetics Cell Saver: Haemonetics Corporation, Massachusetts, United States

This device has been manufactured by the Haemonetics Corporation of Massachusetts since the late 1970s and today enjoys great popularity in the United States. The various models of this collection and cell-washing machine range from totally manual control to totally automated operation. Blood is retreived from the operating field by a double-lumen suction catheter in which it is anticoagulated on contact with heparin (30 000 U/1000 ml) of saline dripped down in the suction tip at 100 ml/h. The harvested blood is diverted into the collection reservoir, where a 180-micron filter removes the gross debris. From there the blood is pumped to a spinning centrifuge bowl, where it is packed and washed with at least 2000 ml saline to remove all the soluble haemoglobin and the RBCs are packed. The effluent containing plasma fractions, platelets, WBCs, free haemoglobin, anticoagulant and debris is discarded. The washed packed erythrocytes, suspended in saline, are pumped from the centrifuge bowl to a transfer bag and reinfused to the patient through a 40-mm filter. If bleeding is extremely rapid the entire process can be accomplished in 15 min. Employing careful aspiration techniques during the surgical procedure by using low suction and keeping the suction tip constantly in the wound, thus avoiding the "slurping" sound caused by the air-blood interface, RBC recovery can be as high as 70%.

The cell saver has been used in over 15000 patients in the United States with no reports of air embolism or major coagulopathy. The unit is extremely mobile and remains next to the surgical field during the entire procedure. It does require a trained technician to operate it safely and efficiently. The software, including suction tubing, costs approximately $150.00.

Dideco: Electromedics Autotransfuser Bt-7958

This is the latest addition to the rapidly expanding field of cell-washed autotransfusion devices. It is compact, easy to operate and extremely mobile, and incorporates a built-in aspiration unit as an intregral part of the system instead of relying on wall suction.

This device has a horizontal working surface with simple control mechanisms. It has power tubing clamps, a safety latch to prevent exposure of the spinning bowl, a large pump head roller, a non-O-ring seal in the centrifuge mechanism, a single-cam chuck and a High side-mounted drainage bag. The pump speed varies between 0 and 300 ml/min, with a faster manual override. The system requires about 2 min to set up. Processing time ranges between 6 and 9 min. The centrifuge speed ranges between 0 and 4800 ± 200 rpm. The cells are washed and suspended in saline. This machine produces high-quality clean red cell suspension, while washing out the anticoagulant, platelets, WBCs, debris and plasma. Anticoagulation is achieved by drippping a heparinized solution into the suction tip, thus inducing a non-clotting state on contact. The software cost is approximately $ 130.00. As in the other cell washer devices, it is mandatory that a trained technician be present to operate this system. We have found this device to be by far the most versatile and most efficient of the cell washers we have tried. The addition of the built-in aspiration unit makes it totally independent of wall suction.

Historical Review

The ancient Greeks believed in the magical properties of blood, and classified it as part of the four humours in the body [11]. Removing blood was one of the main foundations in the treatment of diseases. This practice remained with physicians until the late 1800s. Greek mythology provides us with the first description of blood transfusions when Asclepius gave Athena Gargon's blood [12]. In 1496, the life of Pope Innocent VIII could not be saved by his physician when they attempted to transfuse him with the blood of two young donors. It is not clear whether the Pontiff received the blood intravenously or orally, but in any case both he and the donors died soon after this historic event [11]. In 1667, Lower successfully transfused a patient with sheep blood [11]. Recognizing that therapeutic phlebotomy led to anaemia, Dennis transfused some of his patients with animal blood [11]. Following the death of one of the patients, the practice of transfusions was stopped by the medical establishment in both France and England.

In 1818, Blundell suggested the method of autotransfusion for the first time and also developed a device for blood collection from a donor. He further showed that haemorrhagic shock in dogs could be successfully treated by using blood transfusions from other dogs. He transfused ten acutely anaemic patients with a 50% mortality rate [13]. The first paper actually advocating employing autotransfusion as a therapeutic modality was published by Highmore, an English obstetrician, in 1874 [14]. The first surgical autotransfusion was performed by Duncan in a patient undergoing a lower extremity amputation. The shed blood was collected in a basin containing phosphate of soda for the purpose of anticoagulation [14] and then reinfused to the patient with no apparent ill effects'. In 1883, Halsted reported treating patients with carbon monoxide poisoning by autotransfusing the patient with oxygenated blood [16]. Thies reported the first three cases of intraoperative reinfusion in females with ruptured ectopic pregnancies [17]. In 1916, Lockwood reported the successful use of this technique in patients undergoing splenectomies [18]. After Landsteiner's discovery of the ABO blood groups in 1900 and the subsequent development of anticoagulants, there was a rapid increase in the use of homologous transfusion. The first blood bank in the United States was created at the Mayo Clinic by Lundy in 1935. During World War I, Elmendorf reported the first use of autotransfusion from the haemothorax without anticoagulation [19]. Davis and Cushing reported neurosurgical procedures in which reinfusion techniques were successfully employed in 1925 [20].

By 1931, there were 282 reports in the literature on the use of this modality, with an overall mortality of 2.2% [21, 22]. Tiber, in 1934, reported its use in 123 cases of ruptured ectopic pregnancies and subsequently used it in another 250 cases without a single reaction to the reinfusion [23]. In 1960, Weeks reported three mortalities attributed to autotransfusion where in each case the reinfused blood was present in the peritoneal cavity for more than 3 days and was completely haemolysed [24, 25].

There is some sketchy evidence that British surgeons working in India were using autotransfusion on battle casualties as early as 1865; similarly, German physicians were employing it in treating abdominal and chest trauma cases resulting from exploding grenades [26]. It has been successfully used in cases in which the liver and/or kidneys have been ruptured and blood containing bile and urine was successfully retroinfused.

Autotransfusion was used very little for the 20-year period following World War I primarily because of the rapid development of blood banking which streamlined the use of homologous blood transfusions. Such easy availability of banked blood has caused a meteoric rise in its overall use which in many cases was not indicated. This rapid increase in use also increased the overall rate of transfusion-related hepatitis and other transmittable diseases.

In 1963, Langston et al. reported the concept of preoperative autotransfusion as a viable concept in the overall attempt in reducing the ever-increasing dependency on homologous transfusions [27]. This concept was again introduced by Cuello for use in vascular surgery in 1966 [28].

In 1969, Klebanoff introduced a device which he developed from parts borrowed from the pump oxygenator. This device was tested with good results in Vietnam and was later marketed by Bentley Laboratories as the first modern-day apparatus for the purpose of autotransfusion. Klebanoff also showed that faecal-contaminated blood was not an absolute contraindication for its use in reinfusion [29, 30]. The Bentley ATS 100 was plagued by reports of fatal air emboli and coagulopathies associated with its use [31]. These reports finally caused Bentley Laboratories voluntarily to remove it from the market.

In 1975, Noon et al. [32] reported their experience with a new Sorenson autotransfusion system in which the collected blood was filtered and, using the collection bag as a conduit, the blood was reinfused. Cell-washing as the foundation for a new generation of devices to be used for autotransfusion was an outgrowth of separation techniques and component therapy employed by the blood banks [33].

Hauer, in 1976, reported a 50% reduction in postoperative homologous transfusion given to patients undergoing cardiac surgery by using the Sorenson system when he returned to the patients the unclotted shed mediastinal blood. Thus, the era of postoperative retroinfusion was born [34]. With the high-quality devices now available to physicians for the purpose of reinfusion, the dependency on homologous blood transfusions can be greatly reduced.

Discussion

Autologous blood is of high quality, warm, compatible and most of all available. The RBCs have a normal life span [3], good oxygen-carrying capacity [5], and normal levels of 2,3-DPG. Autologous blood may contain platelets, WBCs and clotting factors depending on the device used for its collection and reinfusion. The blood has physiological levels of serum electrolytes, normal pH and normal acid-base balance. It is therefore not logical to assume that such blood is inferior in quality to banked blood when the latter, at 14 days, has an average pH of 6.7, K^+ concentration of 19 mEq/litre, ammonia level of 470 mg/dl, lactic acid level of 120 /dl and free haemoglobin level of 50 mg/dl and is devoid of platelets, WBCs and clotting factors [10]. The autologous product is warm and thus can be infused immediately without causing a fall in the patient's core body temperature. Also, it causes few if any problems with incompatibility as well as febrile or allergic reaction. The risk of acquiring hepatitis, malaria, syphilis, AIDS or other transmittable diseases is almost non-existent. The chance of transfusing a patient with incompatible blood are also greatly reduced even when facing the chaotic environment inherent to any major disaster.

Contraindications to reinfusion of harvested blood are based on the potential risk of infusing a product which may be contaminated by faecal material, bile, urine or tumour cells. Several authors have shown, however, that it is possible to autotransfuse contaminated blood without lethal effects to the recipient [29, 35]. Other researchers in this field have concluded that when homologous blood is not available, the advantages of infusing potentially contaminated blood may outweigh the disadvantages [2, 8]. Our experience and that of others has shown that a transient bacteraemia occurs following such an infusion with bacterial contamination but that all blood cultures become negative within 24 h [36]. The likelihood of complications from bacterial contamination can be greatly reduced by washing the erythrocytes as well as incorporating additional micropore filters into the infusion lines prior to administration and at the same time using systemic antibiotics as well as incorporating their use in the wash process. It may be oversimplifying the point but we believe that it is safe to assume that it is easier to treat a patient with sepsis than rigor mortis. The risk of reinfusing tumour cells is more a theoretical consideration than a practical one in dealing with mass casualties. Tumour cells have been recovered from filtered blood of patients prior to reinfusion; however, no definite increase in metastasis was noted in patients who received such blood.

The complications of autotransfusion include air emboli reported only with the Bentley [31], which is presently not commercially available except for the software. Coagulation defects may likewise occur in the patients who are autotransfused; however, it is important to keep in mind that these patients may frequently be the victims of DIC from other causes, such as sepsis following massive injuries; they may develop dilutional coagulopathies secondary to inadequate replacement of platelets and fresh frozen plasma. Autotransfusion does not completely protect the patient from such problems, and appropriate component therapy is thus needed, especially in massive blood loss. The possibility of renal failure secondary to increased level of free haemoglobin resulting in autotransfused patients has been suggested by Glover; however, other authors have found no deliterious effect on renal function by free haemoglobin normally encountered in autotransfusion [10]. Renal damage is more likely to occur from unfiltered red cell stroma. It is therefore important to use autotransfused whole blood with caution with renal disease, and when possible it should be washed.

References

1. Brown LA, Debenham MW (1931) Autotransfusion: use of blood from hemothorax. JAMA 96:1223–1225
2. Mattox KL et al. (1975) Blood availability for the trauma patient-autotransfusion. J Trauma 15:663–668
3. Symbas PN et al. (1969) A study on autotransfusion from hemothorax. Southern Med J 62:671–674
4. Symbas PN et al. (1978) Extraoperative autotransfusion from hemothorax. Surgery 84:722–727
5. Ferrara BE (1957) Autotransfusion: its use in acute hemothorax. Southern Med J 50:516–519
6. VonKoch L et al. (1977) A practical method of autotransfusion in the emergency center. Am J Surg 133:770–772
7. Reul GJ et al. (1978) Experience with autotransfusion in the surgical management of trauma. Surgery 76:546–555
8. Davidson SJ (1978) Emergency unit autotransfusion. Surgery 84:703–707
9. Davidson SJ (1981) Correct use of autotransfusion in the emergency patient. ER Reports 2:73–78
10. Glover JL, Broadie TA (1982) Intraoperative autotransfusion. Mass Transf Surg Trauma 2:151–170
11. Wintrobe MM (1980) Blood, pure and eloquent. New York, McGraw Hill, New York, pp 659–683
12. Sigerist HE (1961) A history of medicine. University Press, New York, p 200
13. Blundell J (1818) Experiments on the transfusion of blood by the syringe. Med Chir Trans 9:56
14. Highmore W (1874) Practical remarks on an overlooked source of blood supply. Lancet 1:89
15. Duncan J (1886) On reinfusion of blood in primary and other amputations. Br Med J 1:192
16. Halsted WS (1883) Reinfusion of carbonic oxide poisoning. NY Med J, p 625
17. Thies HJ (1914) Zur Behandlung der Extrauteringravidität. Zentralbl Gynakol 38:1991
18. Lockwood CD (1917) Surgical treatment of Banti's disease. Surg Gynecol Obstet 25:188
19. Elmendorf H (1917) Über Wiederinfusion nach Punktion eines frischen Haematothorax. Muench Med Wochenschr 64:36
20. Davis LE, Cushing H (1925) Experiences with blood replacement during or after major intracranial operations. Surg Gynecol Obstet 40:310
21. Appleby LH (1925) Autotransfusion. Can Med Assoc J 15:36–37
22. Hendry WB (1925) A clinical analysis of 152 cases of ectopic gestation. Am J Obstet Gynecol 10:386–391
23. Tiber LJ (1934) Ruptured ectopic pregnancy. Calif Western Med 41:16–20
24. Weekes LR, Stone E, McCann C (1960) A plea for autotransfusion. Obstet Gynecol 16:715–718
25. Weekes LR (1964) Autotransfusion. J Natl Med Assoc 56:494–497
26. Burch LE (1922) Autotransfusion. Trans Southern Surg Assoc 35:25–35
27. Langston HT, Milles G, Dalessandro W (1963) Further experiences with autologous blood transfusions. Ann Surg 158:335
28. Cuello L, Vasquez E, Rios R et al. (1967) Autologous blood transfusion in thoracic and cardiovascular surgery. Surgery 62:814
29. Klebanoff G (1970) Early clinical experience with a disposable unit for intraoperative salvage and reinfusion of blood loss (intraoperative autotransfusion). Am J Surg 120:718–722
30. Klebanoff G (1978) Intraoperative autotransfusion with the Bentley ATS-100. Surgery 83:708–712
31. Duncan SE, Klebanoff G, Rogers W (1974) Patient experience with intraoperative autotransfusion. Rev Surg 31:121

32. Noon GP, Solis RT, Natelson EA (1976) A simple method of intraoperative autotransfusion. Surg Gynecol Obstet 143:65
33. Gilcher RD, Orr MD (1975) Intraoperative autotransfusion (Abstract). Transfusion 15:520
34. Hauer JM, Schaff HV, Bell WR et al. (1977) Reinfusion of shed mediastinal blood following cardiac surgery: a prospective study (Abstract). Circulation [Suppl] 56:4
35. Griswold RA, Ortner AB (1943) The use of autotransfusion in surgery of the serous cavities. Surg Gynecol Obstet 77:167–177
36. Glover JL et al. (1978) Autotransfusion of blood contaminated by intestinal contents. J Am Coll Emerg Phys 7:142–144

Changes in Important Biochemical Parameters Due to Extreme Haemodilution with Cross-linked Stromafree Haemoglobin Solution

G. Klein, H. Ferber, U. Ottermann, and H. Förster

Introduction

Transport of biological available oxygen in vertebrates is performed by two different principles: physical solution in plasma and chemical binding to the haemoglobin molecule. According to these principles the development of oxygen-carrying colloids proceeds along two different pathways. The fluorocarbons increase the amount of physically dissolved oxygen due to the extraordinary oxygen-solubility of these compounds [7]. Some research groups have favoured the development of stroma-free haemoglobin solutions (SFH). These compounds chemically bind oxygen similar to the natural intraerythrocytic haemoglobin [2, 6]. In particular, Bonhard and coworkers have been able to improve the oxygen-transporting property and the intravascular persistence of these SFH solutions [1, 3]. The former was achieved by pyridoxalation and the latter by intermolecular cross-linkage of haemoglobin molecules. This new type of SFH was called "nhpa", where "n" means polymer, "h" means haemoglobin, "p" means pyridoxalation and "a" means albumin addition for correction of oncotic pressure. This 8.5% nhpa is a research product of Biotest-Pharma, Frankfurt. With this oxygen-carrying colloid we performed extreme isovolemic haemodilution in dogs and examined the changes in different biochemical parameters.

Material and Method

All the investigations were performed in splenectomized beagles ($n = 8$). The interval between splenectomy and our experiment was more than 6 weeks. Details of the exchange procedure are published elsewhere [4, 5]. The animals received a total dosage of 6 g/kg stroma-free haemoglobin. The biochemical parameters were determined the same day using standard analyzing techniques in the laboratories of Prof. Förster.

Results (Table 1)

Lactate

After we had finished our preparations (for invasive haemodynamic monitoring) we found relatively high levels with distinct interindividual differences. The minimum and maximum levels were found to be 5 mg/dl and 46 mg/dl with a mean

Table 1. Changes in important biochemical parameters due to extreme haemodilution with cross-linked stroma-free haemoglobin solution ($\bar{x} \pm SEM$)

Parameter	Preop.	Postop.	24 h postop.	72 h postop.
Lactate (mg/dl)	32.05 (5.33)	36.14 (4.0)	13.86 (3.32)	22.60 (5.56)
Glucose (mg/dl)	85.38 (7.16)	106.14 (5.91)	94.25 (4.24)	111.0 (10.07)
FFA (mmol/litre)	0.62 (0.09)	0.61 (0.17)	1.05 (0.12)	0.59 (0.07)
TG (mg/dl)	69.74 (14.14)	22.9 (5.87)	49.71 (3.0)	102.50 (3.49)
Na^+ (mmol/litre)	148.9 (1.8)	147.5 (3.3)	144.6 (1.7)	146.8 (1.2)
K^+ (mmol/litre)	3.63 (0.07)	3.40 (0.16)	3.64 (0.11)	4.04 (0.31)
Creatinine (mg/dl)	0.93 (0.03)	0.88 (0.07)	1.02 (0.07)	0.96 (0.08)

of 32 mg/dl. During blood exchange, lactate remained nearly constant. During the early postdilution phase it decreased markedly to 14 mg/dl, with a subsequent increase to 23 mg/dl 3 days after the dilution. At all points of measurement we found the above-mentioned distinct interindividual differences of this parameter. But we were unable to find a correlation either with arterial or with mixed-venous pH values.

Glucose

The mean glucose value before we started the haemodilution was 85 mg/dl. During and after dilution we found a slight increase to 106 mg/dl. In the early and late postdilution phase glucose showed no remarkable changes compared with predilutional values. Throughout the whole observation period the highest measured glucose level in all animals was 134 mg/dl. So overall we found that the behaviour of this parameter was remarkably stable.

Free Fatty Acids

Like lactate, the free fatty acids (FFAs) showed distinct intra- and interindividual differences. Apart from slight fluctuations we measured relatively constant FFA levels within a physiological range of around 0.6 mmol/litre. In particular we found no definite pathological values.

Triglycerides

The triglycerides (TGs) also showed distinct interindividual differences, but each animal showed the same reduction trend due to dilution. We measured a decrease from 70 mg/dl to 23 mg/dl in the early postdilution phase. Three days after the blood exchange we found levels higher than predilutional levels but within the normal range.

Electrolytes (Na^+, K^+, Cl^-)

The serum levels of sodium and chloride did not change at all throughout the observation period, remaining stable within the physiological range. Serum potassium showed – apart from a slight dilutional reduction – no significant or even pathological changes.

Creatinine

This important index of renal function remained remarkably stable throughout the whole observation period. We found pre- and postdilutional levels to be about 1 mg/dl. Only one dog developed a slight increase from 0.8 mg/dl to 1.3 mg/dl 4 days after our exchange procedure. But 2 days later the predilutional value was reached again.

Conclusions

Apart from unspecific changes due to dilution we found no significant alterations of any of the above-mentioned parameters. In particular, we were not able to find definite pathological values due to the extreme dilution with nhpa. The remarkably stable serum creatinine levels even at a total dosage of 6-g/kg stroma-free haemoglobin are of special importance.

So this type of oxygen-carrying colloid shows not only remarkable haemodynamic stability during extreme haemodilution [4, 5], but also remarkable metabolic compatibility in our experimental animal study.

References

1. Bonhard K (1982) Basic requirements for intravascular oxygen transport by cell-free haemoglobin preparations. ISH/ISBT Congress, Budapest 1982
2. De Venuto F, Friedman HI (1979) Appraisal of hemoglobin solution as a blood substitute. Surg Gynecol Obstet 149:417
3. Didziak R, Bonhard K (1980) The development of hemoglobin preparations for various indications. Anaesthesist 29:181
4. Klein G, Ottermann U, Dudziak R (1983) Hämodilutionsversuche mit einer neuen polymerisierten Hämoglobinlösung beim Hund: B Sauerstofftransport. Anaesthesist 32 [Suppl]:300
5. Ottermann U, Klein G, Dudziak R (1983) Hämodilutionsversuche mit einer neuen polymerisierten Hämoglobinlösung beim Hund: A Hämodynamik. Anaesthesist 32 [Suppl]:299
6. Rabiner SF, Helbert JR, Lopas H, Friedman LH (1967) Evaluation of a stroma-free hemoglobin solution for use as a plasma expander. J Exp Med 126:1127
7. Schnoy N, Pfannkuch F, Beisbarth H (1979) Fluorocarbone als Erythrozytenersatz. Anaesthesist 28:503

Physical Aspects in Peripheral Perfusion

T. Mostert and W. L. den Dunnen

Introduction

Each living structure originating from an evolution process has a specific mechanism to control the limits of its cell population. One of the most important mechanisms for this control is tissue perfusion. Regulation of perfusion is a way of influencing the quantity of tissue formation. There are lesions which have increased perfusion, leading to hypertrophy and disorder of the structure. The efficiency of blood distribution to the perfusion areas is determined by the timing and synchronization of the blood-pressure pulse and the blood flow. Tissue perfusion, arterial bood transport and respiration are all processes in which the timing, synchronization and the phase shift between the pressure pulse and the flow wave is a very important phenomenon. Nearly all lesions and structural disorders alter the properties of this timing, leading to disturbed perfusion. When partial perfusion in a tissue area is too great it forms a shunt over the surrounding healthy tissue. Absolute diffusion to the cells is dependent on the pressure gradients and duration. Manipulating these timing and pressure differentials is a method of reducing the shunts and improves the efficiency of blood transport. It is obvious that reducing perfusion in tumours will reduce tumour growth; several technique are being developed for this, such as radiation and chemical therapies. But the selectivity of these therapies is still so bad that resection of the affected areas is often inevitable. The pneumatic controlled circulation (PCC) method we have developed is very efficient and selective. It will certainly be a clean method resulting in total restoration of the tissue, and will replace radiation and chemical therapies. Pneumatic-controlled circulation is a technique to control perfusion by application of externally induced cardiac-controlled pressure pulses.

Philosophy

The population of a specific living organism is dependent on the environment. The synchronization and the phase shift of the pressure and the flow wave is a physical property only in a pulsating system. Vegetable life is a non-pulsatile system as opposed to animal life. If in animal tissue continuous blood flow replaces pulsatile flow, this area tends to change in nature, and eczema may develop if it is exposed to the air. This will not mean that the cells are changing but they will be substituted by other organisms. Thus a change in the environment will cause a change in the population. Destroying the vital elements of the microcirculation

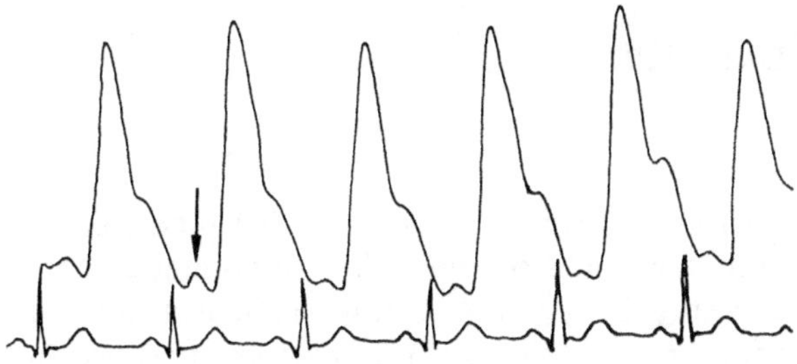

Fig. 1. This photoplethysmogram shows the position of the displacement of blood at the arterial ends (*arrowhead*). The pressure wave is transmitted with the speed of sound in blood

(the contractability of the met arterioles and the precapillary sphincters) causes a non-intermittent perfusion, so eczema will develop if this area is exposed to the air. When the heart ejects blood into the aorta a pressure pulse is transmitted through the arterial system with a much higher velocity than that of the flow wave. The phase shift of the pressure pulse and the flow wave is zero at the level of the aortic valve and increases proportional to the distance. But when it arrives at the distal ends the phase shift always has a specific value. This delay in time between the pressure pulse and the flow wave at the level of the met arterioles and the capillaries in a specific part is the *vascular delay (VD)*. The more rigid or lower the compliance the smaller is the vascular delay. The pressure pulse opens the met arterioles and the precapillary sphincters before the arrival of the flow wave. If the met arteriole or precapillary sphincter is ischaemic and collapsed it will take a specific time to open after receiving the pressure pulse. This time interval is the *perfusion delay (PD)*. It is evident that in the case of altered VD the perfusion efficiency will be reduced and more energy will be needed for proper perfusion. At an early stage of life the VD is equal at all arterial distal ends of the body and the differences increase with old age. Within each cardiac cycle we have two pressure waves at the distal ends. The first pressure pulse, which has a small amplitude, causes slight displacement of the blood to open the microcirculation and so form a low impedance to the blood flow. A low impedance occurs only when the contraction force of the met arterioles and precapillary sphincters disappears during the ischaemic state. The blood flows just through the areas of low impedances so that efficient circulation occurs. This small displacement of blood is detectable with the photoplethysmograph under certain conditions and appears at the same moment of the cardiac ejection (Fig. 1). The second pressure wave at the arterial distal ends is caused by the deceleration of the blood mass. Because the vascular and perfusion delay is specific in the body or parts of the body, new tissue formation is only optimally performed if there are no differentiations in these delays. Every reversible impairment and physical influence alters these parameters. It depends on the origin of the disturbance whether an affection will be finally restored by the body itself or not. For example, decreased vascular delay due to arteriosclerosis reduces the tissue growth while the body is unable to control it.

In contrast, reversible damage to tissue area only will be forced to restore itself according to the specific vascular and perfusion delay. Besides the arterial flow parameters the collateral vessels are important in maintaining the vascular delay for the varying vascular impedances and the lymph meshwork so that the perfusion is maintained during external pressure influences. Perfusion in healthy tissue takes place between the top of the "T"- and the "P"-wave top in the ECG. Thus, during diastole of the heart even the heart itself is perfused.

Pneumatic-Controlled Circulation

Materials and Methods

Let us consider a physical model as in Figs. 2–5. Two parallel tubes, passing through an airtight container, are connected on one side to a common supply. The other ends are left open to measure the separate outflow. Tube *A* is more rigid than tube *B*. This implies that tube *B* will collapse at a lower external pressure (container pressure) than tube *A*. We know that small arterial vessels collapse below a pressure of 20 mm Hg. For that reason we add this pressure to the atmospheric pressure in the container to simulate this effect. We will see that during the systole there is a remarkable flow through tube *A* while the flow through *B* is very slight or nil. During the diastole both outputs rise. This is a simplification of the perfusion in affected areas relative to the surrounding healthy tissue, where *A* represents the perfusion in the affected area. It must be kept in mind that the perfusion takes place during the diastole due to the vascular delay. We establish an intermittent perfusion in healthy areas and a continuous perfusion in affected areas. The constriction properties of the precapillary sphincters and the met arterioles prevent hypertrophy and disorder of the tissue structure. So we may expect that restoring the increased perfusion to an acceptable level relative to the surrounding healthy tissue leads to restoring the differentiations. Reduction of the perfusion by applying an external static positive pressure as shown in Fig. 3 indeed causes a decreased perfusion in the affected areas but will stop or reduce the perfusion in the healthy tissue. Thus there is no relative reduction. Improvement of the perfusion in the healthy tissue by applying an external static negative pressure as shown in Fig. 4 will also increase the perfusion in the affected area. So this is also not usable for that reason but will also cause oedema due to the low mean pressure. The technology of PCC we have developed is shown in Fig. 5. We apply an external positive pressure sufficient to reduce or stop the total perfusion. A negative pressure pulse is induced at the moment of the opening of the aortic valve to open the microcirculation. This causes a slight transport of blood just enough to open the small vessels. This first pressure wave is followed by a second negative pressure wave to decrease the vascular resistance and to make perfusion possible at the most efficient moment. If we now compare the original perfusion in Fig. 2 and during PCC (Fig. 5) then we see that the flow *B* is maintained at the same level. But flow *A* is reduced more or less to the level of the same order of *B*. It is clear that this kind of externally controlled intermittent perfusion allows only tissue formation according to the normal natural physiology. Localization and selectivity is an automatic natural mechanism so that in each area differentiated perfusion will be restored and the interaction between affected areas and healthy areas will be limited.

The clinical application of PCC we can divide into two groups. The first group is the patients suffering from vascular diseases. The PCC controller provides the reduced or missing pulsations at the arterial distal ends. The second group of patients are those suffering from tissue disorders (tumours, affections, wounds, etc.). In all cases the PCC controller has to provide control signals to a pneumatic system to induce the first and the second pressure pulse related to an adjustable delay to the cardiac action. This method is restricted to parts of the body which can be enclosed in a container through a cuff to make it airtight.

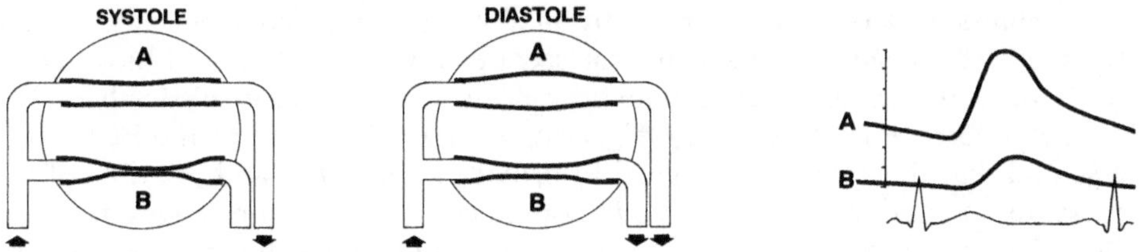

Fig. 2. Static atmospheric pressure

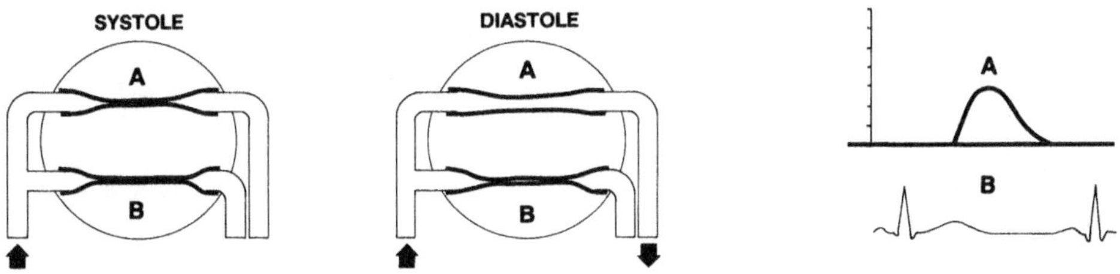

Fig. 3. Static positive pressure

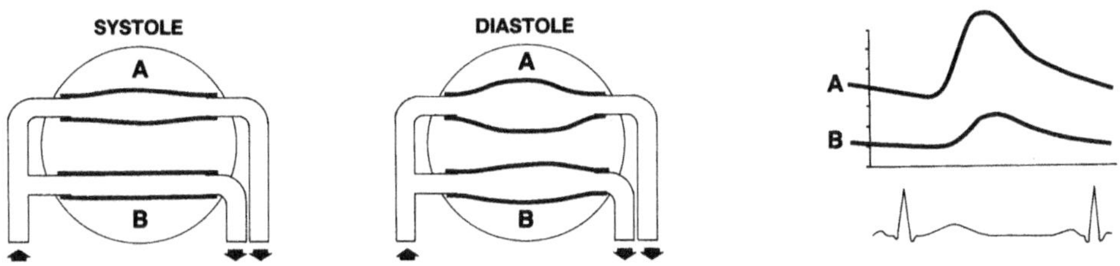

Fig. 4. Static negative pressure

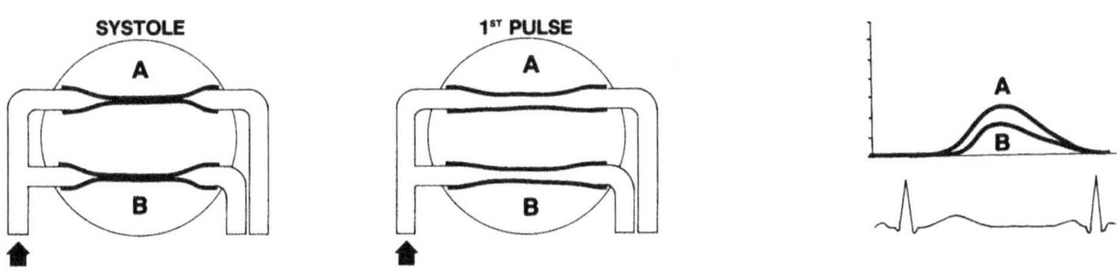

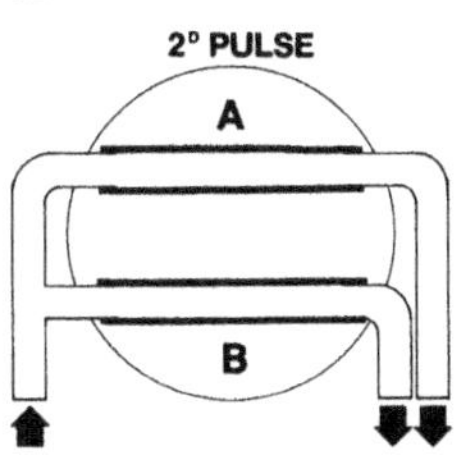

Fig. 5. Pneumatic-controlled circulation

The pressure waves are generated by an electromagnetic-controlled membrane for the first pressure wave and for the second wave by suction and blowing air from and into the container regulated by electromagnetic-controlled valves. The cardiac reference is obtained by triggering on the QRS-wave of the ECG. It is essential that the system is designed to provide a quick rise and fall time of the pressure fluctuations. It is possible to combine the two pressure waves into one. But when the slopes of the pressure wave start and stop at the proper time, the mean pressure in the container is too low and there will be a risk of oedema or skin blisters. A proper waveform of the container pressure with a zero mean pressure is essential to prevent complications.

Pneumatically Controlled Circulation in Peripheral Vascular Diseases

W. L. den Dunnen and T. Mostert

Patient Anamnesis

Pneumatically-controlled circulation (PCC) was applied to seven patients suffering from peripheral vascular diseases and to two patients suffering from lymphoedema of the extremities aged between 32 and 81 years.

Patient 1 was 81 years old. In 1950 he suffered from infected varicose veins. In 1956 he had an anteroseptal myocardial infarction. The same year he was operated on both legs because of varicose veins. In 1980 he had a recidive myocardial infarction. In 1981 he had a cerebrovascular accident with aphasia and right-sided hemiparesis from which he recovered very well. He also suffered from hypertension and was hospitalized because of the poor perfusion of his legs, especially the right leg, which had atrophic changes of the skin and a large chronic ulcer. There were poor pulsations of his femoral arteries. His ECG showed an atrial fibrillation. A lumbar sympathectomy was performed because reconstructive vascular surgery was impossible. In spite of a sympathectomy the ischaemic pain did not cease. The surgeons scheduled an amputation of his right leg.

Patient 2 was 32 years old. Because of a ventral spondylodesis of the lumbar spine her left leg was operated on to obtain transplants from the tibial bone. Since that operation (1982) she suffered from pain in her right leg and poor bone growth. There were atrophic changes of the skin and an osteomyelitis was obvious. The cardiovascular status was normal. She had a normal sinus rhythm on the ECG. Further anamnesis was free from complaint although she stated that she had had vasovegetative instability.

Patient 3 was 73 years old. She was hospitalized because of the pregangrenous status of her right foot. Lumbar aortography showed severe stenosis and atherosclerotic changes. According to the surgical findings a reconstructive vascular operation was impossible. Chemical lumbar sympathectomy was performed. The effect was poor. The ECG showed an atrial fibrillation. X-rays of the chest showed a cardiomegalia. There existed a tendency towards decompensation of the heart which was treated with cardiotonics and diuretics. She had three chronic ulcers on her right foot.

Patient 4 was 62 years old. He was hospitalized because of necrosis of his left foot. Lumbar aortography showed a generalized atherosclerosis with a stop in the left popliteal artery and an obstruction in the proximal part of the right femoral artery. Reconstructive vascular surgery appeared to be impossible. Three toes were amputated. A split skin graft was given but because of the poor perfusion this was unsuccesful. He was scheduled for an upper leg amputation. His ECG showed a normal sinus rhythm and slight ST depression.

Patient 5 was a 62-year-old woman suffering from chronic ischaemic pain in both legs since 1962. In 1963 the diagnosis of Bürger's disease was considered but never confirmed. She was a heavy smoker. The toes of her legs always premained underdeveloped due, to the poor perfusion. In 1972 she had her left foot which was gangrenous, partially amputated. Now she had the same complaints in her right foot, especially the first toe, in which an osteomyelitis existed. Lumbar aortography showed a severe stenosis in the right superior femoral artery at two places. One branch of the trifurcation was totally blocked. A Dotter procedure was unsuccesful. The ECG showed a sinus rhythm with ischaemic changes. There was a tendency towards chronic decompensation.

Patient 6 was a 72-year-old man. He had a pregangrenous right foot. In 1977 he had a fracture of his right ankle joint with thrombosis of the right saphena magna vein. A surgical reconstruction of the arteria profunda was performed in December 1983. After 6 weeks the ischaemic complaints were obvious again and the leg was in poor vascular status. An amputation was already scheduled. His ECG showed a sinus rhythm with ischaemic changes of the ST segment.

Patient 7 was a 78-year-old woman suffering from generalized atherosclerosis and senile diabetes. In February 1983 she underwent a femoral bypass procedure of the left femoral artery, which was succesful. Now she complained of her right leg, in which the peripheral circulation was poor. Because of the poor cardiopulmonary status reconstructive surgery was impossible. She suffered from chronic ulcers near her toes. The ECG showed a sinus rhythm and a small ST depression. She had severe hypertension which was treated with labetolol (Trandate). A chemical lumbar sympathectomy was performed and gave some pain relief.

Patient 8 was a 39-year-old man who suffered from chronic pain due to his oedematous hands and lower arms which, according to the plastic surgeon, was due to impaired lymphous drainage. According to the anamnesis it became clear that the patient had suffered from a vasculatis caused by handling heavy metals during his work (lead and antimonium) for many years. He had no cardiac complaints. Anamnesis was free from complaint. His hands showed severe eczema.

Patient 9 was a 49-year-old obese lady who underwent operations to her legs to reduce the amount of fatty tissue. After these operations she developed a painful oedema of the lower legs which was markedly located distally from the middle of the lower legs. Her anamnesis was free from complaint. She had neither cardiac complaints nor vascular disease. Her ECG showed a normal sinus rhythm.

Methods

Figure 1 shows the experimental setup for PCC treatment of the lower extremities. Before the treatment all patients were given an infusion of Ringer's lactate solution (500 ml). During the PCC treatment further infusion was performed until the preoperative blood pressure was reached again. For this purpose Geloplasma (gelatinous plasma expander, mol wt. = 40 000) was used. The leg (or arm) is put in an hermetically closed acrylic container. After the ECG is connected to the control unit we finally administer beta blockers to reduce heart fre-

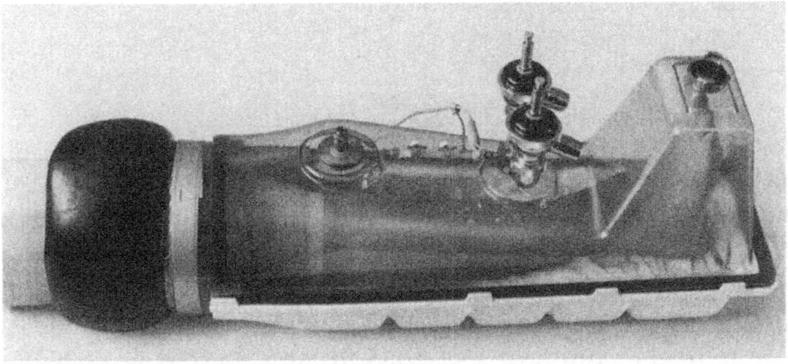

Fig. 1. Experimental setup for PCC treatment of the lower extremities

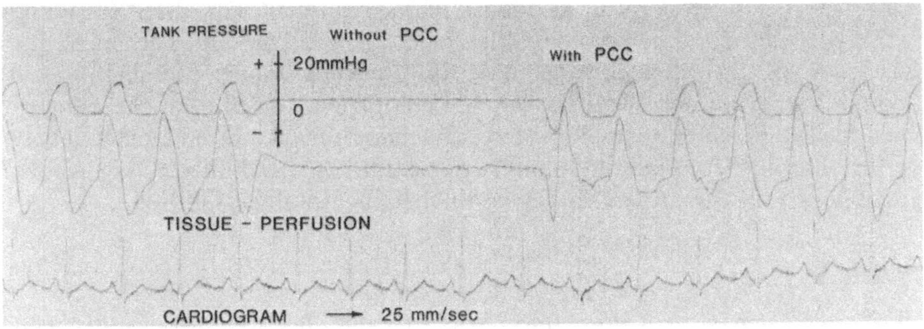

Fig. 2. Typical recordings obtained during PCC treatment (from top): Pressure in container, plethysmogram, ECG trace

quency, which should be around 80–90 beats/min, to increase the efficiency of the treatment. If necessary we administer digitalis to improve the contractility of the heart. A specially designed control unit shows the QRS intervals indicated in milliseconds. This facilitates the setting up of the unit. An audible bleep can be set. The frequency of the audible bleep is related to the heart beat. This provides an acoustic impression of the stability of the heart.

The container is connected to a vacuum and pressure source using electromagnetic valves. During the opening of the aortic valve a low vascular impedance is created in the extremity being treated. Then a subatmospheric container pressure aids the blood flow during the systole. During the diastole the container pressure rises to a slightly positive level. In the case of venous insufficiency a tourniquet with adjustable pressure is placed around the leg just proximally from the container to prevent backflow. A plethysmograph is placed on the skin in several places.

A few patients were given extra oxygen by mask or nose cathether, especially at the beginning of the treatment. Intravenous salicylates and heparin are administered to reduce the complications of possible embolism.

Figure 2 shows the typical recordings we obtained during the treatment. The top trace shows the pressure in the container varying between + and − 20 mm Hg. The second trace is the plethysmogram and the third is the patient's ECG.

Results

Patient 1

Because of his atrial fibrillation synchronization of the pressure fluctuations was difficult. A better perfusion developed very shortly after the first application of PCC. The chronic ulcer at the lateral ankle showed increased perfusion and new tissue growth could be observed. The ischaemic pain ceased and the growth of the nails was obvious 1 week after the first treatment. From the first treatment the patient developed a lower blood pressure and ventricular extrasystoles whenever the pressure fluctuations in the container exceeded 20 mm Hg and went below −20 mm Hg. During the second treatment exsudation of tissue fluid could be observed at several places on the atrophic skin. A few blisters were rising. Although a marked rise in temperature of the leg under treatment was observed simultaneously the untreated leg became colder, especially the lower leg. The temperature (perfusion) of the untreated leg could be improved by smaller container pressure fluctuations. Although the ulcer was not completely healed after the last treatment the patient was dimissed without ischaemic pain and had a permanent better perfusion of his leg. The total number of treatments was limited to six. About 1 year after the last treatment the leg is still in an acceptable condition.

Patient 2

This patient was treated three times. The first time the skin temperature of the leg rose during the treatment from 26.5° to 35 °C. The next two treatments the raise in temperature was less than the first time although the settings were similar. After all treatments the rise in temperature remained from several hours to at least 1 day. During all the treatments the patient complained of a headache which developed during the 1st hour of application of PCC.

During the last treatment the patient complained again of a severe headache and "uncomfortable feelings", so we stopped the treatment. She developed a marked tachycardia (from 76 to 155 bpm) after a short period of severe bradycardia (36 bpm) which was treated with 0.25 mg methyl atropine bromide. Rapid infusion of 2000 ml lactated Ringer's solution and plasma expander was necessary to restore a normovolaemic circulation and an acceptable blood pressure.

Patient 3

This patient was treated four times. Her atrial fibrillation made it very complicated to synchronize the container pressure fluctuations and proper adjustment of the control unit. Nevertheless the ischaemic pain ceased and the perfusion improved, also indicated by a marked rise in temperature of the leg being treated. She also showed a marked decrease in temperature of the untreated leg which could be adjusted in the same way as described with patient No. 1. A slight decrease of the atrial fibrillation was observed after the treatment. The surgeons decided not to amputate her leg because of the improved vascular status and ceased ischaemic pain. About 6 months after the last treatment the chronic ulcers were healed and the patient recovered to an acceptable level. She can walk more than 500 m again without ischaemic complaints.

Patients 4, 5 and 6

These patients were treated five, four and two times, respectively, within 4 weeks. They showed no side effects from the treatment. Synchronization was easily performed. Also in these patients the ischaemic pain ceased within a few minutes of application of PCC. Increased perfusion of the legs was established but the remaining effect after the treatment was restricted to about 5 days so a longer continuation of treatments was necessary. However, this was not possible because of the experimental nature of our research.

Patient 7

In this patient we started with a container pressure fluctuation of between only + and − 10 mm Hg, which was enough to cause a severe attack of cardiac arrhythmia combined with a significant decrease in blood pressure and ischaemic changes of the ECG. When these cardiac arrhythmias developed the PCC was terminated immediately and the ECG became normal. After restart of the treatment these cardiac arrhythmias developed again, which made us decide to stop any further treatment. She was transported to the coronary care unit. There were no signs of myocardial infarction. Her leg showed a significant rise in temperature despite the short duration of the treatment. After reduction of the systemic circulation by the application of a tourniquet around the upper leg, which was treated with PCC, the cardiac arrhythmias disappeared and the blood pressure was restored. The tourniquet was released slightly to guarantee a slow adaptation to increased circulation. Although the treatment lasted only less than ½h, her leg remained warmer for many days.

Patient 8

After application of second time we observed neither decrease in the oedema nor increase in the circulation, so we stopped further treatment. Within 1 month the chronic eczema disappeared from the treated hand while the untreated hand still showed the existing eczema.

Patient 9

The first time of treatment the patient said she had much less pain and "warm feelings" in the leg which lasted much longer than the duration of the treatment.

Table 1. Clinical effects of PCC before and after treatment

Patient	Sex	Age	Pain		Arrhythmias		Number of treatment	First treatment	Last treatment
			Before treatment	After treatment	During treatment	After treatment			
1	M	81	+	−	+	+	6	24/5	18/6
2	F	32	−	−	−	+++	5	14/6	28/6
3	F	73	+	−	±	−	4	10/11	13/12
4	M	62	+	−	−	−	5	20/11	14/12
5	F	62	+	−	±	+	4		23/12
6	M	72	+	−	−	−	2	16/12	20/12
7	F	78	+	−	+++	++	1	20/12	
8	M	39	−	−	−	−	2	24/1	26/1
9	F	49	+	−	−	−	2	24/1	26/1

Two days later the leg was treated again using another setting in which the container pressure rose during the ventricular systole. This caused more pain than during the former setting but the effect on the oedema could not be observed even after applying a synchronous PCC mode. The treatment was primarily meant to stimulate the lymph transport. We could not observe any direct effect.

Table 1 summarizes the clinical effects of PCC before and after treatment.

Discussion and Conclusions

Based on the Matrix Resonation Theory of Mostert we performed this clinical pilot study. Earlier research made it obvious that it was possible to exert an influence on the circulation by externally applied pressure fluctuations as we did on the lung circulation of patients and sheep [1].

The results as outlined in this paper are promising although much research needs to be done to obtain further proof of our theory. However, it is possible to improve the circulation of the extremities by (synchronous) application of pressure fluctuations within the limits of + and − 20 mmHg. If the externally applied pressure fluctuations exceed those limits, severe problems with the whole body circulation can occur especially if the pressure fluctuations are fully synchronized with the patient's heart cycle.

X-ray control of the peripheral circulation showed an increased collateral circulation after a longer period of PCC treatment. Maybe this treatment is a good alternative for vascular bypass procedures or at least can be used to prepare patients for this kind of surgery in the case of the existence of poor outflow tracts. Pneumatic controlled circulation should only be performed under strict supervision of trained personel with continuous monitoring of the patient.

References

1. Scheck PA, Sjöstrand UH, Smith RB (1983) Perspectives in high frequency ventilation. Martinus Nijhoff, pp 122–131

Discussion II

P. Wagner: I have a question to Dr. Faithfull. What do you think the electrodes do to the tissues, and where do you think the electrodes are in the tissues?

N.S. Faithfull: It is impossible to say where you are in relation to a capillary. Therefore, if you stick four electrodes in, some of them are going to be at the aterial end, some are going to be at the venular end, and some are going to be in the middle. And the degree of change is also going to vary with both the positioning and the subsequent flow changes. Just altering the flow will of course alter the PO_2, particularly in what some people call the hypoxic corner. With regard to what the electrodes are doing: Yes they are causing damage. And we are of course not measuring in a cell, we are not even measuring between cells, technically speaking; we are measuring in a little pool of liquid that is sitting there. But nevertheless, this pool of liquid changes its PO_2 very rapidly.

S. Kunke: There are clear oscillations on your PO_2 registration which are synchronous to the heart rhythm. The point is that oxygen microelectrodes do not only measure oxygen tension, they are also measuring mechanical effects. How can you be sure that you really did measure oscillations in oxygen tension? What about mechanical irritations? If you put a microelectrode in a glass of water and shake it even slightly you will have an oscillation.

The myocardium is working, and it is shaking the electrode in its own rhythm all the time. That is why there will always be oscillations of your monitor, whether the oxygen is changing or not.

N.S. Faithfull: I agree, but of course this is an example of a completely unanswerable question. I can partially defend the fact we are looking at PO_2. If the swings in oxygen tension are due to movement, why do we see greater swings of oxygen tension as the PO_2 we are measuring increases?

S. Kunke: This could be because the electrode resistance is lower if higher currents are flowing, and that means that the influence of movements could be higher, too.

E.A. Ernst: You cannot detect oxygen without harvesting oxygen. And so the real crux of the matter is the area of harvest. This is the fight researchers always have: trying to minimize the harvest as far as possible over a large area. The question could only be, what about the harvest effect of your electrode?

N.S. Faithfull: However, we do think we are measuring a certain amout of oxygen.

J. Dorlas: I have a question to Dr. Lapin about air embolism, blood damage and haemolysis. How do you teach other surgeons to work in such a way that the suction does not suck in air and does not slurp? That is the main problem I think.

R. Lapin: Well, the main problem indeed is haemolysis. What you have to do is adjust your suction until you reach the point where it is still sucking but you have no slurping. If you leave the suction sweep in the wound all the time you do not have that air-blood interface, and that keeps the amount of haemolysis down. This is very easy to learn. I think it takes maybe an hour of working with the device, no matter whether you use the Bentley or the Hemonetics one. You should not suck with full vacuum, which would really kill the cells. You can keep a recovery rate of about 70% if you are careful about it. You can even break the clots down by as well without running into coagulopathy problems.

P. Wagner: I noticed that the haemoglobin and haematocrit recoveries over a period of days were about 20%–50%. I guess that implies that a lot of ghosts are reinfused, or why is the Rizzo count so high?

R. Lapin: When we traced the red cells with chromium we concluded that the survival rate was around 89 days. So you really are keeping a pretty good proportion alive. However, the mean was 9% haemoglobin, and we have gone down to a haemoglobin of 1.6% or 1.8% to start surgery. The amazing thing is that if you have good bone marrow you are able to recover at about 0.4 g per day after the first 24 hours.

I have one comment on what Dr. Klein said. His work is extremely important because what he has found in animals we have found in humans. The changes that he has shown are directly related to the acute haemodilution rather than the plasma-free haemoglobin or stroma free haemoglobin. We find in high-risk patients that it is better to achieve haemodilution before surgery. So we can keep the oxygenation high even by keeping it at FIO_2 of 0.8 or 0.6 for 24–48 h without much ill effect. Oxygen delivery and oxygen extraction are considerably better in the diluted state. Your margin of safety in acute haemodilution in the properly selected patient has a tremendous fallout with regard to specifically cardiovascular diseases. And I think that one day we will move from the clinical to the more medium stage production of stroma-free haemoglobin. I think we have very good media for substitution of a lot of things that we now substitute with whole blood.

R. Droh: I have a question to Dr. Klein. I do not quite see how the oxygen can be carried with stroma-free haemoglobin via a physical solution. Because if you have the cell you have a different mechanism for oxygen transport than the one with the free haemoglobin. So this could be understood much better with regard to fluorochemicals than to stroma-free haemoglobin solutions.

G. Klein: The stroma-free haemoglobin is able to bind oxygen chemically in the same way as the natural intraerythrocytic haemoglobin is able to. That means it shows the same sigmoid-shifted dissociation curve as natural haemoglobin. This is possible because the DPG, which is one of the important substances for the shift of the haemoglobin curve, is substituted by pyridoxal phosphate. And this pyridoxal phosphate allows a P_{50} of about 30 mm mercury. This is nearly the same P_{50} as that of natural haemoglobin, and therefore the oxygen chemically bound by the stroma-free haemoglobin is released in the same way as the oxygen chemically bound by the intraerythrocytic haemoglobin. If the partial pressure of oxygen drops towards the peripheral area the amount of oxygen which is released is the same as with natural haemoglobin. So far the mechanism is the same. Oxygen is bound chemically, but in the peripheral regions it is necessary for it to be released by the haemoglobin, and the diffusion of oxygen to the cells is a physical problem of oxygen partial pressure difference.

R. Droh: Yes, but does this stroma-free haemoglobin behave exactly as the haemoglobin in the cells does?

G. Klein: We did not measure the oxygen intracellularly.

R. Lapin: I think the papers that have been presented here present the microcosm of thinking in medicine today, not only in this country but abroad as well. Haemodilution, autotransfusion and oxygen-carrying fluids are the subjects of a tremendous amount of interest for scientists all over the world, because we are beginning to realize some of the problems that have been passed on to blood transfusion. I think the oxygen-carrying fluids are the first step. This material has a tremendous potential for the future, and not because it is a good blood substitute; I think it is a very poor blood substitute. However, on the subject of microcirculatory problems, you cannot find a solution today that has a particle size of one tenth of a micron and is able to carry oxygen on a linear curve that, in contrast to the oxygen dissociation curve, can be shifted either right or left once loaded. Whenever you are in a shock situation or in a haemodiluted situation, strictly speaking the stiffening of the red cell membrane makes it extremly difficult for a 7-micron red cell to penetrate capillaries 3 microns in section. The stiffening of the membrane causes the pooling and devoiding of the microcirculation. Therefore, in such cases as cerebrovascular accidents, myocardial infarction and shock in general, I think a material such as Fluosol promises great progress for the future.

Autotransfusion, on the other hand, takes us down to basic steps. The best blood you can give patients is their own, and therefore all emphasis should be given to reutilizing the patient's own blood. We feel that giving a patient a unit of blood is analogous to giving somebody a liquid organ transplant with all the antigenicity that goes along with it. I think the cases with AIDS in the United States begin to reflect some of our fears with regard to that problem. It is no longer a homosexual disease; in 1984 it had already been transmitted to 73 patients during surgery. So, it is becomming more and more of a problem for surgeons and anaesthesiologists alike. Finally, with haemodilution we got to know exactly where the limit of safety is. I think Professor Erdmann said that up to a haemoglobin level of 5 haemodilution is probably safe. I think that is probably true. It is somewhere between 5 and 7. And I think the fact that patients are not being anaesthetized with haemoglobin less than 10 should really be looked at very critically. We have to find out whether there is any scientitic foundation for that particular stand.

P. Wagner: Dr. den Dunnen, my question relates to the fluid load that was given to the patients. As I understand it, you gave 1 litre saline and then 500 ml of something that sounded like a plasma volume expander. In addition to that, you gave them betablockers. Now it seems to me that this would involve a high risk to the patients, in that it might create pulmonary edema. That may be the explanation of some of the cardiac arrhythmias that you saw. I am wondering to what extent an aged person with a weak heart can be subjected to this fluid load plus beta blockers at the same time. That seems a very difficult thing to me.

W. L. den Dunnen: Without infusions we have much more trouble. Even young people get arrhythmias. But our patients go into intensive care afterwards so the pulmonary pressure can be monitored. And if the pulmonary pressure gets too high we give frusemide.

P. Wagner: Do you observe acute changes just in distribution, or in total cardiac output too?

W. L. den Dunnen: Total cardiac output should increase, but I have not yet measured it.

C. Y. Lin: I think in the United States between 1968 and about 1975 there was an extensive study on the cardiac phase shifting body compression, and actually the programme failed simply because there is a tremendous shift in extracellular space fluid immediately after starting compression. At the same time, it is very difficult to synchronize it in phase.

W. L. den Dunnen: Yes, I agree, it is very difficult, especially when the patient has an extra fibrillation. And a wrong setting can even lead to death; that's true.

M. Wendt: How can you differentiate the effects of your compression and the effects of the drugs?

W. L. den Dunnen: So far we have treated only a few patients where there was nothing to lose and they needed this combined treatment. So I cannot differentiate.

B. W. Lübbers: You showed that the phasic flow increases substantially, but what about the absolute flow in the legs?

W. L. den Dunnen: We talk about plethysmography and its interpretation. The only thing I can say is that we did not actually have flow probes in the arteries; that has been impossible in our experiments up to now. But the legs became warm and red.

D. W. Lübbers: Would it not be possible to weigh the legs?

W. L. den Dunnen: That is possible.

D. W. Lübbers: You need an easy method of monitoring the change you cause in the fluid load in the body. This could be relatively simple to design.

New Aspects of Pharmacological Treatment

Importance of Chronopharmacology in Medicine

B. Lemmer

In all species including man cyclic variations in physiological functions have been well documented. In the past decade the study of circadian (approximately 24-h) rhythms has evolved into a science with implications for clinical medicine [10, 20, 21, 26]. Daily, 24-h or circadian rhythms in man have been shown to exist, e.g. in cardiovascular functions (heart rate, blood pressure, vascular reactivity), in body temperature, in serum constituents including the concentrations of various hormones [cortisol, adrenocorticotropic hormone (ACTH), somatotrophic hormone (STH), insulin, angiotensin, renin, thyroxine, catecholamines], in the functions of the lung (vital capacity, peak expiratory volume, dynamik compliance) in the kidney (renal plasma flow, glomerular filtration rate, urine volume, pH value, electrolyte excretion) and even in performance and mood. Moore-Ede et al. [20] recently pointed out in a review article in the famous *New England Journal of Medicine* that "it is now worthy of note when the rare variable is identified that does not display circadian variations". In Fig. 1 the maxima of some of these rhythms are compiled which were obtained in male healthy volunteers. These rhythms clearly document the periodic organization of the organism and it is therefore not surprising that also the effects of drugs were shown to vary markedly with the time of the day in animal and man. However, as early as 1814 Virey presented a thesis to the medical faculty of Paris in which he described daily rhythms in humans and their implications to health and diseases. He even used the term *l'horlage vivante* to characterize the nature of these rhythms [30].

Within the limited pages of this paper it is only possible to give a short review of the broad spectrum of drugs, the effectiveness, adverse effects, toxicity and pharmacokinetics of which were shown to be greatly influenced in animal and man by the time of drug administration within 24 h of a day. Drugs for which a circadian-phase dependency has been described include cardiovascular-active drugs (α- and β-adrenoceptor-blocking drugs, calcium antagonists, diuretics, reserpine, organic nitrates, etc.), analgesics (non-steroid-anti-inflammatory drugs, opioids, local and systemic anaesthetics), hormones (corticosteroids, insulin, histamine, catecholamines, etc.), neurotransmitters, drugs acting on the central nervous system (e.g. sedative hypnotics, tranquilizers, antidepressants, lithium, neuroleptics), antihistamines and antiasthmatics (e.g. β-sympathomimetics, theophylline) as well as cytostatic drugs [9, 10].

The following presentation will be mainly restricted to analgesic and cardiovascular-active drugs as representative examples in order to highlight chronopharmacodynamic and chronopharmacokinetic drug effects in man and experimental animals.

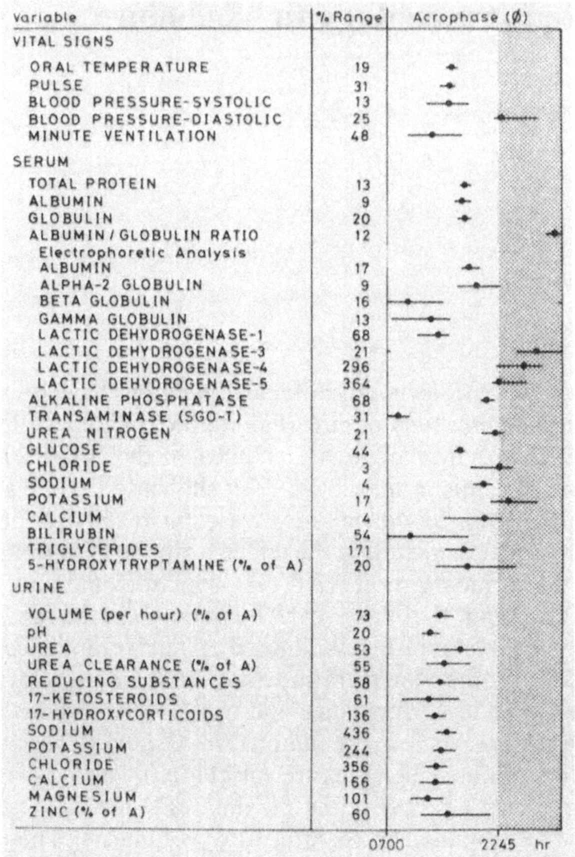

Fig. 1. Acrophase (maximum of rhythm) mapping in 13 healthy male volunteers. (Adapted from Kanabrocki et al. [7])

In healthy humans Reinberg and Reinberg [25] gave evidence that the local anaesthetic effect of lidocaine greatly varies with the time of the day when injecting the same dosage of this drug into the same group of volunteers at different circadian times (Fig. 2). At 3 p.m. the duration of the local anaesthetic effect of lidocaine was about two to three times longer than at 8 a.m. both after intradermal injection in the skin as well as after para-apical application to the frontal teeth. An adverse effect of lidocaine is that it can induce seizures. In mice Lutsch and Morris [16] demonstrated that the percentage of lidocaine-induced seizures varied between 6% and more than 80%, depending on the time of drug injection (Fig. 3). In comparing human and animal experiments it has to be noted that rodents like mice and rats are night-active animals in contrast to day-active humans. This is of great importance in that rodents are used to a great extent as experimental animals to evaluate and quantify drug effects. However, animal experiments are mainly performed in the activity period of man, i.e. during day time, in a period at which night-active rodents are in their resting phase (Fig. 4). Thus, it is indispensable that animal data are compared with human data in relation to species differences in circadian phase. This is clearly demonstrated by the experimental results obtained with lidocaine in humans and in rodents: in both species more pronounced effects of this local anaesthetic drug were observed in the subjective

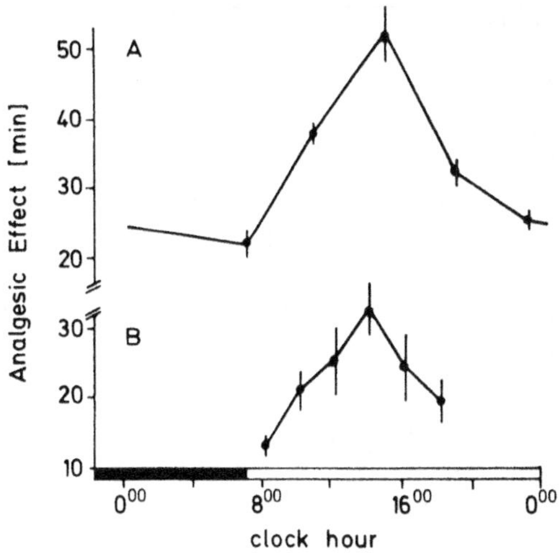

Fig. 2. Circadian variation in the local anaesthetic effect of lidocaine in man. **A**, after intradermal injection of 2 mg in 0.1 ml; **B**, after para-apical injection of 20 mg in 2 ml to the front teeth. (Modified from Reinberg and Reinberg [25])

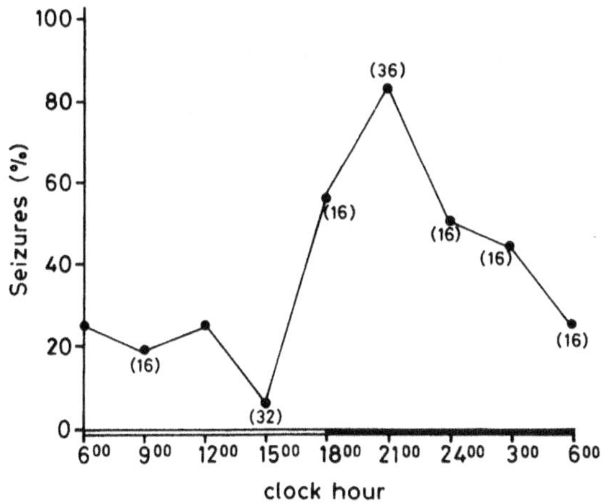

Fig. 3. Induction of seizures after lidocaine (65 mg/kg i.p.) administration to mice at different circadian times. (Modified from Lutch and Morris [16])

activity period of the respective species (Figs. 2 and 3). A circadian-phase dependency has also been observed in the analgesic effect of metamizol in humans [24]. Figure 5 demonstrates that not only does pain perception vary in a time-dependent manner, but that metamizol also has a more pronounced analgesic effect when applied at 3 p.m. than at 8 a.m. or 7 p.m. Thus, the results with metamizol are in good accordance with those obtained by Reinberg and Reinberg [25] with lidocaine (Fig. 2). Circadian-time-dependent variations in the analgesic property of morphine have also been shown in mice [1, 3]. Using the hot-plate test to evaluate the analgesic property of drugs, Frederickson et al. [3] determined the latency of the spring reaction in mice after injection of saline, morphine or the opiate antagonist naloxone. From Fig. 6 it can be seen that also in mice pain perception is clearly circadian time dependent with increased latency, i.e. decreased pain perception, in the activity period of mice (during night), being in good accordance with the findings in man (Figs. 3 and 5). As expected, morphine increased and naloxone decreased latency time in these experiments; however, the circadian rhythm in pain perception in mice was not abolished under either of the opiate agonist and antagonist, respectively (Fig. 6). It is now well known that specific

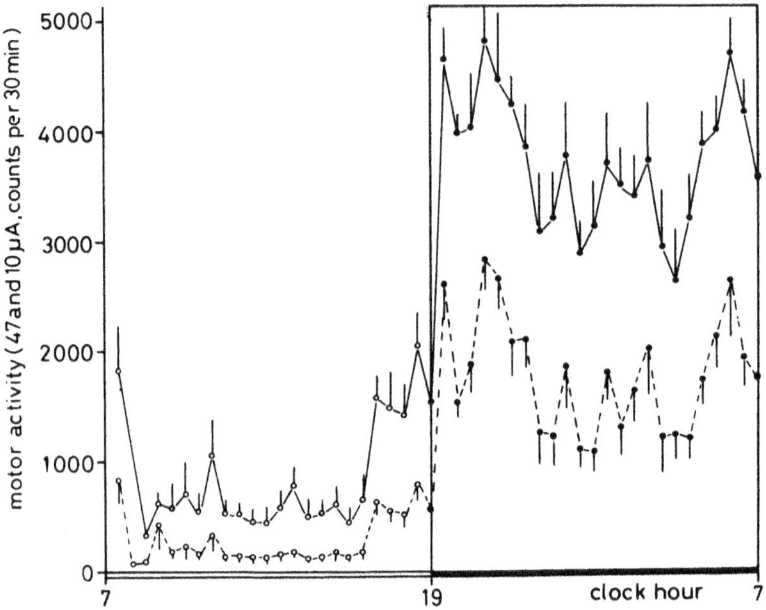

Fig. 4. Twenty-four-hour rhythm in motor activity in rats; total motility and running activity is shown. (Modified from Lemmer and Wenda [13])

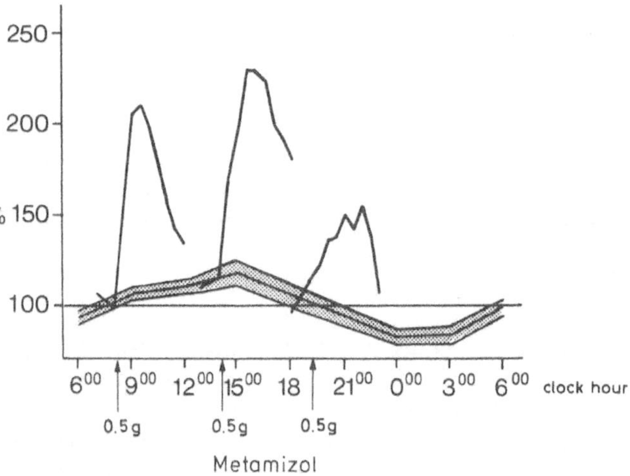

Fig. 5. Circadian-time-dependent analgesic effect of metamizol at the human front tooth; the *shaded area* represents pain perception at control; variations around the 24-h-mean value are shown. (Modified from Pöllmann [24])

opiate receptors exist in the brain of animals and of man and that peptides like endorphines and enkephalins are the endogenous ligands for these receptors. Most interestingly, it has recently been shown in rats that also the concentrations of endogenous endorphines (Fig. 7) and of met-enkephaline exhibit daily variations with increased concentrations in the dark period, i.e. activity period of the rodents [8, 28, 29]. These findings fit nicely with the observations of a decreased pain perception in the activity period of rats as shown in Fig. 6. Furthermore, the data obtained in the animal and human studies presented clearly support the no-

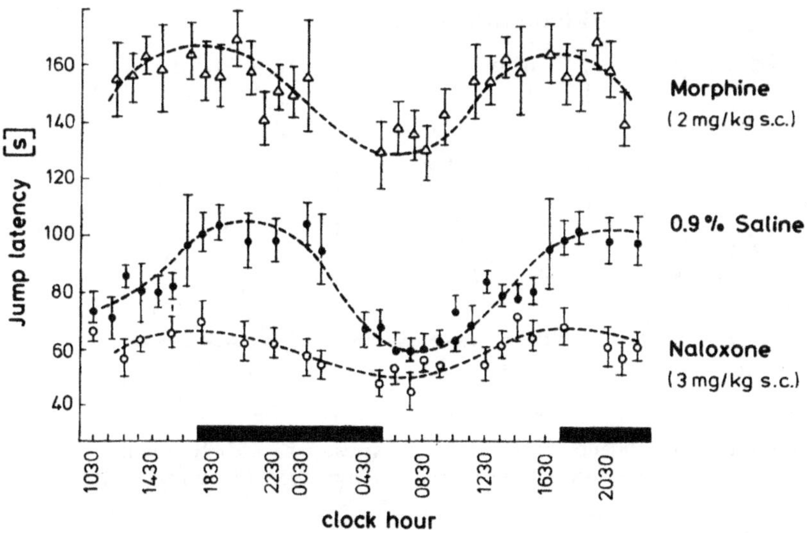

Fig. 6. Twenty-four-hour rhythm in spring latency (hot plate test, 52 °C) of mice under various treatments at different circadian times. (Modified from Frederickson et al. [3])

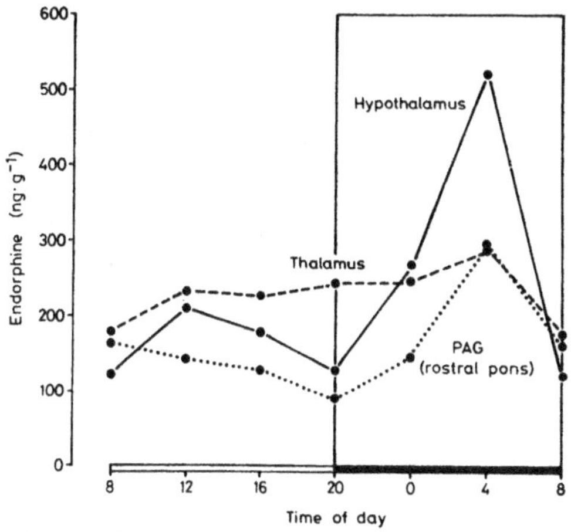

Fig. 7. Circadian-phase dependency in endorphine concentrations in various parts of the rat brain. (Modified from Walker and Mash [28])

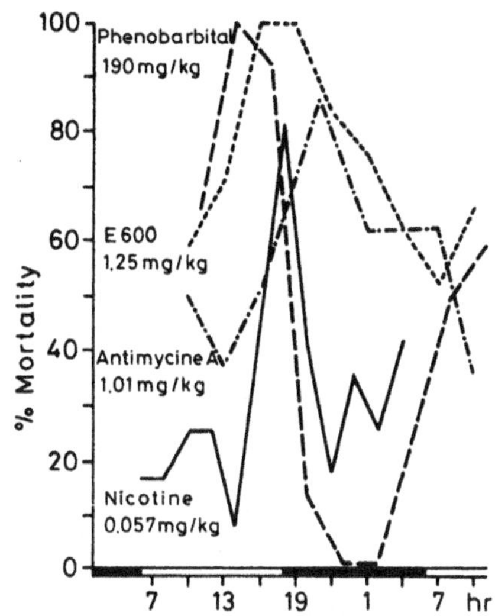

Fig. 8. Chronotoxicity of various drugs in rats. (Modified from von Mayersbach [31])

tion that species-related differences in the circadian phase have to be taken into account when comparing drug effects in animals and in man [10].

As already mentioned, not only do the therapeutic effects of drugs vary with the time of the day, but also toxic effects including drug mortality have been shown to be greatly circadian phase dependent. Representative findings from a great variety of drugs are shown in Fig. 8. In studies on rats, von Mayersbach [31] demonstrated that, e.g. the mortality induced by 190 mg/kg phenobarbital varied between 0% and 100%, depending on the time of drug administration. As early

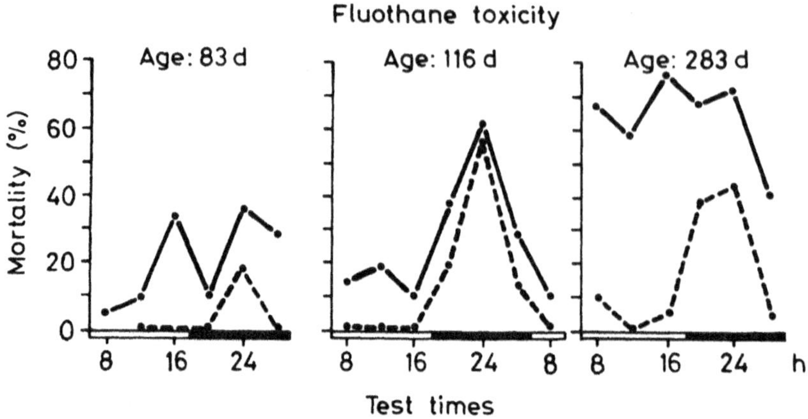

Fig. 9. Circadian-time dependency of mortality on exposure to 3.5% fluothane (——, total mortality; – – –, mortality in 7 min) in male mice of different ages. (Modified from Matthews et al. [18])

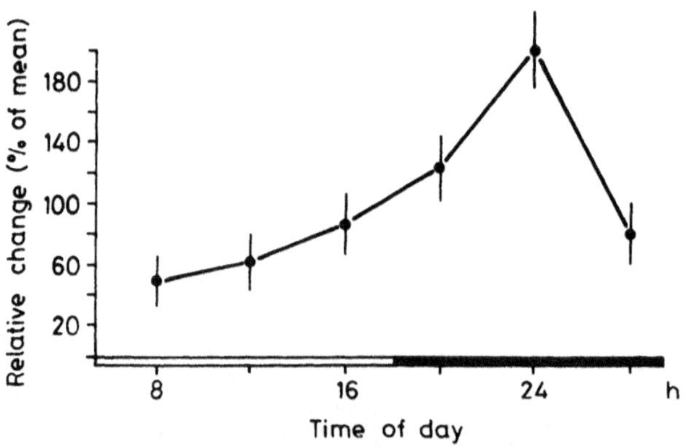

Fig. 10. Relative changes in fluothane mortality; pooled data from Fig. 9. (Modified from Matthews et al. [18])

as 1951 Halberg et al. described that the toxicity of the glycoside ouabain in mice was 60% at 8 a.m. and decreased to 15% at 8 p.m. These data clearly show that LD_{50} values of drugs are – if at all – of very limited information. In rodents the mortality of fluothane also exhibited a pronounced circadian time dependency [18]. Fluothane mortality in mice was not only influenced by the duration of exposure and the age of the animals (Fig. 9), but was shown to be greatly increased when the animals were exposed to fluothane in the middle of the activity period (Figs. 9 and 10). In rats circadian variations in the anaesthetic requirement [minimum alveolar concentration (MAC)] of cyclopropane and halothane with increased MAC values in the early dark period and lowest MAC values in the early light period have been described [23].

Finally, I would like to present some findings on the chronopharmacology of cardiovascular drugs. Daily variations in cardiovascular functions of man were reported as long as 50–90 years ago. In 1898 Hill [4] described the fall in blood pressure during the night and Menzel [19] reported on a 24-h rhythm in the circulating blood volume. Since that time circadian variations in systolic and diastolic blood pressure (see Fig. 1) have been convincingly shown to exist in healthy

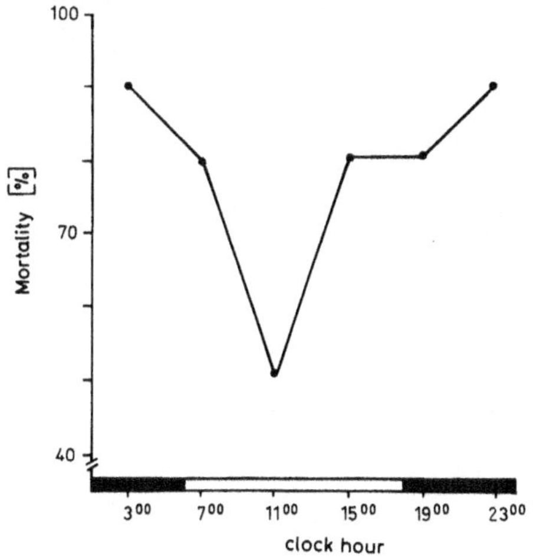

Fig. 11. Circadian-phase dependency of propranolol (125 mg/kg i.p.) mortality in mice. (Modified from Smolensky et al. [27], Lemmer et al. [14])

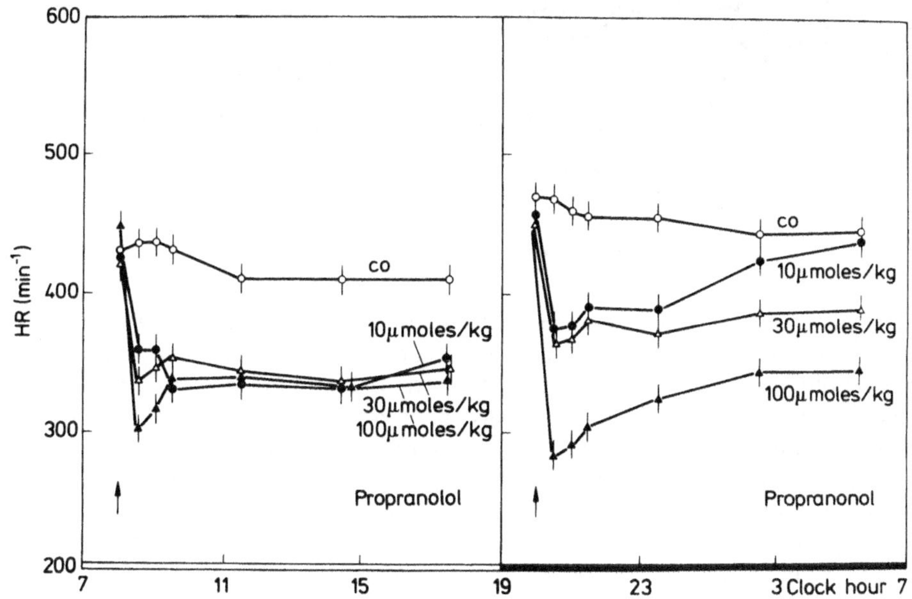

Fig. 12. Heart-rate-lowering effect of propranolol injected i.p. to conscious rats either at 07.30 h or at 19.30 h. (Modified from Lemmer et al. [15])

persons as well as in hypertensive patients [10]. In hypertensive patients as well as in normotensive rats antihypertensive drugs like β-adrenoceptor blockers were shown to have clear-cut circadian-time-dependent effects, with increased drug efficacy in the subjective activity period of the respective species. In Fig. 11 propranolol mortality in rats is depicted [14, 27]. It can be seen that the so-called LD_{50} of propranolol (125 mg/kg) only leads to mortality in 50% of the animals when applied at 11 a.m.(!), whereas at other circadian times propranolol mortality increased up to 90% (Fig. 11). However, mortality on propranolol can be clearly related to the non-specific effect of this drug. The decrease in heart rate and the blood-pressure-lowering effect of β-blockers, on the other hand, are due to the specific blockade of β-adrenoceptors. In Fig. 12 the circadian phase dependency

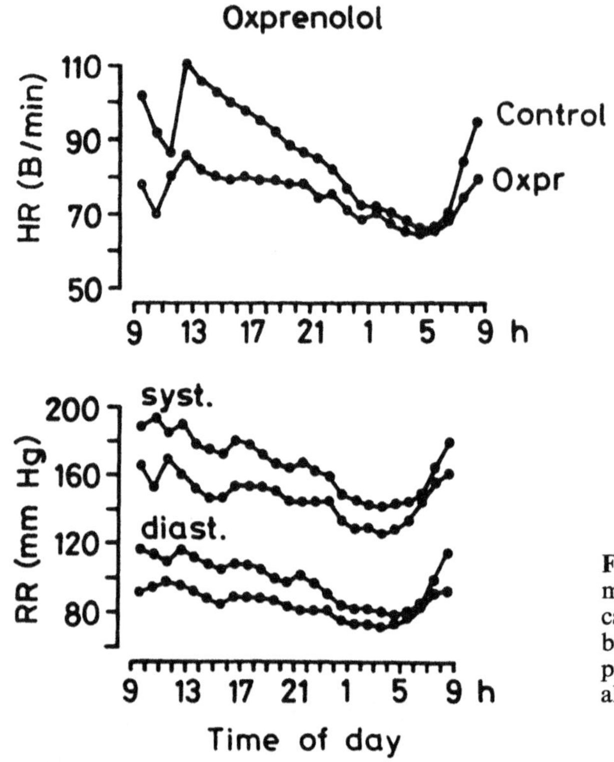

Fig. 13. Effect of a 6-week treatment with oxprenolol on circadian rhythms in heart rate and blood pressure of hypertensive patients. (Modified from Craig et al. [2])

in the effect of propranolol on the heart rate of conscious rats is shown [15]. Propranolol decreased heart rate in either photoperiod; however, in the dark phase propranolol exhibited a dosage dependency as well as a more pronounced heart-rate-lowering effect (Fig. 12). Principally the same results were obtained in hypertensive patients in that the β-blocker oxprenolol decreased heart rate as well as systolic and diastolic blood pressure more pronouncedly in the activity period of the patients, i.e. during day time ([2]; Fig. 13). Thus, in animal and in man the effects of β-blocking drugs were more pronounced in the subjective activity period. What are the mechanisms responsible for this circadian phase dependency in the effects of β-blockers? In general, daily variations in the responsiveness of the cardiovascular system as well as a chronopharmacokinetic behaviour of these drugs can be involved. Experiments on the chronokinetics of various β-blockers in rats revealed that after single-drug administration propranolol (Fig. 14) as well as metoprolol, sotalol and atenolol showed shorter elimination half-lives in plasma and organs when applied in the dark phase compared with the light phase [11, 15]. Since the effects of the β-blockers were more pronounced in the subjective activity period of either human or rat, the chronokinetic behaviour of these drugs is unlikely to be responsible for the chronodynamic behaviour of these drugs. On the other hand, various studies have shown that the responsiveness of the cardiovascular systems display a circadian time dependency. Thus, vascular reactivity to adrenergic stimulation [5] and plasma noradrenaline concentration [22] are increased during daytime in humans and noradrenaline turnover rate in rats is greater at night [12, 15], indicating an increased activity of the sympathetic nervous system in the subjective activity period of the respective species. These data

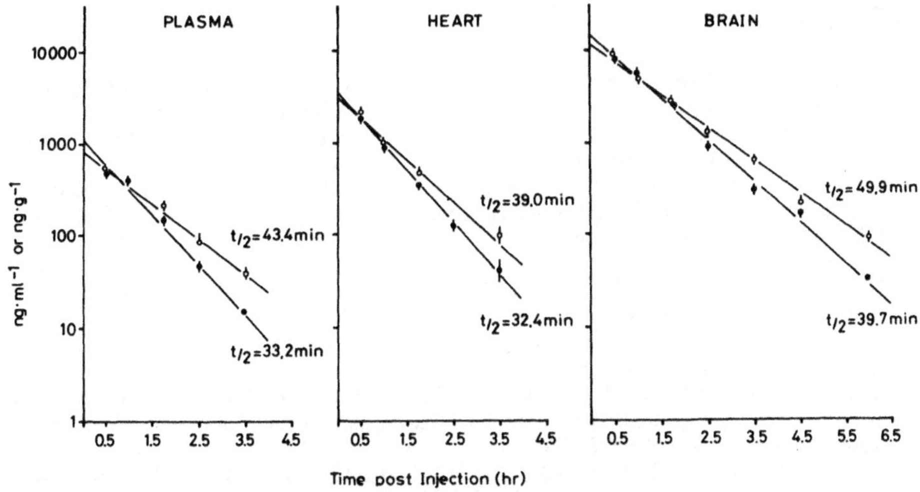

Fig. 14. Concentrations and elimination half-lives of propranolol (30 µmol/kg i.v.) in plasma, heart and brain of rats. Propranolol was injected either at 07.30 h (*open symbols*) or at 19.30 h (*closed symbols*). (Modified from Lemmer and Bathe [11])

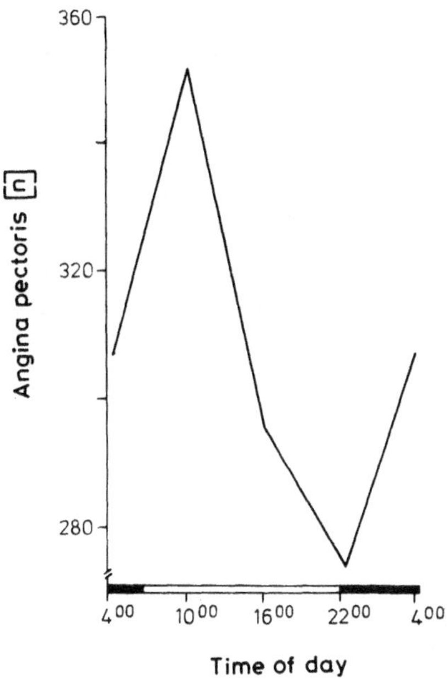

Fig. 15. Circadian rhythm in cardiac morbidity (coronary infarction evaluated by ECG and enzymes) in 1229 patients with coronary heart disease. (Modified from Master [17])

demonstrate that in the period of increased sympathetic tone β-blockers are more effective. In patients with a stable angina pectoris exercise-induced, symptom-limited increase in heart rate and decrease in ST-segment were also greater at 4 p.m. than at 8 a.m. and this circadian time dependency was still observed under β-receptor blockade [6]. These data may help us to reach a better understanding of the mechanisms of regulation of the cardiovascular system in healthy and diseased persons and, furthermore, may explain why coronary infarction is more often observed in the early morning than during the late afternoon ([17]; Fig. 15).

References

1. Bornschein RL, Crockett RS, Smith RP (1977) Diurnal variations in the analgesic effectiveness of morphine in mice. Pharmacol Biochem Behav 6:621–626
2. Craig MW, Mann S, Balasubramanian V, Raftery EB (1978) Blood pressure circadian rhythm in essential hypertension. Clin Sci Mol Med 55:391–393
3. Frederickson RCA, Burgis V, Edwards JD (1977) Hyperalgesia induced by naloxone follows diurnal rhythm in responsivity to painful stimuli. Science 198:756–758
4. Hill L (1898) On rest, sleep, and work and the concomitant changes in the circulation of the blood. Lancet 1:282–285
5. Hossmann V, Fitzgerald GA, Dollery CT (1980) Circadian rhythm of baroreflex reactivity and adrenergic vascular response. Cardiovasc Res 14:125–129
6. Joy M, Pollard CM, Nunan TO (1982) Diurnal variation in exercise responses in angina pectoris. Br Heart J 48:156–160
7. Kanabrocki EL, Scheving LE, Halberg F, Brewer RL, Bird TJ (1973) Circadian variation in presumably healthy men under conditions of peace-time army reserve unit training. Space Life Sci 4:258–270
8. Kumar MSA, Chen CL, Sharp DC, Liu JM, Kalra PS, Kalra SP (1982) Diurnal fluctuations in methionine-enkephaline levels in the hypothalamus and preoptic area of the male rat: effects of pinealectomy. Neuroendocrinology 35:28–31
9. Lemmer B (1982) Chronopharmacokinetics. In: Breimer DD, Speiser P (eds) Topics in pharmaceutical sciences. Elsevier/North-Holland Biomedical, Amsterdam, p 49
10. Lemmer B (1983) Chronopharmakologie: Tagesrhythmen und Arzneimittelwirkung. Wissenschaftliche Verlagsgesellschaft, Stuttgart
11. Lemmer B, Bathe K (1982) Stereospecific and circadian-phase-dependent kinetic behavior of *d,l- l-*, and *d*-propranolol in plasma, heart and brain of light-dark-synchronized rats. J Cardiovasc Pharmacol 4:635–644
12. Lemmer B, Saller R (1974) Influence of light and darkness on the turnover of noradrenaline in the rat heart. Naunyn-Schmiedeberg's Arch Pharmacol 282:75–84
13. Lemmer B, Wenda K (1979) Diurnal rhythms in noradrenaline turnover and motility after reserpine and 6-hydroxydopamine. Pharmacol Biochem Behav 10:361–368
14. Lemmer B, Simrock R, Hellenbrecht D, Smolensky MH (1980) Chronopharmacological studies with propranolol in rodents: implications for the management of COPD patients with cardiovascular disease. In: Smolensky MH, McGovern JP, Reinberg A (eds) Recent advances in the chronobiology of allergy and immunology. Pergamon, Oxford, p 195
15. Lemmer B, Bathe K, Lang PH, Neumann G, Winkler H (1983) Chronopharmacology of β-adrenoceptor-blocking drugs: pharmacokinetic and pharmacodynamic studies in rats. J Am Coll Toxicol 2:347–358
16. Lutsch EF, Morris RW (1967) Circadian periodicity in susceptibility to lidocaine hydrochloride. Science 156:100–102
17. Master AM (1960) The role of effort and occupation in coronary occlusion. J Am Med Assoc 174:942–948
18. Matthews JH, Marte E, Halberg F (1964) A circadian susceptibility – resistance cycle to fluothane in male B_1 mice. Can Anaesth Soc J 11:280–290
19. Menzel W (1940) Über einen 24-Stunden-Rhythmus im Blutkreislauf des Menschen. Acta Med Scand [Suppl] 108:166–177
20. Moore-Ede MC, Czeisler CA, Richardson GS (1983a) Circadian time-keeping in health and disease, part 1. Basic properties of circadian pacemakers. N Engl J Med 309:469–476
21. Moore-Ede MC, Czeisler CA, Richardson GS (1983b) Circadian time-keeping in health and disease, part 2. Clinical implications of circadian rhythmicity. N Engl J Med 309:530–536
22. Mullen PE, Lightman S, Linsell C, McKeon P, Sever PS, Todd K (1981) Rhythms of plasma noradrenaline in man. Psychoendocrinology 6:213–222
23. Munson ES, Martucci RW, Smith RE (1970) Circadian variations in anaesthetic requirement and toxicity in rats. Anaesthesiology 32:507–514
24. Pöllmann L (1977) Über tageszeitliche Unterschiede der Wirksamkeit eines Analgeticums. Dtsch Zahnärztl Z 32:180–182

25. Reinberg A, Reinberg MA (1977) Circadian changes of the duration of action of local anaesthetic agents. Naunyn-Schmiedeberg's Arch Pharmacol 297:149–152
26. Reinberg A, Smolensky MH (1983) Biological rhythms and medicine. Springer, Berlin Heidelberg New York Tokyo
27. Smolensky M, Jonovich JA, Kyle GM, Hsi B (1979) Chronotoxicity in rodents challenged with propranolol · HCl (Inderal®). In: Reinberg A, Halberg F (eds) Chronopharmacology. Pergamon, Oxford, p 263
28. Walker CA, Mash D (1982) Circadian variations of beta endorphin in specific areas of the rat brain. In: Takahashi R, Halberg F, Walker CA (eds) Toward chronopharmacology. Pergamon, Oxford, p 85
29. Wesche DL, Frederickson RCA (1981) The role of the pituitary in the diurnal variation in tolerance to painful stimuli and brain enkephalin levels. Life Sci 29:2199–2205
30. Virey JJ (1814) Ephémérides de la via humaine, ou recherches sur la révolution journalière, et la periodicité de ses phénomènes dans la santé et les maladies. Thesis, University of Paris
31. Von Mayersbach H (1976) Time – a key in experimental and practical medicine. Arch Toxicol 36:185–216

Analgesic Effect of Continuous Intrathecal Beta-Endorphin in Cancer Patients

T. Jin, T. Murakawa, and T. Oyama

Beta endorphin is a peptide consisting of 31 amino acids, isolated from the pituitary gland. This peptide is the most potent endogenous opiate. Prolonged pain relief with single intrathecal administration of beta endorphin in cancer patients has been reported by Oyama [1]. But pain relief did not last for more than several days. Many patients with cancer suffer from severe pain for a long period.

It is difficult to control pain with a single injection of beta endorphin (B-Ep) to the intrathecal space, in spite of the desire to provide pain relief for a long period in these patients. We report the excellent analgesic effect of continuous intrathecal beta endorphin infusion in two patients with cancer pain.

Method

An epidural tube, Portex Mini Pack 18G, was used for the intrathecal catheter. The intrathecal catheter was advanced through the L4-5 intervertebral space and was fixed at the abdominal wall through a subcutaneous tunnel. A Millipore filter was placed between the catheter and the continuous infusion device, Promedos E VI (Siemens). Prodemos E VI is a small, lightweight and portable infusion pump, which was designed to deliver 0.24–12 ml/day, in steps of 0.24 ml/day. The drug reservoir capacity is 30 ml.

Beta endorphin (B-Ep) was supplied by Prof. C. H. Li of the University of California. Synthetic B-Ep was diluted with physiological saline to a concentration of 1 ml/ml. The solution was sterilized by Millipore filtration. The delivery rate was controlled depending on the pain analogue scale score and side effect.

Results

The protocol of our method was explained to the two cancer patients, and their written consents were obtained before the treatment.

Patient No. 1 was a 54-year-old woman with rectal cancer. She underwent Mile's operation in 1982 and was admitted to the hospital on 9 November 1983 for pain over the abdomen and left leg. At the beginning, the pain was controlled with 15–30 mg pentazocine i.m. one to two times a day. Epidural nerve block with 6 ml 0.25% bupivacaine two to three times a day started on 18 November decreased pain sufficiently. However, subsequently, additional pentazocine was needed. From 5 December 2 mg morphine in bupivacaine was injected epidurally, through an epidural tube once a day, but additional pentazocine was needed later.

The pain was localized over the abdomen and the left leg. The intensity of pain was 8–10 on the visual pain analogue scale score when the effect of previous analgesics ended. Her laboratory data were within normal limits except for anaemia. Metastasis to the right lung was noticed in the chest X-ray film. The urinary bladder had been catheterized for dysuria due to bladder invasion. The patient had complained of appetite loss and was required to rest on the bed all day.

On 15 December, we started intrathecal infusion of B-Ep at the rate of 0.96 mg/day. After the start of infusion, the pain analogue scale score was markedly reduced to 0–1 and additional analgesics were not given except for a few times. On the 3rd day, the patient complained of a sensation of uplifting of the body. The delivery rate of B-Ep was reduced, followed by a temporary increase of pain. Therefore, the rate of infusion of B-Ep was increased to 1.2 mg/day. The severe pain which had prevented her sleep at night disappeared. The infusion lasted for a period of 14 days. From 28 December B-Ep was changed to morphine (1 mg/day) because of lack of supply of B-Ep until her death. The pain score was kept at lower levels (1–2) during morphine infusion.

Patient No. 2 was a 57-year-old man. He underwent the low anterior resection for rectal cancer in March 1982. In November 1982, when anal pain appeared, radiation therapy and subarachnoid phenol block were performed, and pain relief was obtained. In November 1983, anal pain reappeared and increased gradually. The patient was admitted to our hospital and was treated with analgesics such as 15 mg pentazocine two times/day and 100 mg indomethacin in suppository form at the beginning. But the treatment was not adequate for pain relief.

The laboratory data revealed leucocytosis and slight anaemia. Otherwise his general condition was good. The pain analogue scale score was about 5, and he could not sleep well for the pain.

A subarachnoid catheter was inserted for injection of 1 ml physiological saline to detect the placebo effect on 28 November. The pain score decreased from 5 to 2, but complete pain relief was not obtained. Next day, the patient complained of severe pain again, and 1 mg B-Ep was injected through the intrathecal tube. The pain score then decreased to 0 for 11 h.

The subarachnoid catheter was connected to a continuous infusion device, Promedos E, on 30 November. The delivery rate of the peptide was 0.96 mg/day at the beginning. The pain score decreased, but the patient still complained of pain. The 2nd day of infusion, delivery rate was changed from 0.96 to 1.44 mg/day. The pain score level 1 continued until 7 December, when the patient developed euphorea, temporary mental disturbance and amnesia. Then the delivery rate was reduced to 0.96 mg/day.

During the course of the infusion, blood pressure, heart rate and temperature did not change significantly. The infusion continued for 12 days.

Complications and Side Effects

Except for the leakage of the solution at the end of the subcutaneous tunnel, complications such as infection, respiratory and circulatory depression were not observed. Transient mental disturbance was noticed in the two patients on the B-Ep course and the delivery rate was reduced.

Discussion

Profound pain relief was obtained, and neither the motor nor autonomic function was affected with intrathecal bolus injection of B-Ep. The use of a single injection of B-Ep to the subarachnoidal space for cancer pain requires multiple spinal punctures and the possibility of mental disturbance and infection. A reduced dose of B-Ep and more stable analgesia than with a single injection were characteristic of this method. We can expect long-term pain relief and less side effects such as mental disturbance and less chance of infection with our method.

The level of B-Ep in the spinal fluid would be low compared with a single injection. Consequently, the concentration of B-Ep diffused to the supraspinal space was lower and the action on the brain would not be stronger than that of a single injection. The effect of B-Ep infusion is thought to be more segmental than that of a bolus injection.

This method appears to have advantages in clinical use over the single injection.

References

1. Oyama T et al. (1980) Profound analgesic effect of B-endorphin in man. Lancet 1:122–125
2. Onofrio BM et al. (1981) Continuous low dose intrathecal morphine administration in the treatment of chronic pain of malignant origin. Mayo Clin Proc 56:516–520

Epidural, On-Demand, Low-Dose Infusion of Morphine and Postoperative Pain Relief

J. Chrubasik

There is no doubt that epidural administration of morphine is superior to systemic administration: lower doses of morphine produce longer-lasting pain relief; and it has been shown that continuous epidural long-term treatment with morphine causes fewer side effects, although tachyphylaxis is unavoidable with epidural, long-term treatment. The aim of the investigation was:

1. To determine whether continuous, epidural, demand-controlled morphine infusion is suitable for postoperative treatment of pain
2. To determine whether tachyphylaxis is produced under the treatment

For continuous morphine infusion, we utilized a four-roller pump (Fig. 1). Morphine solutions of varying concentrations can be put into the 30-ml reservoir. For postoperative treatment, a 0.25% morphine solution has proved to be effective. With the infusion device, the maximum basal rate is 0.06 ml/h. Additional infusions of up to 0.25 ml over 60 or 100 min can be administered on demand.

Table 1 lists the operations undergone by the 56 patients, 35 male and 21 female, between the ages of 25 and 82 years. Patients who abused drugs or alcohol were not eliminated from the investigation. The epidural catheter was applied preoperatively. With 48 patients, the catheter was used intraoperatively to administer the local anaesthetic, mepivacaine, supplementary to the barbiturate, laughing gas and halothane anaesthetics.

Subjective pain was conveyed by a modified Scott's pain analogue scale, no pain being 0, the worst pain being 10. With 50 patients, group I, the analgesic treatment began when postoperative pain reached up to 10 on the analogue scale.

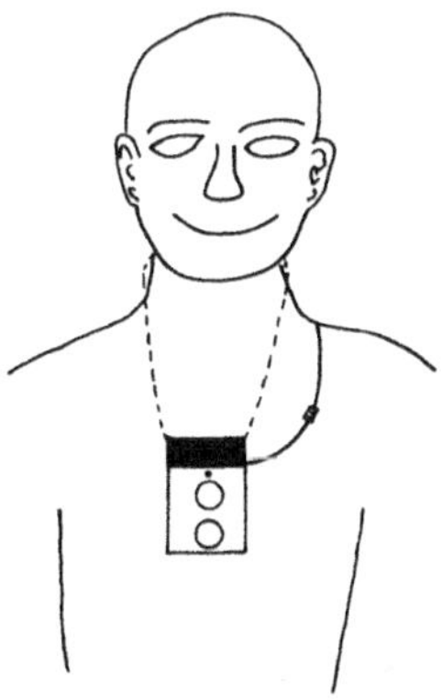

Fig. 1. The externally worn device (11.4 × 6.6 × 2.7 cm) weighs 260 g with the reservoir empty

Table 1. The operations undergone by the 50 patients of group I and the 6 patients of group II

Proctocolectomy	9	1
Colectomy	7	1
Gastrectomy	7	2
Cholecystectomy +cholecochotomy, etc.	8	
Cystectomy	1	1
Palliative abdominal op.	6	
Nephrectomy	1	1
Fascioplasty	2	
Herniotomy	1	
Lymphadenectomy	3	
Exploratory laparatomy	3	
Aortoplasty	2	

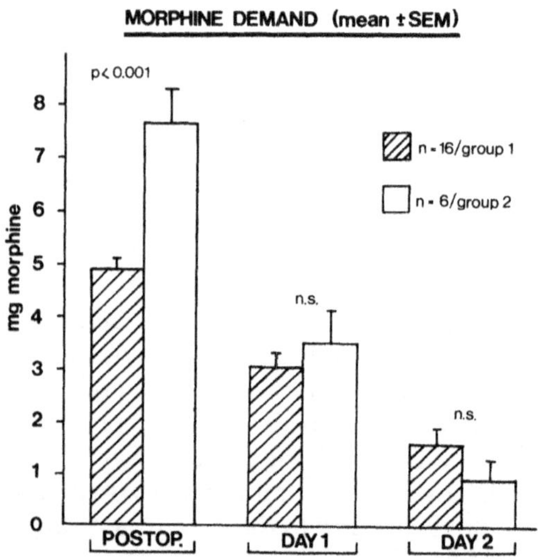

Fig. 2. The mean morphine consumption of group I [$n=16(50)$] after an initial bolus injection of 2 mg morphine and of group II ($n=6$) after an initial infusion of 2.3 ± 0.6 mg, during treatment by continuous, epidural, on-demand infusion of morphine

After an initial bolus injection of 2 mg morphine, a continuous infusion of 0.16 mg morphine/h was administered by the infusion device. Six patients, group II, received a morphine infusion of 0.5 mg/h immediately from the beginning of the operation. Depending on the length of the operation, the patients received on average 2.3 mg morphine until the end of the operation. In accordance with other sources, the operation day ended at 8 a.m. on the first postoperative day; the second postoperative day began 24 h later and ended at 8 p.m. According to how the patients felt, the morphine doses in groups I and II were reduced or supplemented by additional infusions of 0.625 mg over 60 min, administered through the dosing device, or 2 mg morphine by syringe.

Mean morphine consumption of 16 patients of group I and all the patients of group II on the operation day, the first postoperative day and the second postoperative day is presented in Fig. 2. The marked columns show the morphine consumption of group I, which received an initial bolus injection. The blank columns show the morphine consumption of group II, which received a low-dose morphine infusion from the beginning of the operation. While no significant difference in morphine consumption was recorded on the first and second postoperative days, group II required considerably more morphine on the operation day, until 8 a.m. of the first postoperative day. For statistical calculations, the *t*-test for unpaired data was used. Because of this, we resorted exclusively to epidural morphine infusion after an initial bolus injection of 2 mg morphine.

Mean morphine consumption of the 50 patients of group I was 4.8 ± 0.2 mg on the operation day, 1.9 ± 0.2 mg on the first postoperative day and 0.6 ± 0.1 mg on the second postoperative day until 8 p.m. The total morphine consumption over 50 h was 7.1 ± 0.3 mg. In the first 25 h, morphine consumption, 5.4 ± 0.2 mg, was significantly higher than in the following 25 h, 1.6 ± 0.2 mg.

By means of the treatment, pain under conditions of immobility could be continuously kept under 1, and pain under physical stress under 2, on the analogue scale (Table 2). Within 1 h after the beginning of the treatment, analgesia was attained. None of the patients received any analgesic treatment supplementary to the epidural morphine administration.

The pH value in the blood was constantly normal following the operation. The arterial oxygen pressure increased as a consequence of regular postoperative oxygen insufflation from 82 ± 1 mm Hg to 100 ± 5 mm Hg, but subsequently re-

Table 2. Subjective pain, conveyed on a visual pain analogue scale (no pain, 0; worst pain, 10) during epidural, on-demand morphine infusion ($n = 50$) (mean ± SEM)

		Op. day		Day 1		Day 2
	Postop.	8 p.m.	8 a.m.	8 p.m.	8 a.m.	8 p.m.
While immobile	7 ± 0.6	0.7 ± 0.2	0.6 ± 0.2	0.2 ± 0.1	0.1 ± 0	0.0 ± 0
Under physical stress	8 ± 0.5	1.7 ± 0.3	1.3 ± 0.2	1.2 ± 0.2	0.6 ± 0.2	0.2 ± 0.1

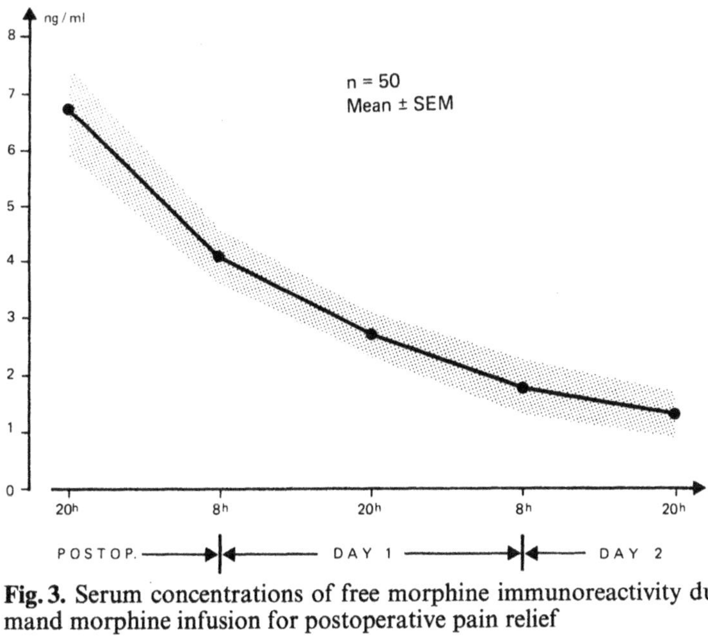

Fig. 3. Serum concentrations of free morphine immunoreactivity during epidural, on-demand morphine infusion for postoperative pain relief

mained in accordance with the normal oxygen pressure, respective of age. The carbon dioxide pressure remained constant, with no indications of respiratory depression.

Blood pressure, pulse and respiratory rate were not influenced by the treatment. Urinary retention was seen in less than 20% of the patients. These patients were among the 46 who received mepivacaine epidurally during the operation. Because the administration of epidural anaesthetics can itself cause bladder disorders, it is unclear whether urinary retention was a consequence of morphine or of mepivacaine. We saw no complications with the catheters.

Figure 3 shows the serum levels of free morphine immunoreactivity corresponding to group I during continuous, demand-controlled low-dose infusion of morphine. Serum morphine levels decreased during the treatment, but there was continuous pain relief nonetheless, in contrast to the situation with continuous treatment by infusions of local anaesthetics.

Our results demonstrate that:

1. Individual, postoperative treatment of pain is possible with continuous, epidural, demand-controlled morphine infusion.
2. Total consumption of morphine can be reduced by an initial bolus injection.
3. Besides causing relatively few side effects, continuous low-dose infusion of morphine produces neither accumulation of morphine in the blood nor tachyphylaxis.

Discussion III

N.S. Faithfull: I have a question to Professor Lemmer. You showed that there was circadian activity in, for instance, the analgesic effect of morphine. Do the respiratory depressive effects and other side effects vary in synchrony, or do they have their own particular rhythm? What do you think about the role of certain receptors in this case?

B. Lemmer: Well, concerning the physiological circadian rhythm in different organs you do not always have the maximum of the rhythm in the active period of the species under scrutiny. So, you really have to investigate each parameter, for example forced expiratory volume and so on, to achieve mapping of these rhythms. It is well documented that there are different shifts in the maxima and minima of circadian rhythms in different physiological parameters as well as in the effects of drugs. In the lung tissue it is very clearly documented that the forced expiratory volume, the tidal volume and the dynamic compliance in normal and asthmatic patients change in cycles with the time of the day. And that for example the effects of orciprenaline and diophyllin are cyclic in their effects according to monitoring at different times of day. The susceptibility of the lung tissue to noxious substances really cycles with the time of day. So for instance more asthmatic attacks occurs at night in human beings. At the same time there is a decrease in catecholamine content and in the cortisol concentration at night. Furthermore, the susceptibility to house dust or to histamine or acetylcholine is increased at night. In asthmatic patients all parameters are changed in such a way that they are most sensitive to every bronchoconstrictor used at night.

P.A. Foster: Is this effect tied to a body clock or is it tied to activity? In other words: if you forcibly changed a person's activity cycle, would you change the response to a different time of a day? To me, the implication here is that we as anaesthetists can change the activity cycle of people. And I do this regularly. I have my people waking up in the middle of the night after long operations or something like that.

B. Lemmer: To answer your question we have to go into chronobiology. We know rhythms, for example in body temperature, which are even present without external time cues, without alternating light and darkness, and independent of activity or rest. Experiments concerned with this have been performed in the USA in the UK, and in Germany at the Max-Planck-Institute (by Ashoff). People were isolated in special chambers for 6, 7 or 8 weeks, without external time cues. They had no information on time of day or date. However, there were still very clear-cut circadian rhythms in body temperature. The frequency was not exactly 24 hours, however, but 24.7 hours. These rhythms therefore are really endogenous rhythms, and it is very difficult to reverse them. On the other hand, metabolic parameters, enzyme activities and motor activity in rats can be reversed very quickly within 4–7 days. They are synchronized by light and darkness, which means they are mainly exogenous rhythms. Within this spectrum you can have all different kinds of rhythms which are predominantly endogenous or exogenous. So, if you want to treat or to study a certain rhythm you first have to reevaluate whether it is mainly exogenous or mainly endogenous. Only then can you draw any conclusions. However, in cancer patients it has been shown, for example, that the DNA rhythm has no phase synchronization to daytime and no phasing to time cues. There are rhythms which cannot be shifted by shifting the light-to-dark or the rest-activity ratio. There are rhythms which are very stable but really free running with no time cues.

On the other hand, there are effects of rhythms on the behaviour and on human emotions. The jet-lag after transcontinental flights demonstrates that this is due to small shifts in circadian rhythms in endocrinological parameters, which have to be resynchronized after such a flight. It takes about 3 to 7 or 15 days to resynchronize to the local time at the particular place. So I cannot give you a general answer. You have to look on the mechanisms of rhythms and the nature of these rhythms.

R. Spintge: Dr. Jin, do you have any explanation for the occurrence of the mental disturbances you observed? Can you refer them to β-endorphin or to the basic disease?

T. Jin: When mental disturbances occurred in the two patients I reduced the rate of delivery from the infusion pump. After this the mental disturbances disappeared. So this was a problem of dosage. We have also seen mental disturbances with morphine. So concerning this side effect I cannot decide which drug has an advantage over the other. It is very hard to control, because with these high dosages we had better analgesic effects at the same time.

R. Spintge: Did you see any problems with infections?

T. Jin: No. We administer antibiotics for 3 days after implantation of the intraspinal catheter.

R. Droh: Dr. Chrubasik, if you took account of the circadian rhythms in programming your infusion pump, do you think this could reduce the amount of analgesic agent needed and at the same time improve the analgesic effect?

J. Chrubasik: No. I think that with morphine we are already at the minimum level. Furthermore, the patient must be able to control delivery of the analgesic on demand.

B. Lemmer: Have you found any correlation between time of day and the amount of analgesic required by the patient?

J. Chrubasik: No, we have not yet analysed our data with reference to this question. The only thing I can say is that many patients require higher doses of analgesics in the morning, probably as a result of nursing procedures, for example. We have seen this especially with our intensive-care patients.

B. Lemmer: You mentioned that nursing procedures could be the reason for a higher requirement of analgesics in the morning. I do not think so at all. On the contrary, it is stated expressly in all the papers from USA and Europe that this is not the reason. The reason is the lowered pain threshold in the morning.

F. Ruetten: Did you see any such side effects as nausea or vomiting with your method? In Rotterdam we had some cases and we had some trouble with these side effects.

J. Chrubasik: These side effects occur much more seldom with continuous epidural low-dose infusion of morphine than with systemic administration of morphine. With respect to respiratory depression our patients are not put in intensive care units or wake-up units. Our patients are normally placed in a normal ward. At the beginning we took a vivid interest in monitoring respiration in the postoperative phase. We have been carrying out animal experiments, and I can show you the morphine level in CSF near the respiratory centre in the brain stem after injection of 2 mg morphine in 10 ml injection volume, which is customary in our university. The morphine infusion did not increase respiratory depression even with the highest CSF level after 2 mg morphine in 10 ml, i.e., over 3000 ng in the respiratory centre. I would therefore recommend you, if you work with postoperative pain treatment, not to use a high volume for epidural or intraspinal postoperative analgesia.

R. Droh: According to the paper presented by Professor Lemmer, I think that in future we will certainly have to pay more attention to the circadian rhythms, in anaesthesiology too. We should no longer accept any studies on the analgesic effect of substances which do not pay attention to the circadian rhythms. Professor Lemmer, during the years of my anaesthesia practice I have often observed that as long as they are of child-bearing age, female patients need less analgesics than male patients. But after the menopause they need the same amount. Are there definitive studies about correlations between the circadian rhythm on the one hand and the cyclic hormonal changes in young women?

B. Lemmer: No, not as far as the amount of drugs needed is concerned. On the other hand, it is quite well known that in the 28-day cycles there are differences in susceptibility to pain. During menstruation we observe migraine attacks more frequently. It would be quite interesting to conduct a study on this, considering the whole time from the first menstruation to the menopause.

Dr. Droh: I could also imagine that the corpus luteum hormone and the follicular hormone have their effect.

B. Lemmer: Unfortunately, there are no studies on the possibility of such effects on the response to a drug. I think this is mainly due to the fact that only biologists and some physiologists have dealt with this matter. Very few pharmacologists have studied these questions, so we are at the beginning of systematic studies in this field. This will certainly also be of great social importance when we take account of the large number of shift workers.

R. Droh: You said biologists have conducted a large number of studies in this field. Are there any studies concerning changes during spring, early autumn or late autumn?

B. Lemmer: There are some studies for instance dealing with the initial situation in hypertension, differentiating between males and females. Blood pressure, whether treated with beta blockers or not, is higher in winter and in spring than in the summer. There are seasonal rhythms and fluctuations and they are easily reproducible. And this is accompanied by an increase in cardiovascular mortality. So, at the seasonal level we have similar correspondences to those I have tried to elucidate on a daily level. Another field relating to the seasonal differences is that of depressive patients. Fluctuations can also be observed in the EEG. Furthermore, we have phase shifting in depressive patients in terms of body temperature and of catecholamine excretion. These phenomena can be normalized with antidepressive drugs. We are carrying out some studies in the USA. So far, we have found that light therapy has the same effect. Light exceeding 5000 lux can remove the depression, including the seasonal fluctuations.

F. Ruetten: Especially in the literature on endocrinology in anaesthesia, it is well known that our anaesthetics have an influence on the hormonal levels. They are acting via the pituitary gland and it may be that our anaesthetics act as neuromodulators. So there is a possibility that hormones produced in the pituitary gland can influence our behaviour and also the requirement for anaesthetics.

R. Droh: I can only confirm this. In the future we should make a point of taking account of these rhythms, the seasonal rhythms and the circadian rhythms. I am quite sure that we will arrive at essentially new findings, for example in pain therapy and other fields.

B. Lemmer: Concerning endorphins and enkephalins, we have almost no information about their influence on circadian rhythms as releasing hormones or inhibitory substances. That might be very important. Now I want to inform you of some studies conducted at Harvard Medical School. The group there infused potassium chloride for one hour in a therapeutic dose range to patients at noon and at midnight. The patients were very accurately monitored for potassium balance for some days before. They found that the relative increase in the serum potassium concentration was much higher when the same dosage of potassium chloride was infused at midnight than when it was given at noon. The reason is reduced renal exrection at midnight. The consequence for the ECG is that the T-wave elevation induced by the same dosage of potassium cloride shows a significantly different effect. The T-wave elevation is much higher at midnight than in the daytime. And that might be of therapeutic relevance.

D. W. Lübbers: I would like to point out that quite a lot is known about this in physiology. Especially the team around Hildebrand discussed correlations between the circadian rhythms in men and the effects of drugs. One conclusion was that these rhythms were not stable during the day, during an illness or during the recovery period. There are fluctuations even in the minute range, for instance, and it can be observed that there are different pharmacological effects even in these short time periods. Rodenfranz and co-workers have also conducted some studies about pharmacological effects related to time of day. These studies clearly show that pharmacological effects can be completely reversed at a different time of day.

Subject Index

Batch number: 10704763

Printed by Printforce, the Netherlands